Dr. Mary Walker

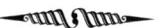

Dr. Mary Walker

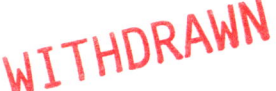

An American Radical, 1832–1919

SHARON M. HARRIS

RUTGERS UNIVERSITY PRESS
NEW BRUNSWICK, NEW JERSEY, AND LONDON

Library of Congress Cataloging-in-Publication Data

Harris, Sharon M.
    Dr. Mary Walker : an American radical, 1832–1919 / Sharon M. Harris.
        p. cm.
    Includes bibliographical references and index.
    ISBN 978-0-8135-4611-7 (hardcover : alk. paper)
  1. Walker, Mary Edwards, 1832–1919. 2. Women physicians—United States—Biography.
3. Radicals—United States—Biography.   4. Physicians—United States—Biography.
5. United States—History—Civil War, 1861–1865—Medical care.   6. United States—
History—Civil War, 1861–1865—Women.   I. Title.
    R154.W18H37 2009
    610.82—dc22
    [B]   2009000781

A British Cataloging-in-Publication record for this book is available from the British Library.

Copyright © 2009 by Sharon M. Harris

All rights reserved

No part of this book may be reproduced or utilized in any form or by any means, electronic or mechanical, or by any information storage and retrieval system, without written permission from the publisher. Please contact Rutgers University Press, 100 Joyce Kilmer Avenue, Piscataway, NJ 08854-8099. The only exception to this prohibition is "fair use" as defined by U.S. copyright law.

Visit our Web site: http://rutgerspress.rutgers.edu

Manufactured in the United States of America

To the Harris Clan—

Jim, Gail, Katie, JJ, Sue, Jimmy, Amy

Contents

Acknowledgments ix

1 "Give me liberty of thought": The Seeds of Radicalism 1
2 Dress Reform and *The Sibyl* 17
3 "The ark of reform": Civil War Surgeon 31
4 Surgeon, Spy, Prisoner of War 53
5 Interlude 75
6 Touring Britain: The Creation of a Public Self 84
7 "A Representative Woman" 100
8 A Crusader's *Hit* 119
9 Women's Rights Unmasked 134
10 The Courtroom, the Legislature, Party Politics 164
11 A Pragmatic Utopia 186
12 Anti-Imperialism and the World Stage 211
13 The Age of Alienation 229
14 The Pioneer Embraced 241
   Epilogue 253

Notes 255
Index 287

Acknowledgments

I wish to thank the many individuals and institutions who have assisted me in bringing this project to fruition. They are many, and I hope I have profusely thanked you along the way, but special acknowledgement is due to a few people whose support has been essential and to the institutions that have graciously allowed me access to their archives and supported my research. Longstanding thanks are due to Susan Belasco, Linda K. Hughes, and Moira Ferguson who supported my study of Walker from the beginning; equally important are friends and scholars who offered encouragement and reviewed materials in progress, especially Theresa Strouth Gaul, Jean Marsden, and the anonymous reader for Rutgers University Press.

I want also to thank the Department of English at the University of Connecticut, Storrs for its support of research leaves during which I was able to complete this project. A National Endowment for the Humanities Fellowship was essential in granting me the time to draft the manuscript, and a University of Connecticut Humanities Institute Fellowship allowed me to complete final revisions; special thanks are due to Richard D. Brown and my colleagues at the Institute in 2007–2008; their keen inquiries greatly aided my thinking during the final stages of the book.

I would also like to thank the following institutions and individuals for permission to use their archives and to publish materials from their records: Syracuse University Library, Special Collections, and Nicolette Dobrowolski; Oswego County Historical Society, and Terry Prior; Drexel University College of Medicine, and Barbara Williams; Special Collections, Penfield Library, SUNY-Oswego; Samuel J. Tilden Papers, Manuscripts and Archives Division, The New York Public Library; Astor, Lenox and Tilden Foundations; Abraham Lincoln Presidential Library, Springfield, Illinois; Manuscripts Division, Rutherford B. Hayes Presidential Center.

Dr. Mary Walker

CHAPTER 1

"Give me liberty of thought"

THE SEEDS OF RADICALISM

The large, rambling Walker house in Oswego Town was already steeped in activity when Mary Edwards Walker was born on November 26, 1832. Her parents, Vesta Whitcomb and Alvah Walker, left Syracuse in August of that year with the vision of establishing a productive home where they could raise their four lively, Syracuse-born daughters—Vesta, born in 1823; Aurora Borealis, 1825; Luna, 1827; and Cynthia, 1828—in a physically and intellectually healthy environment. Oswego Town seemed the perfect place to achieve their dream. They purchased a thirty-five-acre farm on what became known as Bunker Hill Road. The soil was ideal for the growth of vegetables and fruits, there was natural lime-water available, and the acreage was abundant in groves of pine, beech, maple, birch, cherry, butternut, and ash trees. The farm was located only two miles from Lake Ontario and a little over four miles south of the booming city of Oswego. While the growth of Oswego meant an increase in industrial smoke, Oswego Town could still boast pristine air and the quiet life of the countryside. Vesta gave birth to two more children in the early years of their life in Oswego Town: Mary, born in 1832, and two years later, their only surviving son, Alvah Jr.[1]

The limitless future the Walkers envisioned for their children was evident in the names they gave their first four daughters, as if to encourage them to think beyond the usual earth-bound conventions. Alvah had a passion for astronomy, and his love of observing the night skies is reflected in the older daughters' names. If their last two children were named more conventionally, the choice for Mary at least reflected a certain pragmatism on the part of Vesta and Alvah, since she was named after a propertied paternal aunt, Mary Walker (1804–1895). The Walkers' youngest daughter would make the name famous in the annals of America's radical thinkers.[2]

The intellectual environment that the Walkers sought was readily available in the Central New York region of the 1830s, and as progressive thinkers, they added to its vibrancy. Their farm was named "Bunker Hill" because, as Mary later claimed, it symbolized their hope to replicate "the great battle in national salvation" on a personal and cultural level. Alvah and Vesta were originally from Greenwich, Massachusetts, and proud to acknowledge that their families were among some of the early settlers of the Plymouth Colony. Alvah could trace his ancestors in Massachusetts to Widow Walker, who settled in Seekonic around 1643. His great-great grandfather, Philip Walker (?-1679), bought land in Rehoboth in 1660. Philip's youngest son Ebenezer (1676–1741) was the last of ten children. Ebenezer's son and Alvah's grandfather, Abel Walker (1736–1763), served in the Continental Army during the Revolutionary War and thereafter lived in Hardwick; he and his wife, Mary Snow, raised seven children, including Alvah's father, Abel Walker II (1770–1811). Snow's family included four ancestors who had signed the *Mayflower Compact*. Vesta's ancestors could also be traced to the pre-Revolutionary years; some of them reportedly fought in the French and Indian War. Vesta and Alvah's ideas of "national salvation" included a country in which democracy would be more fully enacted, especially with freedom for all of its citizens.[3]

Mary's mother, Vesta Whitcomb (1801–1886), was the daughter of Polly Hinds and James Whitcomb, whose ancestors had lived in New England since colonial times. Vesta's life demonstrates the heritage of a strong intellect and sense of independence. Little is known about her early years. At age twenty she married Alvah Walker (1798–1880) on September 8, 1821, in the Greenwich Methodist Church; she readily uprooted her life and joined her husband in a horse-and-covered-wagon westward trek that would end with a new home in Syracuse and then Oswego Town. Alvah Walker's childhood in Greenwich had been indelibly altered at age thirteen when his father died. As the oldest child, family responsibilities quickly fell to him. Although his formal education ended then, he continued a process of rigorous self-education throughout his life. He took up the trade of carpentry, and his income was a significant contribution to the support of the family, which included seven siblings. When he was nineteen, his mother remarried, and Alvah was able to fulfill his dream of traveling and making a life of his own. An intelligent and thoughtful young man, his talents as a carpenter allowed him to work his way to Pennsylvania, Kentucky, Tennessee, Louisiana, and three years later back to Massachusetts. In late 1820, the twenty-two-year-old carpenter became engaged to Vesta Whitcomb. After their marriage, they determined to travel west, stopping along the way to visit Vesta's relatives in Central New York. Whether it was due to the success of those visits, the time of year, or the good possibility of carpentry work for Alvah in Syracuse, the Walkers decided to settle in the growing city. Alvah quickly found work, and here Vesta gave birth to their first five children. Abel, the first born, died within days of his birth, but their four daughters thrived. The family resided in Syracuse for ten years before moving to Oswego Town.[4]

Transporting their household goods on the packet canal boat into Oswego and then by wagon to Oswego Town, the Walkers settled in the farm's small cottage until they could complete the building of their home, a white frame house with a low roof. The Central New York region was rapidly becoming a hotbed of radical philosophies and social reform movements, including antislavery, suffrage, and health reform. One of their neighbors in Oswego was Gerrit Smith, the largest property owner in the city and a progressive thinker who helped shape the intellectual life of Oswego through his interests in nonsectarianism, abolition, and dress reform. His life would cross paths with Mary Walker's for the next several decades.[5]

Living in Oswego Town rather than Oswego gave the Walkers the independence of distance but the nearness of a bustling center. In Oswego the Walkers could sell the products of their farm and purchase other necessities. Equally important, traveling the four and a half miles to Oswego gave them the opportunity to attend many cultural and political events. By the time the Walkers arrived, Presbyterian, Episcopal, Methodist, Baptist, Congregational, and Catholic churches were well established, and soon Millerites, Adventists, and Universalists would establish meetinghouses in the region. The years from 1830 to 1836 were a boom period for Oswego. The population rose from a little over 2,000 to 5,000 residents; wheat and particularly flour mills flourished; the manufactories' success resulted in a significant increase in the collection of canal tolls after a canal was built connecting the city to the Erie Canal. In 1838 the town proudly built the three-story Market House at the intersection of Water and Bridge Streets. Here the Walkers had access to the post office and customs house; fish, meat, and vegetable stalls were available on the main floor; and they could climb to the second floor to conduct business at the city offices. When they continued to the third floor, they stepped into the multifunctional, one-hundred-foot-long meeting room. Its blue ceiling seemed to open the heavens to its visitors, and they could turn to the windows for a stunning view of the river. In this room, the family could attend theatricals, watch the Oswego Guards' drill practice, or attend the town's annual ball.[6]

By 1850, the city population had reached nearly 15,000. Amid the seventeen or eighteen large flour mills were hotels, churches, and a variety of smaller businesses. Two years earlier the Oswego and Syracuse Railroad had been established, ensuring another important market connection. A writer for the *Water-Cure Journal* suggested that if investors would support the building of more commodious hotels, Oswego might become one of the principal resort areas in the United States. If the city never gained resort status, industrially it prospered. By the 1860s, it could boast the world's largest flour mill as well as cotton factories, tanneries, saw mills, ironworks, and other manufactories. In the years of Mary's youth, it was an exciting and prosperous region. Those features drew creative, progressive individuals who helped to reshape the city's educational and literary endeavors and, ultimately, to be part of Central New York's fermenting radicalism.[7]

Mary Edwards Walker as a child was gifted with intellect, beauty, and an indomitable spirit. Traditionally, these attributes would have cast her as a highly marriageable young woman whose life would be shaped by motherhood and conventional social values, and Mary had her share of suitors. One admirer sent her a Valentine poem, praising her refined taste, raven locks, and a nobility that led to "dreams of fevered sleep"; most important, however, the poem's author asserted, was Mary's "gift of thought." In addition to her intellectualism, two factors led Mary in quite different directions than most females born in the 1830s: her parents' progressive ideas about education, and her own iron will—a will that would give her the courage to travel unimagined paths.[8]

While the Walker house was modestly furnished, books dominated the interior life. The family emphasis on education was distinct, one neighbor recalled: "There was a simplicity, an air of refinement, of culture, an intangible something in its atmosphere that betokened personality. Here lived people with a certain awareness of life as a spiritual adventure." Education for Mary and her siblings began at home; but the education of the Walker children was not limited to formal schooling. The first lesson they learned was that hard work was the primary route to useful rewards, and Vesta and Alvah modeled these values. Their egalitarian marriage embraced the farm and domestic spheres. Vesta and her daughters helped with the chores of planting and harvesting, and Alvah often cleaned the household floors and washed clothes. He was also a talented leather worker who made ladies' calfskin boots and gloves. Alvah was "one of the progressive and forehanded farmers of his day" and an influential member of the Farmers' Club of Oswego, often contributing ideas about cultivating new strains of fruits and vegetables. Although not agnostic like Vesta's famous cousin, lawyer and orator Robert Ingersoll, the Walkers were "free thinkers" in the sense that intellectual interrogation of ideas sustained every aspect of their lives. The Walkers taught Mary and her siblings to question religious tenets in the same way they would probe any other system of ideas. While living in Syracuse, Alvah and Vesta sometimes attended Baptist services, and on other Sundays the Methodist services. The Greenwich Walkers had been Methodists, and Alvah was a church member, but he and Vesta rejected the stark evangelicalism of the Second Great Awakening that was stirring throughout the Northeast. They raised their children with a strong belief in God but not in one particular sect's interpretations. It was a creed that their youngest daughter would embrace throughout her life.[9]

One radically new religious movement of Mary's teenage years was Spiritualism. Influenced by Emanuel Swedenborg's extensive writings on the spirit world that emerged from trances in which he felt he had communed with spirits, Spiritualism was first given its American roots by Andrew Jackson Davis of Poughkeepsie, New York, who published *The Principles of Nature* in 1847. His system of harmonial philosophy emphasized individualism in an era in which the Transcendentalists had made the concept a touchstone for intellectualism. Equally important to the development of Spiritualism in the States were reformers in the abolition and women's rights movements. Many churches were slow to join the antislavery cause, so a significant number of activists turned to Spiritualism. It was also one of the first religious movements in America that encouraged women to speak before mixed audiences. Mary gained an interest in Spiritualism in her youth that she retained throughout her life. Her faith became even less sectarian as an adult; the primary creed by which she lived was an advocacy of "whatever was right and true."[10]

As progressive thinkers, Vesta and Alvah were committed to the eradication of slavery, and their home in Oswego became a stop on Central New York's Underground Railroad. In the early 1830s, Maria Stewart, Fanny Wright, and the Grimké sisters traveled throughout the region lecturing against slavery, and soon thereafter antislavery writings by Lydia Maria Child, Maria Weston Chapman, and many others began to circulate. The Walkers arrived in the Oswego area during the burgeoning era of abolitionism. They occasionally attended the Syracuse Baptist Church where in the fall of 1831 a group of fifteen activists, including Gerrit Smith, announced a meeting for "the friends of the slave." As the group neared the church, they were assaulted by a furious mob and retreated. Although the local press widely condoned the mob's actions, the incident reverberated through the growing community of antislavery sympathizers. Before the end of the decade, three hundred antislavery societies were active in towns across the state. Oswegonians' support of abolition was also recognized in 1849 when Frederick Douglass lectured in the city. It is not known if fifteen-year-old Mary met Douglass at this time, but it is unlikely the Walker family would have missed an opportunity to hear such an important speaker for a cause they believed in so ardently. The year after Douglass's appearance in Oswego, the Liberty Party, which he and Smith had helped to found, held its annual convention in the city, and the passage of the Fugitive Slave Law that year gave rise to increased antislavery efforts in the region. In future years, Mary and Frederick would come to know one another well through the abolition and suffrage movements.[11]

Mary's formal education was also radically shaped by her parents. Determined that their daughters should have as thorough an education as their son and committed to reforming the nation in order to embrace equality in all its institutions, the Walkers decided in the late 1830s to establish a schoolhouse on their Bunker Hill property. With the help of neighbors they erected a building, and Alvah and Vesta founded the region's first free school. They, and later their eldest daughters, served as teachers in the school. The typical curriculum for graduation from common schools in New York State included orthography, writing, reading, and elocution; geography, history, and human physiology; elementary to advanced mathematics; natural, intellectual, and moral philosophies; and drawing and vocal music. The Walkers' free school probably offered many of these areas of study. The exceptional education that Mary Walker received in her youth was evident throughout her life.[12]

During their early formal education, Mary and her siblings gained a new kind of bodily and health education at home as well. Vesta and Alvah were drawn to new ideas about personal hygiene and dress reform, which became major movements in the United States in the 1840s. For the Walkers, dress reform was a health issue. Vesta Walker was severely ill after she gave birth to her first child, and Alvah suffered many illnesses during their Syracuse years; as a result, he became a prolific reader of medical books. He determined through his readings that personal hygiene was the way to a healthy life and that corsets and other forms of binding clothing damaged young females' health. His beliefs were so ardently embraced by his precocious youngest daughter that she became one of the few women in America to embrace the new clothing revolution throughout her life. Health reform for the Walkers was also linked to their temperance and anti-tobacco sentiments. Organized temperance activities emerged in the 1820s, and ministers and physicians alike joined in calling for abstinence from the use of these substances. In 1840, a new direction for the temperance movement arose: "Washington Societies" were organized not by moral leaders but by reformed alcoholics who often dramatically demonstrated on the lecture platform the hellish effects of delirium tremens. Although considered indecorous by some temperance leaders, the Societies greatly expanded awareness of the evils of alcohol abuse. Mary's attitude about the destructive effects of alcohol and tobacco would deepen in the coming years as she studied their physiological effects as part of her medical training.[13]

The growth of several such radical reform movements in Central New York would influence Mary Walker's future as a physician, lecturer, and writer. None was more important, however, than the women's rights movement. One of the primary advantages Mary had over many young women who entered the suffrage crusade was support from both parents. The majority of activists had to endure staunch criticism from their families. As Lucy Stone recalled about her abusive father, "There was only one will in our home, and that was my father's." Mary, however, credited her father with her initial interest in dress reform and both her parents for "support[ing] me in my determination to show the world that I was in earnest, that I had the courage of my convictions." Outside influences were significant as well. Women in New York State were agitating for suffrage several years before the Seneca Falls Convention would draw national attention to the issue. In 1846, for instance, as the state was drafting a new constitution, six women from Jefferson County presented to the constitutional convention in Albany a "Petition for Woman's Rights" in which they argued "[t]hat the present government of this state has widely departed from the true democratic principles . . . by denying to the female portion of the community the right of suffrage and any participation in forming the government and laws under which they live." Taxation without representation, they asserted, denied them "the only safeguards of their individual and personal liberties" and they asked that the state grant women equal civil and political rights. The document is notable for its frank expression of a right to equality, much like the powerful voice that Mary would develop as a suffragist and for which she would be both praised and condemned. She was fifteen when Elizabeth Cady Stanton and a small group of like-minded women organized the nearby Seneca Falls national women's rights convention in 1848. The "Declaration of Sentiments" that emerged as the convention's manifesto observed that "the history of mankind is a history of repeated injuries and usurpations on the part of man toward woman, having in direct object the establishment of an absolute tyranny over her," and the activists established their goal of woman's "inalienable right to the elective franchise" in direct opposition to that tyranny. It was the banner under which Mary Walker would live her life.[14]

As Mary grew into adolescence, many of her free hours were spent studying the medical books that her father had accumulated. She had already developed ideals of aspiration. As yet vague (to maintain high ideals; to develop an independent, genuine career; not to do, think, or say anything simply because everyone else did), they were clearly shaped by her readings. When she read a missionary's letter printed in a local newspaper that detailed the need for women doctors, she began to read voraciously to prepare herself for the evangelical life of a medical missionary. Soon she abandoned the missionary aspect of her goal and devoted herself fully to a detailed study of anatomy. Dr. Calvin Cutter's treatises on anatomy, physiology, and hygiene were her favorite readings at age sixteen. Cutter was an abolitionist, and Mary began to see how reform zeal and medicine could be intimately linked. Cutter's tracts included dozens of engravings that allowed her to study the details of human anatomy. She also read any accounts of coroner's inquests and postmortem examinations she could find. Soon theory was not enough—she wanted to observe an operation. At the time she could not find a surgeon who would agree, but the desire grew with every new text she read. She revealed her interests to her parents, who responded with immediate encouragement. The readings and her parents' beliefs convinced her of the importance of clothing reform, and a new idea began to emerge from her studies: Could she be a physician? All it required was intelligence and a willingness for hard work, both of which she had in abundance. She nurtured the idea as she advanced in her education.[15]

After attending the Walkers' free school, Mary's formal education continued at Falley Seminary in Fulton, New York. Aurora and Luna attended the coeducational seminary from 1845 to 1847. Mary arrived in 1851, the year after the academy's new four-story building was dedicated. She attended the three-term session of 1851–1852. Hungry for the stimulation of advanced study, at nineteen she was also undoubtedly anxious to begin a career, which may explain her attendance for one year instead of the two years her older sisters had completed. The finances of the Walkers were always subject to the precariousness of farming, and that, too, may have been a factor; but most students attended for one year. Three hundred and ninety-five students (220 males and 175 females) were enrolled during the year in which Mary attended. Of that number, only three students (all female) graduated with a two-year degree.[16]

Falley Seminary was not a casual choice for the Walker sisters' education, considering the parents' commitment to new ideas in health issues. The school banned tobacco and alcohol, emphasized personal hygiene, and taught Dr. Cutter's treatises. The "Maine law" of 1851 prohibiting the sale and consumption of alcohol gave new impetus to schools to curb students' alcohol-related unruly behavior. Mary heard Neal Dow, sponsor of the "Maine law," speak in Fulton, and her interest in temperance grew in these years. In her first year at Falley, Mary studied algebra, grammar, natural philosophy, physiology, and hygiene. Six years earlier Paulina Wright Davis had begun a lecture tour to teach women about physiology and anatomy, and water-cure periodicals were bringing new ideas about physiology to their readers; but it was still unusual to have courses on hygiene and physiology in a coeducational school curriculum. Falley proudly noted in its catalog that its library included "numerous means of illustrating the Natural Sciences" and it would offer regular courses of lectures in physiology, natural philosophy, and chemistry. The institution's Executive Board included several physicians. It was the perfect curriculum for a student like Mary with interests in science and medicine. Yet it offered her a more practical education as well. The school's newspaper editor was the daughter of a foreign missionary, and Mary was surprised to have an essay on abolition unceremoniously rejected by the young editor. Mary recalled, "My father had been a very prominent abolitionist and I was very much opposed to human slavery. It struck me as very peculiar that a girl whose father had been a foreign missionary could look with favor on American slavery. That was one of the things which first opened my eyes on this question. I took a stand then and never faltered in my love for American freedom."[17]

After completing the course at Falley, Mary began teaching in Minetto, New York. The boys and girls she taught were drawn to her attractiveness and merriment, but she tolerated no pranks, as one young boy soon learned. In the cold New York winters, the ink bottles often froze, and one morning the boy decided to place a frozen bottle on the stove. When it broke, spewing black ink across the stove top, Mary smacked a ruler across his hands. He was as indignant at being thus treated as the fictional Amy March would famously be, but Teacher Walker held her ground. In reality, Mary viewed teaching only as the financial means to enrollment in a medical college. She was increasingly interested in the new ideas about medical treatments that emerged during her youth and were now gaining ground nationally. While Mary conscientiously fulfilled the requirements of her teaching position, she was also interested in using the classroom as a means of putting into practice her new ideas about hygiene. Her classroom became the future doctor's first laboratory. She also attempted again to observe an operation, asking a local surgeon if she could attend a scheduled removal of a cancerous tumor from a woman's breast, but the surgeon admonished her for displaying "prurient immodesty." Alternatively, she sat with seriously ill neighbors to observe their symptoms.[18]

Following the ideals of her parents, Mary incorporated the theme of dress reform into her views on medical requirements for healthful living. If social proprieties countered her studied opinions, then social proprieties were wrong. While teaching, she began to wear a loose-waist, known as a "Jenny Lind waist" after the young Swedish singing sensation, which was sewn into the skirt of the overdress. She also altered the skirt, raising its length to mid-calf, and added pants beneath the overskirt. When she altered the skirt length again, raising it to the knee, several neighbors verbalized their disapproval. Nor were all of her opponents' attacks merely verbal. One afternoon as Mary was walking along a country road she was observed by a farmer who was outraged to see she was wearing pants beneath a shortened skirt. Mary was a small woman, just over five feet tall and weighing less than one hundred pounds, but this did not cause hesitation on the farmer's part. He gathered a group of boys and they began to chase her, throwing eggs and any object within their reach. While her youth, excellent health, and agility helped her escape (and she proudly recalled years later that she and the farmer had eventually become friends), the incident was only the beginning of Mary's lifelong battle with males who felt free to verbally and physically attack her because of her nonconformity.[19]

After nearly two years of teaching, Mary's dream of a medical education was fulfilled with her acceptance into Syracuse Medical College in December 1853. It was one of the few medical colleges that admitted women in these early years. It is not surprising that she selected an eclectic institution; since childhood she had been steeped in the idea of eclecticism as a form of democratic inquiry. It was the primary basis of her exceptional education: attend more than one church to hear differing ideas about Christianity and draw your own conclusions; listen to a wide variety of lecturers and politicians so as to think critically rather than accept blindly; read widely to bring a well-balanced knowledge to new fields of exploration. Eclectics were part of the Medical Reformers movement of the antebellum era, which included physicians with differing theories of medical practice united by a commitment to liberal reform. While they were interested in exploring all avenues of potential treatment, eclectics drew primarily on homeopathy and herbalism. The American Eclectic Medical Association was founded in 1848, in opposition to the allopathic American Medical Association. Allopaths denigrated eclectics as quacks with no medical standards, and eclectics charged allopaths with being quacks who accepted convention with no scientific investigation into new methodologies. The best physicians on both sides lamented the state of medical training in mid-century America in which medical colleges granted degrees primarily for students' attendance at lectures and less-than-strenuous examinations.[20]

Mary entered the profession just as eclectic medical colleges were engaged in the shift to more rigorous training. While the allopaths' approach would come to dominate American medicine, they were opposed to women in the profession. Equally important for Mary and other reform activists who entered medicine, the AMA was defined by its sense of exclusion and privilege for its members, whereas eclectics emphasized medical therapies for "the common people." Syracuse Medical College was incorporated at the end of 1850 and was certified by the state of New York. It subsumed the eclectic Central Medical College of Syracuse, the first medical institution in the nation to admit women, and Syracuse Medical continued the coeducational policy. One of Central's first graduates, Dr. Lydia Folger Fowler, was appointed professor of obstetrics and diseases of women and children at Central, becoming the first woman medical professor in the United States and a model for women who followed. The handful of institutions that admitted women for medical study in the early 1850s typically had separate curricula or only allowed women to attend selected lectures, often excluding anatomy because it was considered indecent for a woman to view a naked body and an embarrassment for male students to have females in attendance. Many women were fighting to change these standards, but coeducation would not be fully realized in most institutions of medical training for several decades. Elizabeth Blackwell's experiences six years before Mary entered medical college were well known to the public. She was urged by her anatomy professor to forgo attending lectures while the reproductive system was under discussion, and when she began as a resident at the Blockley Almshouse hospital, her male counterparts removed the patients' charts from the wards so she would not have access to their diagnoses and treatments. Mary had experienced the highly unusual situation of a coeducational seminary, and Syracuse Medical's proclaimed philosophy that "nothing should be used as a remedy that will injure the human constitution, and that all means used should have a direct tendency to sustain and not depress the vital powers," undoubtedly appealed to her interest in reform medicine as well.[21]

Medical colleges of this era did not require specific educational preparation before admittance. Acceptance was based on application and fees (and on one's sex). Graduation requirements were completion of two or three winter terms (typically eight to twelve weeks each) consisting of lectures and surgical demonstrations, training in dissection, clinical training in which groups of students visited patients under the guidance of a physician professor, and the successful demonstration of the student's knowledge in an oral examination. The best students sought time outside the classroom with their professors for additional training in anatomical and surgical studies. It was well into the 1870s before any significant changes were enacted on a widespread scale. Mary's medical education was typical for the time: three winter terms of thirteen weeks each, costing $55 per term plus room and board of about $1.50 per week. Each new student was assigned a preceptor, and as Mary's skill and dedication became apparent, Dr. Stephen H. Potter, president of the New York State Eclectic Medical Society and the founding publisher of the *Eclectic Medical and Surgical Journal*, undertook her preceptorship; he became a lifelong friend.[22]

Mary took courses in anatomy, surgery, practice of medicine and medical pathology, obstetrics, women's and children's diseases, physiology, materia medica, therapeutics, pharmacy, chemistry, and medical jurisprudence. It was in the field of therapeutics (treatment of disease) that the various medical philosophies were distinguished. Therapeutics was the invigorating core of medical training in the 1850s, influenced by the progress in physiology and chemistry. Important for Mary's interests was the field's burgeoning attention to diet, hygiene, hydropathy, and other medical regimes that were being developed on a scientific basis. For much of the nineteenth century, hydropathy was an influential aspect of training in therapeutics. The Women's Medical College of Pennsylvania, which would become the most renowned women's medical college in the United States, taught hydropathy as a part of its therapeutics courses and accepted dissertations on the subject; many of its graduates opened sanitariums specializing in hydropathy treatments. Indelibly linked to eclectics' study of therapeutics was that of pharmacy. This course would demonstrate one of the major differences from the teachings of allopathic institutions, where the use of large doses of drugs was commonplace. Eclectics opposed such treatments, preferring to investigate ways in which smaller dosages of drugs (or abstinence from such usage) could be combined with other forms of treatment so as not to "injure the human constitution."[23]

In addition to lectures, Mary was given hands-on experience. Between each term, she moved from the classroom to interning with a licensed physician. A one-year course was all that was required for graduation, but some of the best students, including Mary, remained for advanced study. During these years, she also became a successful subscription agent for the *Syracuse Medical and Surgical Journal*, which was published by the college; she undoubtedly undertook this role to support the eclectic movement but probably to earn extra funds as well. Although in theory eclectics asserted equality, eclectic male students did not always accept their female counterparts as equals. Mary was often told by fellow students that she should marry a doctor, and then if he approved, she could return to her studies. She did make a good friend in another student—Jane M. Clews, who had come from Canada to attend the medical college. Yet when Mary determined to adapt her clothing to a more practical style of a shortened skirt with pants beneath it, other women students did not support her. Clews explained that she agreed in principle but thought they should wait until they had successfully established practices before adding dress reform to their agenda. For Mary, it was a matter of principle, and she would not countenance delay, in spite of negative comments from faculty and students. Her dedication took many forms. Near the end of her medical training, Mary's attention was drawn to the terrible suffering of British soldiers wounded during the Crimean War. She contacted the secretary of war and sought appointment as a physician under the aegis of the British military forces. She may have been influenced, as so many women of the era were, by Florence Nightingale's activities, but she was not interested in nursing. The war ended before she could enact her plan, but the effort foreshadowed the role she would seek in her own country's impending war.[24]

While in medical school, Mary fell in love for the first time. He was a fellow student, identified only as "M.M.G.," and he won her heart by being delighted in her spirit of independence and by pursuing her over a period of several weeks. But as their love progressed, she discovered that he was writing to a young woman from his hometown. Although M.M.G. insisted no discussion of marriage had ever passed between him and the young woman, Mary understood that his correspondent was in love with him. Based on what she termed "principles of justice and self sacrifice" for a woman whose future was dependent on marriage, Mary ended her love affair with M.M.G. (who later married his correspondent). While her decision focused on support rather than competition with another woman, it also allowed her to pursue her studies unencumbered by a lover's expectations.[25]

On February 20, 1855, Mary Edwards Walker was awarded the Doctor of Medicine degree with honors and granted the right to practice medicine and surgery. She earned Censors' Certificates in 1854 and 1855, and the certificates, like licenses late in the century, were an essential requirement for the legal right to practice medicine at this time. On the evening of February 22, Mary experienced one of the crowning moments of her life when graduation ceremonies were held at College Hall. Twelve students received the Doctor of Medicine diplomas that evening. She was one of three students who had formed the Alumni Society; with the motto "Our business is investigation," its members sought to continue their education outside the classroom through weekly meetings in which they engaged in polemical debates, analyzed medical questions, read selected essays, and sought a variety of ways in which to engage themselves intellectually. Because of the high quality of their accomplishments, the three members of the Alumni Society were offered an initial ceremony before the regular commencement began. Albert E. Miller, Mary's future husband, was selected to begin the special ceremony.[26]

Albert's speech offers insights into the values of chartered eclectic medical colleges—and into why Mary was intellectually as well as emotionally drawn to him. We are living in "an age of progress" and reform, Albert told his colleagues and audience members, but reform is not enough. The man who constitutes "the greatest individual of the age . . . is the *liberal* thinker," he asserted, because that man is "free from all prejudice" and breathes the "vivifying atmosphere of science." The hope of the profession was proffered in his conclusion: "Eclecticism . . . is destined e'er long to illuminate the world. Oh! *success to eclecticism*, the *God-send* of the medical mind." Albert's ardency, high standards, and grand ambitions were exactly what Mary avowed for herself in her new role of eclectic physician.[27]

The Society selected J. H. Stebbins to give the valedictory speech for this segment of the commencement, which followed Miller's address. Stebbins noted that, although the Society seemed at first destined to fail, "a few noble minds and progressive spirits, lent a ready and hearty fellowship," and then acknowledged the role that Mary played in the development of the group: "and *woman*, the great pioneer in every philanthropic endeavor, extended her potent aid and sympathy, and through their combined influence and active co-operation, a new impulse was given to our flagging efforts, which has resulted in the awakening of a spirit of investigation which no future discouragements can daunt." The idealism inherent in the Alumni Society's vision of the future was not without an understanding of the difficulty of their undertaking. The Society sought no less than a radical reorganization of society: "All narrow-minded conservatism must give way before a liberal and candid spirit of improvement; and a noble zeal for the welfare of the race, should usurp the place of selfish interests. It requires sound judgment and an unprejudiced mind, as well as indomitable perseverance and determined endeavor; yet not to do this is to be recreant to the claims of truth, the appeals of humanity, and the dictates of conscience." Their creed for medical and social reform, shaped during invigorating weekly meetings, would be the basis for the way in which Mary examined every cause she undertook for the remainder of her life, whether it involved medicine, the law, or civil rights.[28]

Stebbins's speech was followed by a short address from the president, who awarded the members of the Alumni Society special diplomas and then commended the Society for its endeavors. It was, he noted, both "a literary society [that is, the reading of medical literature] for mutual improvement, and for thorough scientific investigation" and that "the habits of investigation here formed would be the key that would unlock the door to the great library of medical practice. Thus they would become *men* and *women* in medical science and literature." When the commencement proceedings were published in the *American Medical & Surgical Journal*, the editor commented that the recognition given to Walker, Miller, and Stebbins was an impressive scene never to be forgotten by those present.[29]

The ceremony then turned to the regular commencement events. Mary had the distinction of presenting the first speech. She addressed the challenges, the many "ignoble obstacles," that faced a woman who pursued medical training. A moving representation of both her exhausting endeavors and her hopes for the future, the speech reflected the difficulty she still felt as a woman taking on the role of physician. Both Miller and Stebbins had freely used "I" in their speeches, but Mary shifted from the individual to the generic woman physician and to the third person form of address. Few women in America at this time understood themselves to be intellectuals, and the shift to third person collective was a means of softening her own claims and projecting solidarity with other women. "'Get wisdom, and with all thy gettings, get understanding,' has made an indelible impression upon her mind," Mary asserted about the woman physician, "and every effort to efface it, brings a *new* proof of its indelibility. She has resolved to avail herself of the only means whereby she can acquire wisdom, which is, intellectual toil." Mary did not shy away from the question that always arose about a woman physician—that bodily knowledge would taint her as a woman. To "Know thyself," she asserted, is commanded in the Bible, but "how can she be acquainted with herself, unless she possesses a knowledge of her self intellectually, not only, but physically." Nor did Mary sidestep the lack of liberty that shaped her own and all women's lives: "She has of late cried as loudly for liberty as did Patrick Henry—her language is—my chains of circumscribed thought *must be sundered*. 'Give me liberty' of thought or give me death!" Observing that she was charged with "criminal curiosity" for pursuing medical studies, she drew upon a lecture by DeWitt Clinton, the renowned New York political leader, to challenge such claims: "*Knowledge never debases.*"[30]

This was one of the first public speeches Mary presented, and as she reminded the audience, the request for herself, Miller, and Stebbins to speak was a surprise that came with short notice. In the newness of her position and the haste to prepare her first speech, she sometimes pushed her metaphors to extremes, but turning to her professors and her peers, she captured her heartfelt appreciation of faculty who did not resist having a woman in their class: "we appreciate the courtesy extended to us as *ladies*, and shall ever remember with gratitude, the noble, philanthropic hearts, that granted us scientific privileges, equal with gentlemen, which, although they might belong to us, have not until recently been enjoyed—and even now, only in a very few colleges. . . . We earnestly hope that you may be successful in all your efforts to promote reform in medicine,—may your anticipations be realized, and may you reap a full reward for all your toil." When she addressed her peers, her voice gained a confidence of equality and experience that had been refined through the debating skills she learned by participating in the Alumni Society. She defined her colleagues' time together as "pleasant and profitable," and then charged them with the responsibility of being "competent to discharge all the duties pertaining to the profession with satisfaction to others, and honor to yourselves." She commanded the students in the audience who had not yet finished their studies to recognize "that their privileges cannot be estimated too highly." As one of only a handful of women in the United States to receive the medical degree, she understood that such an education was, indeed, a privilege of the few. She concluded with a poignant farewell to her colleagues: "But the time to part has arrived. The hand must be taken for the last time. The eyes by which the emotions of the soul are so clearly read, must take their last look. The 'good bye' that has been so often breathed must be repeated. Highly esteemed, and never to be forgotten professors and fellow students, all Farewell!" It was more of a farewell than the graduates may have realized at the time. The college had been founded by a group of notable physicians and teachers, many of whom would go on to distinguish themselves at other medical colleges, but funding was always a challenge, and when Dr. Potter was lured to Cincinnati at the end of 1855, Syracuse Medical College closed. The eclectic medical reform movement, however, would survive into the early twentieth century.[31]

Earning a medical degree was a major accomplishment, but it did not necessarily insure a successful practice. Most of the earliest women physicians struggled to establish private practices that would afford them a livable income. One of Alvah's sisters, Harriet Walker Hall, settled with her family in Columbus, Ohio, and with the family's encouragement, Mary set out for Columbus. Dr. E. W. Stockwell of Cincinnati wrote a letter of recommendation as to her skill as a physician to aid her in setting up practice. Her time in Ohio was short, however. Mary and Albert Miller had kept in touch after graduation. A man of intellect, charm, and eloquence, Miller seemed a suitable life partner for Mary. Although decades later she would insist M.M.G. had been her one true love, she entered her marriage believing it was both a love relationship and a commitment between two like-minded reformers. They worked closely together for two years during their formal studies and in developing the Alumni Society, and the separation of several months while Mary was in Columbus obviously kindled their romantic attachment. Albert set up practice in Rome, New York, and shortly after Mary returned to New York they became engaged. Her three surviving sisters (Cynthia died in 1849 from unknown causes) had all married by this time—Vesta to Willet Worden, Aurora to Lyman Coats, and Luna to Wickham Griswold—and undoubtedly Mary entered into her engagement with Albert expecting, like her sisters, to be forming a lifelong bond.[32]

They were married on November 16, 1855, in the Walker family home, ten days before Mary's twenty-third birthday. Rev. Samuel J. May presided over their marriage. May was well known to the Walker family. He was a liberal Unitarian, an abolitionist, and a longtime supporter of women's rights. Mary wore a dressy version of what was becoming her usual style of apparel in these years: a shortened skirt over pants. Their ceremony reflected Mary's strong feminist values. She would not include the word "obey" in their vows, as she believed antislavery should extend to marriage, and she was supported in her request by Reverend May. Equality was essential to marriage for Mary: "How barbarous the very idea of one equal promising to be a slave to another, instead of both entering life's great drama as intelligent, equal partners! Our promises were such as denoted *two* intelligent beings, instead of one intelligent and one chattel—'to love and cherish each other as long as both shall live.'" The marriage was announced in the local papers, and because of their profession and Mary's growing regional reputation in dress reform circles, notices also appeared in the *New York Medical Journal*, the *American Medical and Surgical Journal*, and Amelia Bloomer's dress reform journal, *The Lily*. One change brought about by Mary's marriage may have remained a mystery to her at this time. Although Alvah Walker was a progressive thinker and supported Mary's desire for a profession, he was not without certain conventional ideas. His will was written to leave most of his property to his son, an annual income to his wife, money to his two married daughters, Aurora and Luna, and to Mary Walker "on the day of her marriage."[33]

Mary and Albert's union was to be an egalitarian marriage and professional partnership, and the sign over their door at 76 Dominick Street declared their joint practice of "Miller and Walker, Physicians." They maintained separate offices on the ground floor; each had his and her own clientele, and Mary drove her own horse and carriage to call on patients. Initially, she intended to treat only women and children, but she was asked occasionally by women patients to be their family physician and began treating a few male patients.[34]

Situated at the foothills of the Adirondacks, the town of Rome was developing quickly in these years; like Oswego, its connection to the Erie Canal made it an important industrial site, and its production of metals would soon earn it the sobriquet of "Copper City." In 1859, Mary and Albert moved their residence and practices to larger rooms at 60 Dominick Street. The combination of woman physician and dress reformer was unusual even in this region of radical thought. In these years Mary was still experimenting with the dress-over-pants style of clothing. She had ten to twelve outfits, with several different skirt lengths. "No matter the length of skirt I wore," she later recalled, "somebody considered it his or her Christian duty to tell me that I ought to wear some other length." Soon Mary experimented with additional changes in her attire. "After a while I wore a marine skirt, made of a sort of transparent fabric; then I got up the courage to take my petticoats off altogether. I wore the loose sack from some time after this."[35]

A part of Mary's support system in these years included other dress reform advocates and women physicians, many of whom would remain lifelong friends. Though few of the women physicians were located near her, they corresponded as best they could with their busy professional and domestic schedules. One of her correspondents during her early years in Rome was her medical school friend Dr. Jane Clews, who had returned to Canada to practice with an established male physician in Bowmanville. Clews's letters reveal the challenges that young women physicians in the 1850s faced when they tried to break the medical barriers. Persecuted by relatives and isolated in the small community of Bowmanville, Jane wrote to Mary for strength and a sense of community. Asserting she was inspired by Mary's perseverance, Jane wrote, "onward onward is my motto." Their new professional experiences were the most important aspect of their correspondence. In one letter Jane noted that she had just returned from a snowy twelve-mile round trip to see a patient. She recalled that Mary had always loved to watch the falling snow, and she proclaimed of her house call, "I had a good time." The isolation was difficult, however, and Jane decided to look for a position in a large city where she would have better support and perhaps the chance to marry. She demanded of Mary, "Say it is better since you are married."[36]

Within two years another woman physician friend would aid Mary in her new role as a writer, and these professional friendships were an important source of support in the years to come. Mary was establishing a solid reputation among her patients. Harriet Harris wrote a letter of appreciation to her in April 1857; Harris had suffered a long illness with chronic pain, but "Doctor Walker has positively cured me," she proclaimed. Harris considered Mary now to be a "Beloved friend," equal in the "love and respect" Harris held for her own sister. Everything on Mary's horizon seemed blessed: she had achieved her extraordinary goal of becoming a physician, she was established in private practice, she had married a man who accepted her radical ideas about equality and who was her intellectual equal, and she was beginning to develop her interests in reform activism and writing. But looming equally large on the horizon were a national catastrophe in which she would play an important role as a woman physician, and a personal catastrophe that would forever reshape her life and her ideas about marital relationships.[37]

CHAPTER 2

Dress Reform and *The Sibyl*

Mary Walker wanted to be famous. She dreamed of it in her youth, and she proclaimed in her commencement address that she and her colleagues should seek "greatness in usefulness" as their highest priority but also should write their "names on the highest tablet of fame." Her desire for public recognition was well known among her friends. As Clews wrote to Mary, since "you are an aspirant after fame[,] I am with you." While Clews feared that fame meant notoriety, Mary saw it as an acknowledgment of intellectual achievement. Although "notorious" would be the term by which many critics identified Mary's national standing in the coming years, she had an extraordinary belief in herself and her abilities that was confirmed by her admirers. Her fame would chart every possible facet of public recognition, from curiosity and scandal to admiration and national treasure. Her greatest fame would come from her seven-decade crusade for women's rights.[1]

In the 1850s Mary began to realize that her love of literature and writing was both a means of gaining a wider audience for her radical beliefs and an avenue to fame. Literature had been an integral part of the Walker family household. In Mary's youth the Central New York region became increasingly famous due to the writings of authors such as James Fenimore Cooper and Washington Irving. Periodicals flourished in the region, and Oswego itself produced a literary magazine, *The Oasis,* in the mid-1830s. Family scrapbooks of literature were common among educated families, and the Walker family scrapbooks reveal the wide range of materials that was available to Mary and her siblings as a means of advancing their liberal education. In addition to religious selections, the scrapbooks were rife with poems about temperance, antislavery, equality, and the maltreatment of Native Americans. The importance of education was highlighted. Not least important among the politically oriented poems were selections such as "Fashion," which exposed the financial burdens of dressing in fashionable female clothing. Mary's love of poetry is evident in the many quotes that pepper her writings, and she was moved to make her own experiments in the genre. One poem, written after the Civil War, reflects on the desire to live into old age and then pass into "fields Elysian—/ ... Through quiet transition." Nothing in Mary's life would be through quiet transition, but in 1857 she was about to add a new avenue of endeavor, one that would shape her life for the next six decades. The transitional avenue was writing, but it was dress reform that would be the driving force of her ideals and her growing fame. For Mary, dress reform was the link between her love of medicine and her belief in women's equality.[2]

Her commitment to women's rights would have made the suffrage movement one of the most likely avenues for these endeavors. She was well acquainted with the leaders of both suffrage and antislavery groups, but her heavy schedule of medical training, moving to Ohio and back to New York, marrying, and establishing a practice limited her overt political activities in the mid-1850s. By 1857 when she was ready to become more active, the women's rights movement was in the throes of crisis. Many of the leaders—including Stanton, Stone, and Rev. Antoinette Brown Blackwell—were pregnant or nursing newborns, and their collective activities flagged. Further, much of the time they did have was being directed toward antislavery efforts. Legal decisions, such as the *Dred Scott v. Sanford* case that allowed slave owners the right to their "property" even in free states, caused major splits in the woman's suffrage organizations. With dissension rising, funds diminishing, and leaders exhausted, the 1857 national convention was cancelled. Thus Mary determined to devote herself at present to the dress reform cause.[3]

Dress reform evolved over several decades. Many women who were part of the westward movement or who, like Mary and her sisters, lived on a farm had learned quickly that practicality made the wearing of pants a necessity of physical labor. These early changes in costume received little public attention or criticism. Women such as George Sand and Rosa Bonheur began in the 1840s to alter their clothing choices, and while they were loudly condemned in the popular press they were also seen as exceptional women who had little relation to the sex in general. Dress reformers asserted that liberty of body and mind were inseparable. Elizabeth Smith Miller, daughter of Gerrit Smith, brought dress reform to national attention in the spring of 1851 when she began to appear publicly in "Turkish trousers" (billowing pant legs that tapered to a tight fit around the ankles) and a skirt shortened to about four inches below the knee. She created a sensation because no necessity of physical labor precipitated her actions. Miller's cousin, Elizabeth Cady Stanton, joined her in wearing the reform dress, and their mutual friend, Amelia Jenkins Bloomer of Homer, New York, quickly embraced their actions. In the June 1851 issue of her temperance magazine, *The Lily*, Bloomer published an explicit argument about the physical dangers of conventional clothing: women's dresses "distorted spines, compressed lungs, enlarged livers, and [resulted in] displacement of the whole abdominal viscera." Because Bloomer had the power of the press in which to make her arguments, the new female attire quickly became known as the Bloomer dress, although many variations were created by reformers.[4]

In spite of cartoonists' satire and condemnation from many newspaper editors, a significant movement for dress reform was born. Allopathic physicians largely insisted that women remain dressed in conventional clothing, but many eclectic, homeopathic, and hydropathic medical practitioners supported the new style for women. Most of the major figures in the suffrage movement donned the reform dress in these years. Two important advocates were Dr. Lydia Sayer, who began wearing a reform dress in 1849, and her soon-to-be husband, John S. Hasbrouck, of Middletown, New York. When *The Lily* ceased publication in 1856, Sayer and Hasbrouck were determined to continue the cause. On July 1, 1856, they published the first issue of *The Sibyl: A Review of the Tastes, Errors and Fashions of Society*, a periodical edited by Dr. Sayer and devoted primarily to dress reform. The idea of the journal was born at the first meeting of the Dress Reform Association (DRA), held in Glen Haven, New York, in February; *The Sibyl* became its official publication. Mary's and Dr. Lydia Sayer Hasbrouck's mutual commitment to medicine and dress reform formed a long-lasting bond for the two physicians, and Hasbrouck began to recruit Mary as a contributor to her publication. The pages of *The Sibyl* reflected both the publisher's and the readers' wide range of political interests. *The Sibyl*, like the DRA, was adamant that what constituted propriety for women in American culture was exactly what needed most to be reformed: "*Resolved*, That, in advocating Reform in Dress for Woman, our object is not to advocate for her positions of singularity, eccentricity, immodesty or to get her out of her 'appropriate sphere;' but to enable her to act with that freedom needful to find out what her 'appropriate sphere' is."[5]

Well-known women who abandoned or criticized the dress reform movement were subject to considerable criticism from *The Sibyl*. The Bloomers had been quickly associated with exoticism, and Susan B. Anthony, Stanton, and Stone felt the extreme level of criticism they received for wearing the dress had martyred them for the cause. Suffragists confronted the same kind of attacks about their work for the vote, but clothing made it more personal, and there was a discomfort with the attention that the reform dress brought to their bodies. However, Mary and Lydia Hasbrouck believed that far more than appearance was at stake: clothing extended to all aspects of women's equality. Anthony proclaimed during her advocacy of the reform dress, "I can see no business avocation, in which woman in her present dress *can possibly* earn *equal wages* with a man." Thus when Hasbrouck reprimanded the women who were abandoning the movement for having so "little faith" and such a "lack of energy" for true reform, she was doing so in the belief that women's full equality was being undermined.[6]

The journal engaged many other women's rights issues as well. While Hasbrouck praised the very popular Fanny Fern for satirizing the latest fashions for women, she and her readers were quick to chide Fern for a satiric attack on women physicians. Fern denigrated the female physician as incapable of rationality and professionalism: "A female doctor! Great Esculapius! Before swallowing her pills (of which she would be the first), I should want to make sure that I had never come between her and a lover, or a new bonnet, or been the innocent recipient of a gracious smile from her husband." In an editorial, Hasbrouck declared, "Fanny Fern has uttered many good thoughts on women and society, but a late dash of her pen on 'Woman Physicians,' should brand her forever as one to be scorned by her sex, and all true spirits seeking for society's elevation and purification." The challenges faced by women physicians were common subjects in the periodical from its inception. Women physicians interested in reform published letters and articles on a variety of subjects in *The Sibyl*, including conditions for women at coeducational and women's medical colleges. Regular contributors included Dr. Fidelia R. Harris of Wisconsin; Dr. Ellen Beard of the Glen Haven Water Cure center in New York and editor of *The Reformer* (when she married in 1859, she and her spouse published their marriage protest in *The Sibyl*); and Dr. Harriet Austin of Dansville, New York, who would become president of the National Dress Reform Association (NDRA) in 1860. Mary's involvement with organized dress reform afforded her many lifelong friends, especially other women physicians.[7]

The Sibyl contained poetry and occasionally fiction, but it was primarily a publication for the articulation of reform goals and thus essays and letters to the editor—often with extended responses from Hasbrouck—were its primary genres. The literary works related specifically to the ideals of reform, with poetry by well-known figures such as Alice Cary and John Greenleaf Whittier. The integration of autobiographical narratives was common in the journal as a means of sharing the experience of wearing a reform dress. Anti-tobacco arguments, temperance, suffrage, and women's economic disparity were also explored in the pages of *The Sibyl*. Hasbrouck wrote impassioned editorials against businesswomen's taxation without representation, and in favor of going en masse to the polls attempting to register to vote as the best way to enact change.[8]

Writing did not come easily to Mary as a child, but her grandfather and father kept lifelong daily journals and she and her sisters were encouraged at a young age to do the same. Mary began her journal when she was quite new to the process of writing: "I was so small that I had not been attempting to write but a short time and when I wanted to read my journal over, I used to go to one of my sisters to decipher my writing parts of which I could not read myself. My mother was amused at this but I remember how she suppressed her smiles because she knew keeping such a journal I would improve my writing." During the Civil War, Mary's father would again encourage her to return to journal writing so her extraordinary experiences would not be lost to history. "I attempted to do [so] for a time," she recalled, "but there was so much to be written and I was so weary that I abandoned it after a brief time." Diary keeping may have been abandoned, but when it came to political writing and the reform causes to which she devoted her life, her pen flowed.[9]

Mary's first contribution to *The Sibyl* in January 1857 was a brief letter to the editor confirming interest among residents of Rome and neighboring communities in the upcoming dress reform convention in Canastota. Although stiffly formal, the letter nonetheless reveals patterns in Mary's style that would develop as she became more experienced as a writer. Using the formal "we," she reported, "We expect there will be a good attendance of those who are richly provided with common sense, intelligence, and decision of character" and that the convention would "tell well" for reformatory principles. Her second contribution to *The Sibyl* continued her role as reporter, this time covering the January 7 convention. She produced a detailed account of the gathering, its participants, and its evolving policies, including the agreement not to demand only one style of reform clothing. She had been one of the speakers, along with Gerrit Smith and others. Through her work for dress reform over the next few years, Mary came into contact with like-minded individuals who embraced multiple reform agendas. Some were old friends, such as Rev. Samuel J. May, Smith, and Stanton; others were new acquaintances, including Angelina Grimké. Hasbrouck was delighted to have recruited such a promising writer for the journal, and she added a note in the issue thanking Dr. Walker for her contributions and her efforts to increase *The Sibyl*'s circulation.[10]

During this year Mary also began a third part of her career that, like medicine and writing, would last until her death: lecturing. Her reputation as a dress reform lecturer spread quickly. Soon her own activities were the subject of reports in *The Sibyl*, where she was praised for her "very easy and graceful manner" and her "familiarity with the science connected with her profession." Although this era also saw the beginning of public ridicule of her attire from newspaper editors, the positive responses to her lectures and the encouraging words of Hasbrouck and others were effective. She increased her lecturing schedule and began to submit short letter-articles to *The Sibyl*. Her first two contributions, "Synopsis of a Sermon, By Rev. A. S. Wightman" and "A Bloomer in the Street," offered critiques of someone else's argument. This format allowed Mary to develop her writing style and to hone her skills in argumentation. In the early months of 1859, Mary began to publish her own arguments on a variety of subjects, and for the first time, she used a strong and assertive "I." She was able to balance a sense of outrage and injustice with a reasoned examination of motivations and solutions. For instance, in late 1858 Mary Morris Hamilton and other female managers of the Ladies' Mount Vernon Association announced that they were using their $500,000 in funds to purchase and restore George Washington's home. Women's rights activists across the country were outraged that women would use such an enormous amount of money to further recognize a man who had been accorded innumerable honors rather than using it to aid the advancement of their own sex. Elizabeth Cady Stanton wrote a letter of protest to Hamilton, urging her to use the money for women's education. In February 1859, Mary published her analysis of the association's decision. She too argued for the funds to go toward women's education, adding that if Martha Washington could speak, "she would beg women not to rob themselves." She suggested the money be used to erect "one grand national literary female college, where every opportunity for improvement could be afforded to women that is now given to men. This would indeed be an honor to the nation. . . . How much more noble to educate the immortal mind, to build intellectual monuments that are self-moving and progress, that cast no shadows of a somber hue, but shed a halo of light around them." She found some solace in the situation, however, as the responses to the Association's goal signified that women were agitating to find a means of directing their energy for the sex's advancement.[11]

Mary learned her ideals not on the public stage but in that enlightened household on Bunker Hill Road. No better reminder of that fact could have been given to her than the letter to the editor that followed Mary's article. It was written by her mother, who also wore the reform dress, and was titled to emphasize her own outrage—"Let your Women Keep Silent." Vesta followed events that were unfolding in her hometown of Greenwich, Massachusetts, where a woman had recently stood during a Presbyterian prayer meeting and spoke about her faith. The "act was considered so sinful," Vesta wrote, that the minister cancelled the meeting. Ironically, only days later the minister and male leaders of the church wondered how they might improve "the low state of religion." One of the leaders suggested they encourage women to take an active part, but the idea was squelched by the minister, who asserted "that the Bible forbade women speaking in public!" Vesta's letter reveals the spirit that nurtured her youngest daughter's beliefs in the right to speak her mind.[12]

Mary's next contribution to *The Sibyl* opened a new area of interest for her—the law. The sensational Sickles-Key murder trial engrossed the American public. In the early nineteenth century, reporting about murder trials was typically a two-pronged process: exposing the horror of the events, and, most importantly, creating a sense of mystery around the idea of the crime itself. The mystery centered on the argument that murder was an incomprehensible act, one to which meaning could not be assigned because it was inhuman in and of itself. Thus murderers became moral monsters against which readers could assert their own normalcy. Mary would accept some of these premises—that someone who murdered another person was not representative of the common sinner but a moral aberration—yet like her sister women's rights advocates, she challenged the idea that such crimes must be shrouded in mystery. Meaning could, indeed, be drawn from the act of murder when it was connected to the marriage relationship.[13]

On Sunday afternoon, February 27, 1859, Congressman Daniel Sickles shot Phillip Barton Key on the street in front of the Sickleses' home in Washington, D.C. The congressman's rage had been festering for weeks as he came to believe that his wife was having an affair with Key. The intrigue of a murder in response to a marital affair would have garnered sufficient press on its own, but the fact that Sickles was a congressman and that Key was the district attorney for the District of Columbia and son of Francis Scott Key inflamed public interest. Sickles's attorney argued that his client could not be held responsible for his actions because he had been driven insane by his wife's infidelity. This insanity claim became a point of national debate. As *Harper's Weekly* observed, "the public ear, it seems, can not be satiated with details of the catastrophe." Such reactions also justified feeding that appetite. The widely read weekly sympathized with Sickles and proclaimed, "the public of the United States will justify him in killing the man who had dishonored his bed." Such a case allowed for a salacious and titillating discussion of sexual relations, and *Harper's* was willing to assume Mrs. Sickles's guilt—"a fact of which it appears that there can be no doubt"—before the trial even began. In the weekly's reports over a period of two months, Sickles was depicted as a gentleman whose actions were justified, who "maintained a very proper deportment," and was a loving father. A few weeks later, two full pages were devoted to a flattering biography of the defendant.[14]

As the trial itself approached, the reportage moved from fervor to frenzy. In the early weeks of newspaper coverage, Teresa Bagioli Sickles received little attention from the press except as the fallen woman. Daniel Sickles obtained from his wife a written confession, but suspicious of the circumstances under which it was produced, the court refused to enter the document as evidence in the trial. However, it was printed the next day the *National Police Gazette*. Teresa Sickles purportedly confessed that the house in which she met with Key was owned by "a colored man," which to a mainstream audience added to the immorality of her actions. The confession allegedly included such details as "I undressed myself. Mr. Key undressed also" and concluded with an acknowledgment that Daniel had given her "repeated orders" not to let Key visit when he was away from home. In spite of the court's ruling that the confession was not evidence, defense references to it left the jury with no doubt that infidelity was the defendant's justification for the murder. Finally, in May, the verdict was rendered: not guilty. It was the first successful insanity defense in U.S. courts. In reality, none of the participants was without blame. If Key's reputation as a "ladies' man" was made evident during the trial, Daniel Sickles's was not. But after the verdict was recorded, even the supportive *Harper's* ran an item decrying the exclusion of evidence of Sickles's own infidelity. The prosecution certainly could have found any number of witnesses, since Daniel Sickles had been known to wander through the Albany Assembly chamber in company with a woman who ran a local bordello. As one diarist of the period remarked, "One might as well try to spoil a rotten egg, as to damage Dan's character."[15]

It was the double standard employed by the national press that compelled Mary to write an extensive analysis of the case. As Mary observed in her opening assessment of the "Sickles and Key Tragedy" in April 1859, "Much has been said concerning this lamentable tragedy, but in none of the quill parlances, have we seen any true sympathy manifested for Mrs. Sickles." Mary was particularly disturbed by the ways in which women had joined in the chorus condemning Teresa Sickles. Where, she asked, is the hand of charity to "help her out of the moral ravine—not to *sisterly* say, that she might have been one of the brightest stars in the moral world, if she had been surrounded with a train of more favorable circumstances," but neither to condemn solely. It was a carefully crafted argument, not condoning infidelity but pointing out that Teresa Sickles was emblematic of the cultural insistence that women were responsible for morality in U.S. society. As Mary's critique of the condemnation of Teresa Sickles moved more broadly to woman's situation in society, she mocked the censure of Sickles for breaking the oath to "'love, honor, and *obey*'" her husband that had been expressed in a woman's letter to the *New York Express*: "A *woman* advocating women being self bound life slaves to masters!" she exclaimed. Could anyone have been married so long that they would accept the idea of "an intelligent being [turned] into a *chattel*"? She also wondered why Daniel Sickles was not condemned for tyrannically demanding that his wife write out a confession and, especially, for then exposing her indiscretion to public view by giving the court and the press access to the document. If he did not care about the shame and infamy brought upon his wife, she asked, did he never think about the consequences for his daughter?[16]

Equally disturbing to Mary was the *Express* writer's insistence that Teresa Sickles was "'*more* culpable than Key, because she led him along.'" As a physician, Mary had insight into the diversity within marital relations, and it allowed her to argue that nothing suggested Teresa Sickles lured Key into an affair; one could just as well suggest that "the crime consequent upon Mrs. S. and Key's intimacy, was one of *force* . . . and of threats of exposure afterwards." In reality, the most likely scenario, given Daniel Sickles's well-known record of extramarital affairs, was that "Key probably thought that it would be no worse for him to ruin the character of Mrs. S., and then boast of it, than it was for Sickles to boast of *other* conquests." How, then, could Teresa Sickles be more culpable? "Never," Mary wrote, "until women as a mass are better educated physiologically—until they are considered something besides a drudge or a doll—until they have all the social education and political advantages that men enjoy; in a word, *equality* with them, shall we consider vice in our sex any more culpable than in men." The tragedy was not only that a murder was committed, but that women's ignorance was celebrated: "I would that ladies who have no time to read had sense enough to throw aside their embroidery, and read Mental Philosophy, Moral Science, and Physiology; and then go to a smith's and have their dressical and dietetical chains severed, that they may go forth free, sensible women, 'slow to judge, and slower to despise.'" In this last twist, Mary brought her critique full circle: the letter-writer to the *Express*, had she been educated to true knowledge instead of to patriarchal bondage, would not condemn Teresa Sickles but would offer charitable sympathy, and work to see that other women did not fall prey to an education that sees charm as woman's greatest attribute. She signed the article, "Yours in charity for our own sex."[17]

Mary believed marriage was a sacred commitment, but she held liberal ideas about the need for equality in marriage and did not believe that it could only be sanctified by a church ceremony. In August 1858, for instance, she and Albert hosted an unconventional wedding in their home in Rome. Lucretia Bradley, "the far famed aeronaut" and lecturer on phrenology from New London, Connecticut, married Algernon Sidney Hubbell, a well-known orator from New Haven. It was a "Friend's ceremony," but the couple was "married, by themselves." Supporting the Bradley-Hubbell ceremony signified Mary's belief that marriage was a personal endeavor and not one to be regulated by the state. She also was interested in other women who led unconventional lives, including Lola Montez (1821–1861). Montez was widely known as a dancer and as mistress of Bavaria's Ludwig I. She toured the United States in the early 1850s and shocked San Franciscans when she performed the erotic "Spider Dance." Mary owned a copy of the *Lectures of Lola Montez, Including Her Autobiography*. In some ways the two women could not have been more different—Montez lived primarily off her beauty and Walker her intellect—but Mary had just embarked on her own career as a lecturer and may have hoped to draw guidance on what appealed to Montez's audiences. She appreciated that Montez discussed an "intellectual kind of beauty" as well as physical. Montez talked about "preposterous fashion" and bewailed the popular but "health-destroying bodice," asserting that fashion should be to "preserve the health of the human form." Mary may well have felt that the text spoke directly to her, as Montez used the generic name of "Mary" to describe the growth and maturation of a woman from her teens to adulthood. Montez's attention to "Heroines of History" appealed to all women who were attempting to advance women's causes, but her account of George Sand undoubtedly drew Mary's ardent attention, especially since Montez understood that Sand wore pants "from no mere caprice or waywardness of character, but for the reason that in this garb she is enabled to go where she pleases." Sand was described as a highly intelligent woman who talked earnestly on great subjects, and it must have thrilled Mary when Montez remarked on Sand as a representative of women reformers' search for freedom of mind and body: "like most of the reformers of the present day, especially if it is her misfortune to be a woman, is a target placed in a conspicuous position to be shot at by all dark unenlightened human beings, who may have peculiar motives for restraining the progress of mind; but it is as absurd in this glorious nineteenth century, to attempt to destroy freedom of thought, and the sovereignty of the individual, as it is to stop the falls of Niagara."[18]

Mary refused to remain silent about issues that were supposed to be too "delicate" for women but which impacted their lives in the most intimate and life-changing ways, including pregnancies of unmarried women and abortion. She published two substantial commentaries in August and September of 1859 calling for the building of a state-run foundling hospital. She called on *The Sibyl*'s readership, in support of their unmarried sisters and the children they bore, to pledge funds and thereby demonstrate to the state the need for its cooperation in the project. Although the essays were subtitled "A Hastily Written Whisper to Every Woman," the publication and frank discussion of the topic was anything but a "whisper." Citing poet Bayard Taylor's remark on New Yorkers' conservatism, "If some benevolent millionaire should propose to building [a foundling hospital] in New York, pulpit and press would ridicule with the red hot shot of holy indignation," Mary agreed, but added, "we cannot believe that the intelligent, the noble, the philanthropic powers of the press, that sway the world of mind, will come out against what their extensive knowledge of the necessities of the world demands." It only hurts the children of unmarried parents and encourages criminal acts such as abortion when Americans try to ignore the fact that "the world is as it is," she declared.[19]

New York State laws, which Mary cited, allowed abortions in two instances—if it "shall have been necessary to preserve the life of such woman, or shall have been advised by two physicians to be necessary for that purpose." Although the law prohibited physicians from any act that would "produce miscarriage," Mary observed, women were going to find a way to have an abortion "regardless of future consequences, while there is no provision made for her, where her misfortune may not be maliciously published to an unsympathetic world," unless alternatives such as a foundling hospital became available. She was treading into dangerous territory. For decades, the term "female physician" had been used to refer to abortionists; the most notorious female abortionist, Madame Restell (Caroline Lohman), was from Mary's home state. Lohman was brought to trial in the 1840s in a case that drew wide public attention and made the connection between women healers and abortionists prevalent in the public mind. When women in the 1850s sought to attend medical colleges, critics often charged that they were simply attempting to become abortionists. But Mary's concerns about abortion and its often dangerous consequences for women were well founded. Since legitimate physicians were barred by law from performing safe abortions, women had only unlicensed and sometimes incompetent abortionists to turn to for aid—and they were doing so in significant numbers. Abortion had become epidemic in America by the 1850s; in New York City, stillbirths and abortions had increased in the last decade by 140 percent. Following the beliefs of the day, Mary asserted that children born outside of marriage were prone to a life of poverty and crime; but she sought to change cultural attitudes. Instead of seeing these women as sisters who need sympathy and assistance, she observed, women are restricted by cultural attitudes that condemn both the respectable and the "fallen" woman. "Can it be," she asked, "that an intelligent woman fears 'the world's cold frown' in doing a humanity deed? . . . Could all of the infanticides, the abortions, the poisoning of other men's wives, and the innumerable wrongs resulting from what a Foundling Hospital would prevent, be presented to the reader, what a long list one year would show in the State of N.Y. alone!" To change circumstances, she directed readers to support the construction of a foundling home. Mary's understanding of these issues was crafted on the medical battlefield, and her comments in this article are revealing of the life of a woman physician at mid-century:

> Few see into the heart of society unveiled as the physician does, and it is impossible for any one to do so as unmistakably, as a female physician. There are no class of persons that are confided in as the physicians are. Thousands of people believe that all their thoughts and acts are unmistakably read by doctors, and the physician is priest before whom more confessions are made, than before any ordained divine. More confessions are made to physicians, than even to deity. The very whisperings of conscience meets the physician's ears.[20]

In September Mary published a second article on the subject. Responses were forthcoming in "quite a number" from women who were willing to serve as agents.

This is "emphatically 'woman's sphere,'" she declared, suggesting that subscriptions could be increased by a systematic organizing of their actions. "Each town or city agent can appoint assistant agents, in other wards or school districts, thus expediting the matter, so that the state may easily be canvassed by the first of January. All Ladies' Societies should be called upon, and solicited to pledge themselves to furnish a certain number of articles for bedding." Undoubtedly Mary envisioned herself as physician and director of the hospital. It was not only a cause dear to her heart; it was typical of the ways in which early women physicians found the means to successfully survive and perhaps even prosper in their chosen profession. Mary would have been well aware of the New York Infirmary for Women and Children that Drs. Elizabeth and Emily Blackwell founded just two years earlier. To establish a hospital of her own would have given Mary that same possibility for success, and it was the first of several such institutions she would attempt to establish throughout her career. The foundling hospital was never brought to fruition, partly because of lack of support from the state and partly from two events that were simmering and about to radically change Mary's life: explosive revelations about her own marital relations, and the impending Civil War, which would require all of the state's and the country's money to support.[21]

———

In the summer of 1859 notes in *The Sibyl* from Dr. Hasbrouck to Mary began to suggest that she was not meeting deadlines, and she was suddenly absent from dress reform conventions. Part of her new-found sense of self certainly came from her successful public activities, but it was also shaped by her private endurances. In March 1860, Mary placed a notice in the *Rome Sentinel* announcing the relocation of her medical office to 48 Dominick Street, above Shelly's Clothing Store: "The Doctor expresses her gratitude to the Romans for their liberal patronage, and solicits a continuance of the same." The newspaper's editor added words of support, "Those who prefer the skill of a female physician to that of a male, have now an excellent opportunity to make their choice."[22]

Months earlier Mary was devastated to discover that her husband was involved with at least one other woman. She confronted Albert about his "vileness" and demanded a divorce. Unrepentant, he suggested she forgo a divorce and claim "the same *privileges*" of extramarital relationships. Angry and humiliated, she insisted he leave. Mary's brother-in-law L. J. Worden arrived at the house just as the scene was unfolding. As Albert dashed past Worden and into his carriage, he told Worden, "in a *meaning* and *mean* manner" as Worden discerned it, to attend to Mary. When Worden entered the house, Mary was weeping, filled with pain and outrage at Albert's infidelity and open-marriage proposition. She told Worden in this moment of rare openness about her marriage "that people who thought her *so happy* knew little of her *wretchedness*."[23]

She was determined to obtain a divorce while maintaining her professional life. Even in her smaller offices, the first few months of operation cost her more than she took in because of the expenses incurred in moving and in purchasing supplies. Over the next few years she would discover, through reports from independent court-appointed referees, that Albert had numerous affairs, fathered at least one child with another woman, was arrested for seducing a female patient, and generally led a life of debauchery, all the while maintaining his community standing as a physician. Although they were now living separately, Albert would haunt Mary's life and thwart her attempts for a divorce for the next nine years. In 1860 New York State's divorce laws were among the most restrictive in the nation. Only adultery was accepted as a basis, and the costs of filing were repressive. Although legal, divorce was still a social disgrace, even among many women's rights activists. But Mary was determined.[24]

In spite of her personal difficulties, Mary attended the NDRA convention in Waterloo in May. Had her personal situation been different at this point, she would likely have risen to the presidency of the organization, as she was already a vice president and was asked at the evening session to take the chair in the current president's absence. She offered input on the resolutions and business policies of the association, but she declined to take the chair even in a temporary capacity. She was already planning to leave the state, and her participation in the organization she loved had to wait until she could sever her relationship with Albert. She had the necessary grounds for divorce in New York; yet Mary knew that the state required a five-year waiting period before a granted divorce became final. She decided to try to expedite matters. In 1843 Iowa had revised its laws to authorize a divorce when "it is apparent to the satisfaction of the Court that the parties cannot live in peace or happiness together, and that their welfare requires a separation between them." Believing she met the standards and hoping quickly to end all connections to Albert, Mary left her medical practice in Rome and her burgeoning career as writer and lecturer and moved to Delhi, Iowa. She resided with the House family, old friends who had lived in Oswego. A. E. House was a lawyer and judge, and he generously advised Mary on Iowa laws. The editor of the Delhi newspaper, who wrote an editorial in support of her reform dress after the nearby Dubuque press satirized her attire, asked her to write an article for the paper, but when she produced details of her "own doings," as he put it, he refused to publish it. No woman, he believed, could at the age of twenty-seven have been a teacher, medical student, physician, and dress reform lecturer.[25]

Deciding to use this time for self-improvement, in the fall of 1860 she enrolled at the newly founded Bowen Collegiate Institute in nearby Hopkinton with the goal of studying German. She had begun teaching herself German while in Rome and now wished for advanced study. But the institute was foundering financially. Although it had advertised German as an area of study and accepted her enrollment fees, there was no one to teach the course. Mary threatened to take Bowen to court if they did not offer the course as advertised and, perhaps worse for the struggling school, let it be known publicly that they could not fulfill their promises. It was the kind of insistence on rightful actions Mary would always take in such situations; but at this moment in her life she was tired of feeling she had been misled and her anger boiled over. As a reprieve from the tension of her dispute with the administration, Mary attended an evening meeting of a debate society organized by several young men in Hopkinton. She thoroughly enjoyed the debates and asked at the end of the session to become a member. A vote was called, and she easily won admission. She was also invited to participate in the debate scheduled for the following week. When Bowen's director of women students, Miss Cooley, heard about the evening's events, she ordered Mary not to participate in the forthcoming debate. It was ludicrous, Mary felt, for the school to attempt to control her evening hours, so she ignored the charge and participated in the debate. The moment would have passed without notice if Cooley had not insisted that Mary be suspended from the institute for disobeying her direct order. It was a power struggle between two strong wills. This time Mary had met her match.[26]

When publicly informed of her suspension, Mary gathered her belongings and left, and most of the young men left with her. They quickly decided to make a blatant protest. Forming a procession with Mary in the lead, they marched through several downtown streets, garnering exactly the attention they hoped to receive. The result was that the men were also suspended. They soon asked to return, however, and insisted Mary be able to join them. Cooley refused; the men returned, but Mary was expelled. It was not a trivial issue for Mary. She was already a paid lecturer, she had followed the bylaws of the organization and been admitted by its members, and therefore the denial of her right to participate was unjust. It was the first of many public protests over denial of women's rights that Mary would initiate in her lifetime. In the end she may have been expelled, but she gained a small group of supporters in the community. Waiting for the divorce to progress, she was pleased to be able to work occasionally with a local physician, Dr. Cunningham, but it was a frustrating time at best.[27]

In spite of the new laws of Iowa, Mary did not receive a divorce decree in the state. While living in Delhi, she corresponded with B. F. Chapman, an attorney in Rome. She had not told Chapman when she left Rome that she intended to seek a divorce, but she eventually revealed her plans to him. He responded quickly by sending her a five-page abstract of recent New York State divorce case decisions. As Mary quickly realized, the state courts had repeatedly refused to accept out-of-state divorces. Chapman was a trusted friend, and she heeded his suggestions. Painful as it was, the education in legal matters that accompanied Mary's drawn-out divorce proceedings served her well in the future. For now, she packed her bags and returned to New York.[28]

Only months before her separation from Albert, Mary published "Women Soldiers" in *The Sibyl*. It would be her last article in the magazine for nearly eighteen months. By September 1859 when the article appeared, the country knew it was moving toward war. John Brown's raid on the federal arsenal at Harper's Ferry in

October and his subsequent hanging would be a critical turning point toward war for Northerners. Dr. Hasbrouck began to use her editorial power to speak out in favor of abolition in *The Sibyl* as well. The timeliness of Mary's article coincided with ongoing discussions in the magazine and on the lecture platforms at women's rights conventions of the injustice of women's taxation without representation. Conservatives, Mary noted, always respond to this argument with the tired charge, "Shoulder the musket and go to the battle field . . . just as though every one that had political rights must of necessity be a warrior." It is time, she added, that "such ignorant conservatives" hear the truth: "women have gone to the 'battle field,' fought and died in their country's cause, been willing martyrs, and you have not heard of them! Women have helped to gain the elective franchise that you to-day enjoy, and now you thrust her away from the polls, as though she were not worthy to enjoy what she has fought for by your sire's side." She attacked what she called opponents' "butterflyism," the denigration of women as incapable of such service. The voice of indictment she developed in this essay was one she would call on for the rest of her public life:

> But Mr. or Miss Conservative, you say that only very young and inconsiderate women ever expose themselves to the fury of the cannon's mouth or anywhere else out of their sphere. You are not as ignorant as you are malicious, for you wish that you could trample on all women, and you try to convince yourself that there is not, nor ever has been any women who aspired to notoriety in any other direction, than owning a "love of a bonnet," "queenly robes," "white arms and necks," &c.

After citing women from various countries who had fought in righteous battles, she concluded that conservatives would be proved wrong: "they will see many such 'instances of Bloomerism' in our own country, among our 800 Bloomers, if war should break out and need such service. Yours in rendering to woman honors due. Dr. Walker." Her alliance of Bloomerism with the warrior spirit embraced a transition in the definition of Bloomerism to that of a militant force. As the Civil War began, Mary would reject the musket, but she would shoulder her medical bag and "go to the battle field" with an ardent commitment to the Union cause and an insistence on her right to serve her country as a physician—not as a nurse, which the military would have preferred. It was a daunting challenge to the gendered code of the nation, and it was an act that would forever place her in the public consciousness.[29]

CHAPTER 3

"The ark of reform"

CIVIL WAR SURGEON

In April 1861, war began in earnest. Mary was entering the most extraordinary years of her life, years that would catapult her into the fame for which she had longed; but her first battle was the arduous legal process of seeking a divorce from Albert. She retained her friend B. F. Chapman as her attorney, and the court appointed an independent referee, D. D. Walrath, Esq., to determine the validity of the charges of adultery against Albert. On September 16, the state supreme court granted Mary a divorce. The court's decree included Walrath's assertion that "all the material facts charged in the complaint are true, and that the said defendant has been guilty of the several acts of adultery therein charged." Albert had used his lecturing career, begun about the same time as Mary's, to engage in liaisons with numerous women he met while traveling throughout New England. The most unusual aspect of New York's restrictive divorce laws was also rendered: the adulterous spouse was prohibited from remarrying during his ex-wife's lifetime, but she was free to remarry. Albert was also ordered to pay $100 for Mary's legal costs. Although the divorce was granted, the five-year waiting period meant an incomplete resolution. Still, Mary could now pursue her own endeavors without the humiliation of an openly promiscuous husband.[1]

While waiting for the court's decision, Mary closely followed developments in the war. Her sentiments were rendered in a poem, "King Cotton," that she recorded: "What *groans arise*, what *blood* is spilt, / What bitter lamentation: / And shall such sufferings have no end? / Such misery be eternal? / Shall enlightened people still defend / A system so infernal?" Having determined that her medical training was the asset she could best contribute to the war effort, Mary began preparations to close her medical office and offer her services as a physician to the Union army, refusing the preferred method for women physicians of serving as a nurse. The Second Battle of Bull Run in late August had overwhelmed the nation's capital with wounded soldiers, and Mary concluded that she was needed most in Washington. In addition to her support and concern for the wounded soldiers, she spoke out against the rape culture of slavery, an issue rarely mentioned publicly by white women: "the interests of the cruelly-abused coloured women had the strongest claim" on her endeavors, she declared, and she "was confident that the God of justice would not allow the war to end without its developing into a war of liberation." Two weeks after completing her divorce actions, she was in the capital, ready to serve her country.[2]

Her country, however, was reluctant. The military had never contemplated accepting the services of a woman physician, even though medical personnel were already in short supply. Volunteer male physicians were contracted as acting assistant surgeons and given the rank and pay of lieutenant; they served under the regular military physicians who were in charge of hospital and battlefield services. Mary went directly to Secretary of War Simon Cameron to request appointment as a surgeon. Equally unnerved by her appearance in a reform dress and by the idea of commissioning a woman, Cameron promptly rejected her request. Undaunted, Mary set out to visit a number of the relief hospitals to seek work as a surgeon. She quickly settled on the Indiana Hospital, one of the largest hospitals in Washington at the time. It was set up in the unfinished U.S. Patent Office. The makeshift hospital's surgeon in charge, Dr. J. N. Green, was attempting to treat 100 severely wounded men. He warned Mary that his predecessor had died from overwork, but she accepted the challenge. Green wrote to Surgeon General Clement A. Finley, requesting he appoint Mary as his assistant surgeon. She took the request directly to Finley, supplied her credentials—and was just as promptly turned down.[3]

Still determined, Mary met with Assistant Surgeon General Robert C. Wood, who had no objections to the appointment, but since Finley had already declined, insisted there was nothing he could do. Frustrated but unwilling to abandon the idea of serving as a physician, Mary returned to the Indiana Hospital and offered to work with Green as a volunteer surgeon. Green established her duties as if she had been regularly appointed and offered to give her part of his salary, which she declined. Through her work at the hospital, Mary became only the second woman to practice as a physician in Washington; the first had been her friend Dr. Lydia Sayer Hasbrouck, who had a practice in the city in the mid-1850s. At this time Mary also met Dr. J. M. Mackenzie, a Sacramento physician who had come to Washington to treat the wounded. Mackenzie wrote a letter of recommendation for her, with the required testimony as to a physician's moral character; as a woman—and one who defied convention by traveling without a male escort and wearing a reform dress—this testimony was doubly necessary for Mary. In spite of Mackenzie's recommendation that she was "well versed in the science of medicine" and that her "unbounded patriotism and love of humanity" would aid the wounded, no commission was forthcoming and she remained a volunteer.[4]

It was a daily challenge to treat patients because of scarce supplies. The medical staff consisted of Drs. Green and Walker as surgeons, three women nurses, and several male nurses. They slept in the building, on beds tucked into alcoves. A routine was soon worked out whereby Mary had some breaks during the day and took the night cases in order to allow Green time to rest. Mary proudly noted in her war recollections, "I examined and prescribed and continued the treatment of these hundred patients" each night. She thrived in spite of the conditions and demands of her position. Occasionally she accompanied patients to their homes, and these breaks from her hospital duties allowed her to see new places in the region. Even in the midst of war, she could not contain her excitement at seeing the South for the first time, as she revealed in a letter to her family in Oswego: "I suppose you all expected me to go to war, and I thought it would be too cruel to disappoint you, and have accordingly made my way to 'Dixie Land.'" She traveled to Virginia on several occasions, including by steamboat to Alexandria. The city's abandonment struck her; "all the wealthy people have gone farther South since the trouble commenced." More surprising was the scene at Camp William: "As far as the eye can reach it was one connected city of tents up and down the Potomac." But when she turned to personal issues in the letter, she guarded her marital history: "No one," she commanded, "is to be allowed to read any of my *written matters or letters*. I wish that to be distinctly understood, as there is nothing in any way that concerns any of you."[5]

Mary now took the time to explore the Patent Office; though not yet completed, it had already accumulated an array of artifacts. Her brother and father were inventors, and she knew they would delight in the collections of the Patent Office: "thousands of every kind of patent, from patent medicines, to frames for peas to run on, to steam boats and engines." By mid-November the hospital managed to reduce the number of patients to eighty, and added a dispenser to prepare the medicine prescribed by the two doctors. One of Mary's duties at the hospital was to examine patients for smallpox before they could be admitted. Washington was rife with the disease, and nearly nineteen thousand soldiers would die from its ravaging effects during the war. As the disease spread among the troops in the fall of 1861, the surgeon of the U.S. Volunteers established a hospital for smallpox patients, and Mary, who had been inoculated, directed soldiers with the disease there. On November 5 Dr. Green again requested that she be appointed assistant surgeon, writing directly to Wood: "This is to certify that Mrs. Dr. Mary E. Walker has rendered me valuable assistance during the past five weeks as assistant in this hospital and I commend her as an intelligent and judicious physician." Again the request was denied. As she continued her duties, her presence at the hospital became known among soldiers' relatives, many of whom wrote directly to her when they needed assistance. Elizabeth Conklin of New Jersey, for instance, wrote in December. Her husband had been arrested on assumption of desertion, and she asked Mary to intervene, as Conklin was feeling desperate: "My babes is all the time sick. I haven't resieved any help since my husband was Arrested." Conklin's was among dozens of similar letters that Mary received in these months, and she made every effort to locate the soldiers and report their condition to worried relatives.[6]

While working in the hospital, Mary met governors, congressmen, and other national leaders, and soon her reputation began to spread far beyond the District. One event, which "somewhat amused" Mary, was indicative of the way in which the more conservative among her sex shunned her for the choice of alternative clothing and career. Dorothea Dix visited the hospital. On first encountering Mary, Dix appeared troubled. Only later did the doctor learn that "a part of [Dix's] mission was to try to keep young and good looking women out of the hospital;" that a young, attractive woman physician would examine men's bodies was particularly shocking to Dix's sensibilities. Mary was equally appalled at Dix's pretensions: Dix "walked through the hospital in a manner that it is hard to describe. When she saw a patient who was too ill to arrange the clothing on his cot if it became disarranged and a foot was exposed she turned her head the other way seeming not to see the condition while I was so disgusted with such sham modesty that I hastened to arrange the soldier's bedclothing if I chanced to be near when no nurses were to do this duty." Mary's sense of the young nurses she met was that they "proved to be efficient and worthy in all regards." Yet Mary attempted to soothe her sense of alienation from Dix, recognizing that she was "a good hearted woman and had been years before of great service in lunatic asylums where she had helped to do away with cruelties to patients.... For this the country should be grateful to her."[7]

Mary's attention at the time, however, was directed toward a much more pressing situation. Demoralization was endemic among troops. Frederick Law Olmsted of the Sanitary Commission filed a report on the problem after the battles at Bull Run, where the majority of Mary's patients had been wounded. Olmsted described the soldiers as "sullen, fierce, weak and ravenous." For those soldiers who required hospitalization, the situation became much worse. Mary made every effort to spend what time she could with each patient, and she was frequently rewarded by their gratefulness. As she moved through the ward, she was conscious of the effect her presence could have on the men: "there seemed to be such a gloom pervading the ward that I put a smile upon my face and tried to say something pleasant to every one in the ward." One day she picked up a photograph case on the stand beside a young soldier's bed. "I suppose the sweetest face in the world is in that case," she remarked. He replied, "Yes, you open it and you will see the sweetest face that I ever saw." Opening the case, Mary discovered a looking glass.[8]

Although additional surgeons were added to the hospital's staff, the emotional toll of working under these conditions remained great. "There were cases where [soldiers] had been wounded in the arm or leg, and in the most pitiful manner that made it very difficult for me to suppress my emotions," Mary acknowledged. "They would ask me if that leg would have to come off, if that arm would have to come off, telling me that ... they would rather die than lose a leg or lose an arm.... I did not want to be unprofessional and say anything to any other medical officer's patients that would seem like giving advice outside of a council; but as I had a little experience and observation regarding the inability of some of the ward surgeons to diagnose properly, and truthfully I considered that I had a higher duty than came under the head of medical etiquette." Yet as a volunteer Mary had to be cautious. Amputation was the most controversial medical issue of the war. During the Crimean War, the British surgeon general had opposed all amputations; his pamphlet had been distributed to U.S. Army surgeons by the Sanitary Commission at the beginning of the Civil War. By December 1861, however, the policy was reversed and a second pamphlet on the subject was distributed in which amputation was recommended when there were serious lacerations of the limb or a compound fracture. While soldiers' lives were of concern, so was expediency. The debate would continue throughout the war—and after. Amputations during the war years were brutal and typically completed in ten to fifteen minutes because the physician needed to move on to other patients. The mortality rates for amputees explain Mary's concern— nearly 60 percent of leg amputations done at the knee resulted in death, and for hip-level amputations the number rose to more than 80 percent. Mary observed two surgeons who seemed to amputate more for their own practice than from necessity. Such practice was "utterly cruel," she declared.[9]

Disgusted with herself for participating in one of the questionable surgeries, she made a decision: "It was the last case that would ever occur if it was in my power to prevent such cruel loss of limbs." She began a process of double checking a patient's wounds whenever she heard that one of the suspect doctors intended to remove a limb. If she thought the surgery was unwarranted, she counseled the soldier that surgery was his choice, though she also told soldiers not to reveal that she had counseled them. In later years she insisted that "many a man today has for it the perfect and good use of his limbs who would not have had but for my advice, to say nothing about the millions of dollars in pensions that would have been paid without all the suffering, had I not decided it my solemn duty to the soldiers instead of carrying out etiquette towards my medical and surgical brothers. If there ever was a time when that grand golden rule should have been carried out to its uttermost, it was in cases like these." Several soldiers wrote after the war to thank her for saving their limbs.[10]

Mary's experience as a reformer and fundraiser for *The Sibyl* was now put to good use. Supplies were dwindling even as more patients arrived, so in her free hours, she wrote to Relief Societies in nearby states with lists of items that were desperately needed at the hospital. There were moments when the hospital demands waned, however, and Mary used these opportunities to undertake a variety of activities. Washington was not an easy city for an unescorted woman to navigate. Walt Whitman described the capital in the early years of the war as "mad, wild, hellish," full of the well-intended but also profiteers. Mary was fearless, but not naïve; she carried a gun on most of her travels. It was a dangerous yet invigorating environment that satisfied both her patriotism and her adventurousness. At one point she escorted a seriously wounded soldier on his trip home to Ravenna, Ohio, and she continued her war efforts there by giving a benefit lecture for the Soldiers' Aid Society.[11]

Mary's reputation for helping soldiers was now well known. Thus one evening after she returned to Washington, she was approached by the mother and wife of a Lieutenant Wren who was bivouacked near Bull Run. Wren, they told Mary, was seriously ill, and they feared he would die; his only child was also ailing. With few exceptions, women were not allowed to travel to the front lines, but the Wrens insisted that Mary "could do anything" and asked her to go the front lines, secure a leave of absence for him, and accompany him back to Washington where they were boarding in a house on K Street, N.W. Mary agreed without hesitation and did not wait for the requisite pass. She simply set out the next day on her own. As she reached the far side of the Potomac, a guard stopped her. She repeated to the guard the heart-wrenching story of the lieutenant's condition and his family's fears. Her skills as an orator held sway, and the guard let her pass.[12]

Mary boarded the train at Alexandria and rode to the end of the line. She had another five miles to travel, and conditions were not conducive for a woman traveling alone. Roads battered by troop movements spread out in several directions from the station, and she had no means of knowing precisely where the lieutenant's camp was located, but through conversation with members of a relief association, she discerned a likely direction and borrowed their saddle-horse. Mary related: "I knew it was dangerous riding through the country there where both armies were skirmishing at different times, no one knew when; but as I was determined to go to Lieut. Wren, I was ready to run all kinds of risks to keep my word good." The Civil War years were often depicted as a culture of honor; Mary had been trained to such attitudes from childhood, and the war's emphasis on honor and one's word became embedded in Mary's sense of herself and her strident construction of morality in subsequent years. She eventually located the camp, where she negotiated with officers to find Wren a place in an ambulance. She and her patient arrived at the station late at night, and the only available space for them was on the floor of a boxcar; but with the help of candles she secured before leaving, she was able to treat Wren en route. In Alexandria, she enlisted the train's conductor to arrange for an ambulance to take them to a boat, which carried them across to the Seventh Street wharf. From there she solicited aid from strangers to get the lieutenant aboard a streetcar, lying across a seat, until they arrived at their K Street destination. By this time it was so late at night that they were the only passengers on the streetcar. Mary could not carry the lieutenant by herself, so she convinced the conductor to halt the streetcar long enough to help her carry the patient to his home a few feet away. "I need not express the delight felt by all parties upon the lieutenant's arrival home," Mary said with pleasure at accomplishing her goal.[13]

In January 1862 Mary found time to write a short piece for *The Sibyl*. "What Can Woman Do?" detailed her own activities, encouraged readers to continue wearing the reform dress, and complimented Hasbrouck on having begun to openly support abolition in the pages of the journal even when it cost her subscribers. It would be six months before she could again find time to write, and most of her subsequent publications in *The Sibyl* were relatively short letters to the editor.[14]

With several surgeons now assigned to Indiana Hospital, Mary turned in earnest to the idea of being contracted by the army. To assure her work was widely known, she shifted to visiting various hospitals in the Washington area where she assisted in surgeries and dressed wounds. When she saw needs that could not be met by the overworked medical officers, she went directly to authorities and pled for the necessary changes. One day when she was at the post office she was approached by a stranger who gave her a handful of paper scraps addressed to "Lady Dr. Walker, the soldier's true friend." The notes came from inmates at the Forrest Hall Prison in Georgetown who claimed to have been erroneously arrested as deserters. A large group of prisoners met with Mary when she arrived. They immediately overwhelmed her, talking at once, telling their stories, and insisting she take a statement of their case to officials. For six hours she wrote out the accounts of those who seemed to be wrongfully imprisoned; when she rose to leave, the prisoners cheered loudly and thanked her. Mary knew that rumors of an attack on Washington itself were circulating, and the government desperately needed more men for its defense. She exacted a promise from the prisoners to defend the city if she could arrange for them a return to their regiments; then she met with War Department officials, gaining agreement for her plan. However, when the threat to the city subsided, she was dismayed to learn that the government did not keep its part of the bargain and returned many of the men to the prison. Some of them probably had deserted, but a significant number of those with whom she talked were too wounded to return to the front or had unexpired leaves of absence. She wrote an argument on behalf of those men, noting that many of them had been arrested simply so their pursuers could be paid the fees for capturing deserters. Northerners would not condone "such outrages," she proclaimed. Secretary of War Stanton agreed with the plan to return the soldiers to their posts or homes, and to ensure the men were treated well, Mary wrote twenty-five letters to corps commanders asking that they honor the fact that the charges of desertion had been removed at Washington.[15]

As no medical commission was forthcoming, Mary undertook a change in direction. Witnessing so many kinds of battle-related injuries increased her concerns about medical treatment under wartime conditions, so she decided to study new treatments being offered at the Hygeio-Therapeutic College in New York City. It was common in these years for physicians to take second degrees as a means of advancing their training, and this medical college appealed to Mary for several reasons. Foremost was its medical philosophy—hygiene studies were the cutting edge of medical science at the time. Equally important was the fact that Lydia Sayer Hasbrouck was one of its earliest graduates, and the institution established itself as a headquarters for dress reformers when they came to New York. It also had a woman professor, Dr. Huldah Page, and advertised itself as admitting women and men "on precisely equal terms." By the time Mary arrived in 1862, the institution had graduated nearly two hundred students, half of whom were women. The Hygeio-Therapeutic College was chartered in 1857 by Dr. Russell Trall. Trall had initially trained as an allopath, but he came to believe that the allopathic reliance on drugs was both ineffective and harmful to the body. The major focus of his new methodology was hygienic, and he was responsible for distinguishing the field of hygienics from hydropathy. Hygienics was a part of Mary's training at Syracuse Medical College, but few physicians yet paid serious attention to the issue. Allopathic physicians largely dismissed such concerns; during the war, battlefield hospitals were built with open latrines surrounding them, allowing any number of diseases to infiltrate the hospital environment, and surgeons used unsterilized knives on patient after patient. Thus, tens of thousands of soldiers died from disease and surgical infections. Mary viewed the Hygeio-Therapeutic College as offering her better preparation for her wartime medical practice. The course length was twenty weeks, but Mary and two male physicians were able to take a shortened course because they already held medical degrees.[16]

In addition to the usual medical college system of lectures, Mary participated in clinics at Bellevue Hospital. She completed the term and received a diploma on March 31, 1862. Among the sixteen graduates were two colleagues with whom Mary would remain close friends—J. F. Preston Day of Osawa, Iowa, and Ellen Beard Harman of Aurora, Illinois. Medical school theses in these years varied widely at all institutions, with theses on serious medical issues such as the brain, nervous systems, and pneumonia but also on topics such as the duties and responsibilities of physicians and women as physicians. Among Mary's co-graduates at the Hygeio-Therapeutic College, this wide variation was also acceptable, with graduates addressing topics from respiratory cures to non-traditional subjects such as woman as reformer. But the most unusual thesis was written by Mary: "The Secessionists." At the graduation ceremony, the theme of reform prevailed; later toasts were made to Dr. Trall as "the greatest philosopher of the age" and to "Women Physicians—living protests against injustice, and noble examples of energy, capability, and usefulness." Trall followed Mary's career throughout the war. Shortly after the conclusion of the conflict, he proclaimed, "she has been one of the greatest benefactors of her sex and of the human race." Trall's influence on Mary was long lasting. He gave a lengthy lecture on drugs and tobacco as poisons to members of Congress and physicians at the Smithsonian Institute in 1862. Mary's parents had been anti-tobacco, too, but Trall's ability to put that issue into medical terms became integral to her own medical philosophy.[17]

In July, Mary sent a letter to *The Sibyl* in which she confirmed her commitment to dress reform: "There will never be any progress if all are to wait until a sufficient number embark in the ark of reform so as 'not to be conspicuous.'" Suffragists who proclaimed they could not tolerate the criticism brought upon them by wearing a reform dress received her sharpest rebuke. Lucy Stone attempted to justify her abandonment of reform clothing with the assertion that women's "miserable style of dress is a consequence of her present vassalage, not its cause," which, to Mary's mind, should have made it all the more important to physically as well as intellectually represent the refusal to accept that vassalage. Some suffragists attempted a compromise: Elizabeth Smith Miller shifted to wearing an ankle-length reform dress, and Elizabeth Cady Stanton wore the Bloomer only while at home. Well before the war, they abandoned it publicly. Yet Stanton was always uncomfortable with her decision. She lamented, "Such is the tyranny of custom, that to escape constant observation, criticism, ridicule, persecution, mobs," she returned "to the old slavery and sacrificed freedom to repose." Mary's concluding comments represented her unfaltering sense of duty to fight for clothing and all freedoms:

> Whoever will not choose their field of labor and place themselves in positions to surmount obstacles that will result in some benefit to civilization, will be compelled to meet those which will be annoying, and health and comfort destroying, without gaining the sweet reward of having accomplished anything to compensate for the time and energy expended. It is literally impossible for one with any force of character and humanity to remain "in the background," when convinced by knowledge and reason, that their mission is evidently one that will result in great good to those whose necessities demand what they have not the power to gain for themselves. For such let us labor. Virtue is as much higher than innocence as angels are higher than mortals.[18]

In October, Mary returned to Oswego. While there, she presented a series of lectures on her extraordinary experiences at Indiana Hospital and in the nation's capital. A draft of the "On Washington" lecture reveals the ardency of her abolitionist values, beginning with her opening lines: "What changes have been wrought in the last 72 years, & had not slavery cursed our land there would have been still greater strides visible here, in the march of civilization and everything good that is connected with it—." Her passion rose as she discussed the Smithsonian's weekly lectures on abolition:

> Our best, & most radical speakers that the country affords, were invited to lecture, & a large number accepted who would not dared to have spoken in public in the city of Washington, before this war commenced—Never was more radical sentiments uttered in regard to slavery & all of our National affairs than were uttered in this hall, & yet they received the most deafening applause—At the very mention of the name of Cohn Barow, the Chattels Martyr, or of John C. Fremont, who would have been the best working Gen. of the north—the applause was long & loud, & actually amounted to screams in some instances—Shall a people *filled with* such enthusiasm yield to a hoard of slave drivers? Shall our capital city with all of its fine buildings & everything indicative of a Nation's prosperity be forever guarded to keep rebellious children from thrusting out her loyalists or destroying them? Let it not be said! but raise to the conflict the star-spangled banner on every plantation & there let it wave—let it wave!!!!!!!!!![19]

Mary returned to Washington in the early fall and settled into rooms at 52 Morton Street. In December she sent another letter to Hasbrouck on dress reform and soldiers' bravery, and she was soon in the thick of the war herself. A battle was raging at Warrenton, Virginia, and she left for the battlefield to offer her surgical services. On arrival, she discovered a group of ill and wounded soldiers who were without any medical care, lying on the floor of an old house. Many of the men were severely weakened from the effects of typhoid fever, and the military officer in charge told her, "If there is anything you can do for these men, for God's sake do something," as he had been ordered to move his troops to another battle site the next day. She was appalled at the lack of supplies; only a bucket of water and a cup were available. The Confederates' battlefield hospital had been located in that same area shortly before Mary's arrival, and the enemy had already confiscated every item of possible use from nearby homes. Mary finally found one woman who had secreted a large basin from the Confederates. She paid a silver dollar of her own money for the basin and back at camp tore apart the only long nightdress she had brought with her into one-foot squares to serve as towels. Giving them to a nurse, Mary ordered her to be sure to use a clean basin of water for each patient unable to wash himself.[20]

With the soldiers better situated, Mary directed her steps to the army's headquarters where she informed Major General Ambrose Burnside, commander of the Army of the Potomac, that the men must be sent to Washington immediately as they could not be properly cared for under the present conditions. Burnside agreed and prepared authorization papers for Mary to take the patients to Washington. On November 15, she and her wards left on the train. There were 120,000 men encamped near Warrenton, and it was a dangerous environment. Union leaders were expecting the Confederate army to raid the area between Warrenton and Alexandria at any time, and the system of moving the wounded by train was too new for the officers to know whether the Confederates would target it. The train was made up of six freight cars and one passenger car, carrying people such as Congressman Henry Wilson on official business. It was inefficient in size and space for the number of wounded; some patients without life-threatening wounds had to be placed on top of the cars, in spite of the cold November weather.[21]

The train proceeded only a short distance when it stopped in an isolated area. Most of the wounded were doing as well as possible, but two men were near death. Mary carried a small booklet with her so she could record the names and addresses of the dying in order to notify families (it also contained her own identification in case of death). One of the men died before he could reveal his name. She quickly moved to the other patient; barely able to speak, he uttered only his name and hometown before dying. Increasingly impatient with the train's delay, Mary sought the conductor, who informed her there was no officer on board to authorize him to make the trip to Washington. Since she had authorization from General Burnside to go to Washington, Mary commanded the conductor to proceed, and they finally were on their way. "I could not help suppressing a smile," Mary later recalled, "at the thought . . . that in reality I was then military conductor of the train that bore one of the law-makers of the nation not only, but its citizens and helpless defenders." Senator Wilson would later become vice president of the United States in Grant's administration, and Mary always delighted in recalling that she had been given authority over such an eminent figure. Officially, Mary's duties ended when they reached the capital, but she had one more task awaiting her before she could conclude her business: "I gave the information regarding the deaths of these two soldiers to a representative from the War Department, then I wrote a letter addressed to the soldier at his home, and wrote on the outside for his relatives to please open. I gave to them a history of the brave life and of the death of the soldier, signing my full name." To inform survivors whether or not their loved one had effected a "Good Death"—died in spiritual grace—was essential to the culture of the war, and the duty often fell to surgeons or fellow soldiers. Twenty years later, Mary discovered that her letter had also helped verify the soldier's duty during the war and thus his father had been awarded a pension.[22]

Mary was back in Washington only a few weeks when the Union army suffered a brutal defeat at Fredericksburg. The news of nearly 13,000 Union casualties sent a ripple of shock throughout the North. Since Warrenton, Mary had given up wading through the unending channels of the military for an appointment; if there was a battle with high casualties, she set out for the field. General Burnside respected her medical skills, and she soon arrived at Fredericksburg's makeshift hospitals even though she came under fire as she neared the city. Accounts of the battle's aftermath detailed the dreadful cries of the wounded, "weird, unearthly, terrible to hear and bear." Walt Whitman was there, tending his brother George who had been wounded. Whitman saw at Fredericksburg "what well men and sick men and mangled men endure," an environment that Mary had endured on various battlefields over the past year. She was told by military surgeons to take any cases she wished. The wounds she saw at this site were of the worst sort, but they also fascinated her as a physician. One patient had a piece of his skull the size of a dollar coin blown away by a shell shot. "I could see the pulsation of the brain," she wrote, "and when he talked I could see a movement of the same, slight though it was. He was perfectly sensible, and although I never saw him after he was taken to Washington, I learned that he lived several days."[23]

In battlefield medical care, creative resourcefulness was a necessity for treating the wounded as even the most basic care was sometimes lacking. On May 8, Mary was given a military pass to move to Aquia Creek so she could aid in the transport of the wounded to hospitals in Washington. She observed the soldiers being carried on stretchers down to the bank of the river where they were loaded onto boats. Aides invariably started head first with the soldiers, unaware of the damage this could cause. "There seemed to be no one to manage that part of it," Mary observed, so she "stood close to the edge of the water and as soon as they were close enough so that I could order them I did so, directing them to immediately turn around and take them feet first. It is almost needless to say that for men who were wounded so that they were obliged to be taken on stretchers . . . taking them down head first would have produced pains in the head if not serious congestion of the brain on such a warm day."

Mary traveled at one point with Quartermaster L. M. Painter and his wife and their relative, Dr. Hetty K. Painter. An 1860 graduate of Pennsylvania Medical College, Hetty was a cousin of John Brown, had a son in the Union army, and had signed with the army as a nurse. Mary and the Painters stopped at Piedmont, Virginia, where they discovered that a makeshift hospital had been set up in a church but no medical officer was available. The two women physicians set off immediately for the hospital; they found soldiers with fevers and little food. In addition to treating them, Mary scoured the area, able to secure a peck of cornmeal by trading a pair of her boots for it, and eventually the soldiers began to recover. As they improved, they began to loot the neighborhood, at one point stealing a side-saddle to present as a gift of appreciation for Mary's medical care. The saddle belonged to the Misses Shaklett who owned a house and several buildings in Piedmont, including the church in which the hospital was housed. When the sisters discovered the theft, they abused the thieves with "such earnest English," as Mary put it, that the men threatened to burn the Shaklett house. Unable to reason with them, Mary announced that she would sleep in the house with the sisters every night and be burned as well if the soldiers set it afire. The Painters joined her, and eventually calm was restored between the Shakletts and the soldiers.[24]

After her work at Fredericksburg, military surgeons with whom Mary had worked again attempted to secure a commission for her. Dr. Preston King informed the secretary of war that Mary was acting as "physician and surgeon in the Hospitals and in attendance upon the sick and wounded of the volunteers," but his request that she be commissioned was denied with the assertion that there was no "authority of law for making this allowance to you." Her work garnered only rations and a tent for sleeping on the rare occasions when she had time to rest. Army records describe her as having "labored day and night" to treat the wounded. She had largely given up her medical practice to offer her services during the war, and she would not be relegated to the status of a nurse; so she altered her clothing to signify her status as a physician. Military surgeons wore a green sash so they could be quickly identified on the battlefield, and Mary added the sash to the dark blue uniform she had designed for herself. Gold stripes ran the length of the outer part of the pant legs, and she wore an officer's greatcoat. If the War Department would not recognize her status, she proclaimed it herself.[25]

A reporter for the *New York Tribune* observed Mary's work as an army physician and published an account of it in December:

> She is a native of New York, has received a regular medical education, and believes her sex ought not to disqualify her for the performance of deeds of mercy to the suffering heroes of the Republic. Dressed in male habiliments . . . she carries herself amid the camp with a jaunty air of dignity well calculated to receive the sincere respect of the soldiers. . . . . She can amputate a limb with the

skill of an old surgeon, and administer medicine equally as well. Strange to say that, although she has frequently applied for a permanent position in the medical corps, she has never been formally assigned to any particular duty. . . . We will add that the lady referred to is exceedingly popular among the soldiers in the hospitals, and is undoubtedly doing much good.

Such commentaries spread news of Mary's wartime activities across the country.[26]

On January 1, 1863, President Lincoln issued the Emancipation Proclamation. Mary joined other abolitionists in celebration at the National Antislavery Society gathering for its Twenty-Ninth Annual Subscription Anniversary, at the Church of the Puritans in New York City in February. Mary was becoming known as a political force in Washington, one who worked with military and political leaders to benefit the soldiers. She was also in attendance at a reception held in the Executive Mansion in the spring, where she met the president and Mary Todd Lincoln. These annual democratic receptions included government officials, diplomats, celebrities, and the general public. This was Mary's first attendance; it was a ritual she continued all of her life as an act of patriotism, and her presence always received national coverage. She found the president to be "cordial" and Mrs. Lincoln "lively and pleasing."[27]

By early March, spring rains soaked Washington. Only the main thoroughfare was cobbled, leaving residents immersed in mud-filled streets. Suddenly the reform dress gained praise. Mary wrote to Dr. Hasbrouck, satirizing women whose fashionable, long-skirted dresses swept through the mud. This prelude allowed her to turn to the real focus of her letter: what it meant to be a pioneer in a cause. It was one of her most revealing statements on the subject:

> As it has been in all ages, so is it now: those who live principles must live them against the opposition of the world for a long time; and "few there be" who are able to surmount all the ignoble obstacles that are incident in such a course. The cutting of chains of professed friendship—the failure of equals to fully appreciate merit—the thousand and one of the "little things in life" that make such a large proportion of "life itself;" sometimes weigh so heavily on the spirit, that "scarce the firm philosopher can" walk alone!
>
> But . . . it is far better to feel that we are meeting and enduring in a cause that will benefit our suffering sex, long after we have passed away from their causes than to feel that we have lived to no purpose.
>
> It matters not whether future generations of women shall "rise up and call us blessed." . . . The goal gained will be just as precious, and in any case, we shall feel that we have only performed our duty in setting a physiological example to our own sex, (who have a right to look to physicians for such examples,) and proving ourself "a good divine, by practicing what we preach."

Mary's words deeply affected her colleagues in the movement. Despite having to miss several conventions, she was reelected a vice president of the NDRA at its convention in Rochester later that month.[28]

At this time Mary also rendered her hometown a poignant service. She sent a long letter to an Oswego newspaper, noting that she had been to the convalescent camp near Fort Barnard, Virginia, and discovered a large group of wounded soldiers from Oswego. She listed the status of dozens of men from the region, informing readers of each soldier's condition and to what hospital he had been taken. Mary offered her services to soldiers in many ways beyond medical care. Young William Clawyer of the New York Volunteers found it impossible to navigate the legal workings of the military. "This is my Case Just as it is," Clawyer wrote to Mary, "and i would like to have you to Cleare my Case if possible." Many other letters came from family members seeking Mary's help, and officers also wrote her for various kinds of assistance. Captain Alexander Springsteen wrote from Camp Casey, Virginia, in November asking her to find one hundred pair of mittens with fingers for his troops: "I know of no one except you on whom to make a '*Special Requisition*' and expect it to be filled." Springsteen led the 2d U.S. Colored Troops, and he knew that Mary would make every effort to see that the African American men fighting for the nation would be well cared for if at all possible.[29]

In April Mary penned a long letter-article for *The Sibyl*. "Woman's Mind" captured both her frustration with the limitations placed on women and the value she placed on her own intellectual abilities. Like other women's rights activists, she believed that the Jacksonian era of so-called democracy was a gendered one; Elizabeth Cady Stanton described American republicanism as an "aristocracy of sex" that required the subordination of women. Mary's letter demonstrated the force of argument she too was bringing to women's rights advocacy. Too many women of intellect, she asserted, are unappreciated by their male friends and relatives, some of whom are incapable of understanding "superior minds." "Woman's Mind" was her manifesto for the woman intellectual:

> Woman's mind is capable of the profoundest reasoning, and it matters not where she is placed, how she is circumscribed, she reasons still; and although women as a general rule are not in the habit of explaining all the how's and why's; all their conclusions are arrived at through a course of reasoning, and the process of reasoning could be explained step by step, as well as men's reasoning operations, if they were in the habit of expressing themselves on such points.
>
> I have a woman's mind, and know that all my conclusions are obtained through the reasoning powers and not through instinct. Let no man dare say that woman jumps at conclusions through instinct, for no man is capable of fathoming a woman's mind; for woman reasons by telegraph, and his stage coach reasoning cannot keep pace with her's. Woman's mind is an emanation from deity, and man's mind very probably emanated from the same source,

and the difference in the minds of the sexes is owing in part to the weight and roughness of the clay, that is, the message bearer or soul clogger of the mind.

Ultimately, she concluded, a man's appreciation of a woman's intellect depended on his own level of intelligence.[30]

The war's horrendous cost in lives and in the spirit of men who survived was becoming increasingly evident to the American public. In May, the Union defeat at Chancellorville added to Northerners' morose state, but conditions were desperate on both sides. When Confederate prisoners taken at Chancellorville arrived in Washington, Mary published her impressions in the *Oswego Times*. President Lincoln was among those waiting at the Sixth Street Wharf. She noted his "careworn cheeks" and dramatically captured the fatigue and impoverished status of the prisoners: "Some had a piece of ingrain carpet for a blanket, some had no hats, but wore a turban made of a handkerchief, while those who had hats or caps looked as though they had served them since 1860; some had no shoes or stockings; some no coats, and nothing but a woolen shirt about their waists." In less than a year she herself would know the hunger and fear of being a prisoner of war.[31]

During the hot summer months in the capital, Mary maintained a medical practice as best she could under the trying circumstances, worked at the Corps Hospitals whenever possible, and spent numerous hours negotiating with the government on behalf of soldiers. Her attention turned to several soldiers who had been jailed for five months without a trial. Taking their statements to the War Department, she demanded immediate trials. A court martial was convened, and in one of the cases Mary served as the defendant's attorney, which she believed was the first instance of a woman serving as an attorney in the capital. She lost the case, but appealed it to Judge Advocate General Joseph Holt on the grounds that testimony from a witness who could provide the soldier with an alibi had been excluded from the court's report. Holt reversed the court's initial finding, granted the soldier back pay, and at Mary's request allowed him thirty days' leave to return home to Michigan. The case was a key stimulant to her growing interest in the law.[32]

She was also invited by the Union League of Washington to present a lecture on her experiences working with the Army of the Potomac. On August 18, 1863, Mary joined William ("Wild Bill") Cody on stage, and related her war experiences. In the early fall, Mary's work on behalf of the Union was again celebrated in a front page article in the *New York Tribune*: "Since the commencement of the war, a slight, girlish figure, costumed in a bloomer dress of blue cloth, has been constantly seen in the various hospitals of the Capital, performing with great skill surgical operations, prescribing for the sick, or soothing them with smiling words." The reporter traced her battlefield work as well, noting that she "has won there an acknowledged reputation for professional superiority." The newspaper again chastised the military for failing to appoint Mary to a regular position or (with notable indiscretion) pursue her interest in serving as a spy for the Union army. The article concluded, "What 'ism' is more absurd than Conservatism? If a woman is proved competent for duty, and anxious to perform it, why restrain her?" *The Sibyl* reprinted the *Tribune*'s comments with an editorial from Hasbrouck praising Mary's efforts and suggesting that if Mary needed pecuniary assistance the readers should donate toward her cause. In the next issue, Hasbrouck revisited the subject, arguing that New York politicians who were offering no assistance "to aid women to a full and free political recognition" should read Mary's latest letter. "Read, men of this district, and ponder where your duty lies!" Mary's letter followed: "I sat up until after midnight helping to write the transportation orders on the furloughs of the New York soldiers the Saturday night previous to election. I feared many would not get there in time to get their tickets to go home and vote the Union ticket, and I went and volunteered to help. I had the thanks of hundreds of soldiers; so you see I helped others to vote if not allowed to myself." Mary and other abolitionists were dismayed when Horatio Seymour was elected to the governorship of New York in 1862 instead of James Wadsworth, the Republican Union candidate and an abolitionist. Seymour had campaigned on a platform rooted in fear-mongering that freedmen would commit brutal acts "of lust and rapine." Mary recognized that Seymour had succeeded to the governorship largely because tens of thousands of New York soldiers who were stationed outside the state were not allowed to vote, and she intended to help defeat Seymour's party this time by insuring that soldiers had furloughs so they could vote—even if she could not.[33]

By the fall of 1863, Mary was despairing of any appointment from the army, but when another brutal battle in mid-September resulted in masses of wounded soldiers, she returned to the battlefield. Rosencrans' Battle at Chickamauga was the worst defeat yet for that area of the war, resulting in nearly 16,000 casualties. Mary worked at the Chattanooga battlefield hospital, where she met General George H. Thomas, who observed her medical and organizational skills as she took charge of several wards by order of the surgeon in charge, Dr. Salter. In one ward, she had sixty patients and oversaw the work of assistant surgeons, and in another she assisted with surgeries. It was an important experience for her, and the contact with General Thomas would prove invaluable in the coming months.[34]

Salter asked Mary to continue working with him, but she wanted an official appointment in order to go to the front, and she devised an alternative plan. On November 2, three days before Thomas was appointed commander of the Army of the Cumberland, she laid out her plan in a letter to Secretary of War Stanton:

> Will you give me authority to get up a regiment of men, to be called *Walker's U.S. Patriots*, subject to all general orders, in Vol. Regts.?
>
> I would like authority to enlist them in any loyal states, & also authority to tell them that I will act as first Assistant Surgeon. Having been so long the

friend of soldiers, and their friends, I feel confident that I can be successful in getting *re*enlistment of men who would not enlist in any other persons Reg., also some from *prisons* who were parolled, and supposed there "would be no harm in going home until exchanged." Some of the latter have but a few months to serve. I propose to enlist them "for the war."

Hoping to hear from you soon to receive the *order* solicited,

I await your reply—

In haste

Dr. Mary E. Walker

It was an unprecedented proposal for a woman.[35]

While waiting for a response, Mary wrote what was to be her last article for *The Sibyl*, which suspended publication before the war's end. "Positions that Women ought of Right to Occupy" was timely and influenced by her own dissatisfaction with the many closed doors she faced. Although arguments had been set forth that women's social progress must be set aside during wartime, she believed the war ultimately would help to demonstrate women's abilities as they undertook unforeseen new demands. Men must forego the idea of a separate "women's sphere," she declared: "Either let her have her choice as to what occupation shall be her's, or be gallant and give your 'inferiors' in strength and abilities an opportunity to live easily and accumulate money for her labors as you are doing, that she may be independent pecuniarily." Women must be allowed to work outside the home—and to be respected for such activities: "I confess I have not such a depth of reasoning powers that I can persuade myself that it is any more unfeminine for a woman with natural affections to go from home and act as clerk in some business-office, while her children are at school, or cared for by a competent servant, than it is for an uneducated woman to leave her children in school, or with no care, and go and clean business offices the same length of time." Equally incomprehensible was men's willingness to have a laundress travel with their regiments but not a woman surgeon. Turning the question of respectability from her own endeavors to those of the men who were blocking her, she could not contain her anger: "This war would have closed long since if women had been properly employed; but, Mr. Men, if you will not do it now, and give noble, patriotic women positions of trust and usefulness—if you withhold them simply because they are women, you will protract this war until so many men will be killed that women will be in power, and will have their God-given rights to fill every sphere that they wish to; for woman aspires to nothing that she is not capable of doing." The "tyrannical spirit" of men who thwart women's ambitions, she concluded, "is a disgrace to any one born under the Stars and Stripes."[36]

Mary also engaged in a new form of activism in these months. One day she observed a public disturbance around a woman who had fallen in the street. A police officer informed her that no city hospital would admit the woman because, by being alone in the city, her reputation was open to speculation. The

Washington-Alexandria area purportedly housed 7,500 prostitutes during the war, and women without male escorts were instantly suspect. Learning that the capital city had no women's residence, Mary moved into action, turning to suffragists for assistance. A few evenings later, some of the earliest speeches on woman's franchise in the city were made at the Odd Fellows Hall on Seventh Street and again at the Union League Hall on Ninth Street. At both venues, Mary sought permission at the close of the meeting to appeal for funds to establish a "respectable woman's home." Mary gained support from city leaders as well and established a house for women opposite Ford's Theatre. She sought the assistance of General Edward R.S. Canby, assistant adjutant general in the secretary of war's office, for cots and bedding that were being discarded from hospitals; she hired a matron; and she met with the chief of police so his officers would know to direct women to her home. With the house ready, she posted a notice in local newspapers:

> LODGING ROOMS FOR HOMELESS WOMEN—Dr. Mary Walker has the pleasure to inform those females who are homeless that she has secured respectable rooms where they can remain over night, *free of charge*. Let no woman who is nearly out of means "perish in our streets" hereafter. She will also hear the cases of prospective mothers who are without homes and means to take care of themselves, and begs leave to inform all such who will *endeavor to lead better lives* that they need not commit suicide, or murder innocents, for they shall be cared for and their misfortunes not be published to the world, for, Russia-like, your names shall not be asked. We shall have a temporary "Foundling Hospital" for the present, supported by voluntary contributions, and we wish to know how many are in want of such a home during the period that they are unable to labor. We have the *lodging rooms* ready and shall have the "Foundling Hospital" soon. The rooms now ready are near her residence, and those wishing lodging will call, *if possible*, before seven o'clock P.M.
>
> M. E. Walker, M.D.
374 Ninth street

She clearly envisioned this moment as an opportunity to establish her long-desired foundling hospital and to aid unwed pregnant women as well as soldiers' families.[37]

But supporters did not want "fallen" women in a home for "respectable" women. Mary was able to convince city leaders to give her two rooms in the City Hall where she could interview the "friendless females," arguing that because the police were housed at City Hall, they could easily bring the women to her there. She had to compromise, assuring everyone that her goal was "that the most respectable women should not be compelled under adverse conditions to stay in a room, even for part of a night, with those with whom it would be an offense." The house on Tenth Street became a lifeline for women who came to the city alone during the war, but Mary soon realized housing alone was not sufficient. It was often impossible for women to know at which hospital their loved ones were being treated; no system of public notification was available, record-keeping was sparse, and the only recourse was to walk or, if they could afford to, take streetcars across the city trying to locate their relatives. To solve this dilemma, Mary arranged with Major General Daniel H. Rucker of the War Department's Quartermaster's Bureau to have an ambulance and driver report to her each day to take the women to the various military hospitals.[38]

Mary was pleased with the initial success of her plan, but she could not run the home on her own. To create a women's association to aid in her efforts, she published a notice calling for a meeting of women willing to assist. A small but determined group of women responded, and the first Women's Relief Association in Washington was founded. Four women, three of whom were physicians' wives, helped establish the organization. Mary served as the WRA's first president. Once she felt other members understood how to run the home, she turned over the presidency to another volunteer and served as secretary and medical officer. When the Tenth Street house became too small for its purposes, Mary opened her own home on Ninth Street for the association's use as well, whether or not she was in the city.[39]

In January 1864 Mary went to New York to add her support to the struggling Woman's National Loyal League, founded by Stanton, Stone, Ernestine Rose, Lucretia Mott, Angelina Grimké, and others. It advocated full civil and political rights for women and African Americans when the war concluded. In the spring of 1864 Sen. Charles Sumner would present their petition—with 400,000 signatures—to Congress, but the organization only survived until late summer. The League was in debt for much of its existence; to fund its activities and pull itself out of debt, it sponsored weekly lectures at the Cooper Institute by famous individuals who would attract large audiences. Wendell Phillips and Frederick Douglass donated their services, and Mary gave a speech on women's rights, the war, and human nature. As she often did in these years, she concluded the lecture by quoting a poem that reflected her sense of the precariousness of the era in which they were living: "We are living, we are dwelling / In a grand and awful time, / In an age on ages telling / To be living is sublime." She was back in Washington a week later, attending meetings of the WRA and seeking support from other women.[40]

During this time, Mary learned that Secretary Stanton had rejected the request to establish her own regiment. Unwilling to accept his decision, she wrote on January 11 directly to the president:

To His Excellency,
Lincoln, President, U.S.A.:
   Whereas, The undersigned has rendered much of valuable service in her efforts to promote the cause of the Union, not only in acting as an Assistant Surgeon at various times in hospitals and on the field, but in originality and urging several measures that are of great importance to Government, one of

which is the Invalid Corps, she begs to say to His excellency that she has been denied a commission, solely on the ground of her sex, when her services have been tested and appreciated without a commission and without compensation and she fully believes that had a man been as useful to our country as she modestly claims to have been, a star would have been taken from the National Heavens and placed upon his shoulder.

The undersigned asks to be assigned to duty at Douglas Hospital, in the female ward, as there cannot possibly be any objection urged on account of sex, but she would much prefer to have an extra surgeon's commission with orders to go whenever and wherever there is a battle that she may render aid in the field hospitals, where her energy, enthusiasm, professional abilities and patriotism will be of the greatest service in inspiring the true soldier never to yield to traitors, and in attending the wounded brave. She will not shrink from duties under shot and shells, believing that her life is of no value in the country's greatest peril if by its loss the interests of future generations shall be promoted.

Mary E. Walker, M.D.

Douglas Hospital was one of the temporary wartime facilities. The Sisters of Mercy served as nurses in the facility, and Mary knew that if Lincoln did not want her on the battlefield, the female ward of Douglas Hospital with nuns as nurses would be less offensive to conventional sensibilities.[41]

President Lincoln's reply, handwritten on the bottom portion of Mary's letter, was carefully worded. The work of women for the war effort was essential, but he also did not intend to make a special appointment for her. "The Medical Department of the army is an organized system in the hands of men supposed to be learned in that profession and I am sure it would injure the service for me, with strong hand, to thrust among them anyone, male or female, against their consent," Lincoln wrote. "If they are willing for Dr. Mary Walker to have charge of a female ward, if there be one, I also am willing, but I am sure controversy on the subject will not subserve the public interest." It was a true politician's rejection. Lincoln knew that the appointment of a female physician would create great national debate over women's war efforts and their role in society in general. His every action at this point in the war was rife with controversy, and he was unwilling to take on more criticism to satisfy the desires, however patriotic, of one woman.[42]

Finally, Mary turned to Congressman John Franklin Farnsworth for assistance. Farnsworth had risen to the rank of brigadier general, but he had left the army in March 1863 due to battle injuries. He was an estimable ally for Mary to use in her battle to serve as a physician, and he wrote a letter of recommendation for her to Assistant Surgeon General Wood, who had long thought privately that Mary should receive an appointment. This time Wood interceded on her behalf, directing her to report to Chattanooga for the standard Medical Board evaluation of a physician's medical skills before being contracted. Arriving with the support of the assistant surgeon general of the United States should have given Mary significant standing, but the Medical Boards wielded considerable power on their own. On March 8, Mary went before the Board of Medical Officers of the Department of the Cumberland. Dr. G. Perin was the director of the army medical staff in the region. Like most regular corps physicians, Dr. Perin and his associates did not like contracting non-military physicians, though the war's length and number of casualties left them little choice—it did not mean, however, that they had to accept a woman physician. After the war, Perin scathingly claimed that the Board examined Mary and found her abilities so feeble that they questioned whether she had really had any medical training; he asserted that they concluded her skills were "not greater than most housewives possess." Of course, if she wished to serve as a *nurse*, the Board was willing to recommend her as qualified for that position. When Perin's post-war assessment surfaced, Mary was furious at the claim, writing to President Andrew Johnson to clarify the record. She had not been examined by Perin but by Dr. George Cooper's Board, although to much the same result: "the examination was intended to be a *farce, & more than half* the time was consumed in questions regarding subjects that were *exclusively feminine* & had no sort of relation to the diseases and wounds of *soldiers*." The male physicians had a great deal of fun at her expense, refusing to take her seriously as a physician and discussing only those medical skills that related to the female body, undoubtedly in an attempt to embarrass her. When they refused to assign her, she explained, "I intimated that I would see Gen'l Thomas."[43]

Sexism played a large part in the treatment Mary received from these medical officers, but there was a long background of professional conflict that was playing out in the war years as well. Physicians trained in allopathic medicine had been politically astute in their pre-war campaign to designate themselves as "regular" physicians and anyone who was not an allopath as a "non-regular." It was a loaded rhetorical manipulation that soon pervaded public discourse. The popularity of homeopathic and eclectic physicians also played a role in the defensive gesture of forming the American Medical Association. When the war came, the U.S. Sanitary Commission was, controversially, the oversight organization for recruiting physicians for the Medical Department, and the AMA's allopathic physicians were given enormous influence through the Commission. They used their methodological differences to cast aspersions on non-allopaths who sought commissions in the service. The power of the alliance of allopaths and the Sanitary Commission was demonstrated most fully when Surgeon General Clement A. Finley was replaced in April 1862 as a result of his opposition to the Commission's power. Thus the Board's treatment of Mary was exacerbated by her sex but was part of a general pattern of exclusion.[44]

One independent perspective that survives from these early weeks in March is that of a reporter for the *Cincinnati Commercial* who signed his name only as "Montrose." He reported that after Mary met with Perin, "For several days the fair surgeon practiced in the hospital where she displayed marked skill." Ironically,

Mary was often misidentified by observers and physicians alike as a "regular," suggesting that in these years the differences were as much political as medical. Finally, General Thomas wielded his authority as commander of the Army of the Cumberland and intervened on Mary's behalf based on his own observations of her medical skills from the Chickamauga Campaign. On March 14, 1864, overruling the Medical Board's negative recommendation, he assigned Mary as a contract surgeon to the 52nd Ohio Volunteers. It meant she would be paid the equivalent of a lieutenant's salary, which was $80 per month. Perin was thus forced to send the order: "In compliance with the directions of the Major General Comdg. you will report without delay to Colonel Dan McCook, Comd'g. 3rd Brig. 2d Div. 14th A. C. [Army Corps] now on duty at Gordons Mills." The action grated on Perin's sense of authority, which he vindicated in part by addressing the order to "Miss" rather than "Dr." Walker. After the war, he would have his revenge; but for now, Dr. Mary Walker was at last a contracted acting assistant surgeon with the United States Army, the only woman to attain that position during the Civil War.[45]

CHAPTER 4

Surgeon, Spy, Prisoner of War

Before Mary left for her first assignment as a contract surgeon, she resigned from her position with the Women's Relief Association. After serving as the founding president, she worked for two months in a variety of capacities, including secretary, member of the finance committee, and as the association's physician and surgeon. Her work with impoverished patients in these months led to her lifelong commitment to serve as physician to the laboring classes. She helped to secure 25 cots, 70 blankets, and a good supply of sheets, pillowcases, and other items for the WRA, as well as initially paying the rent on the house. In the six weeks between Christmas 1863 and the first week of February 1864, the WRA supplied 350 lodgings and 450 meals to soldiers' families and others. Their efforts were significantly aided when the renowned activist Anna Dickinson gave a lecture to help the cause. So Mary was surprised in late February when some WRA members criticized her for deciding to resign her positions. She wrote a letter of explanation to the *National Republican*, a Washington newspaper that reported often on WRA activities. Arguing that she donated her time and labor as a physician, she bluntly stated, "I cannot afford to donate any more at present." She found it necessary to pawn the gold watch her parents had given her for her eighteenth birthday in order to continue volunteering her medical services to soldiers, and her impending departure for the war front would result in long absences. She observed that there were now others capable of directing the organization, and those others were "directly or indirectly being supported by Government." There was a bitter note to this point; four of the five women running the organization were married to male physicians who were on the government payroll, while Mary had to volunteer her services at the Indiana Hospital and on the battlefield. But she concluded the letter on a more positive note. "My heart is still with the cause, but my energies must be in another direction." Those energies now focused on preparations for her assignment with the Union army.[1]

Before leaving Washington, Mary corresponded with a number of people she met during her years in the city and in the battlefield areas to which her profession had taken her. The custom of exchanging cartes de visite was popular throughout the country. As Oliver Wendell Holmes remarked, card portraits "have become the social currency, the sentimental 'green-backs' of civilization." Mary was fascinated with visual representations, and she would soon become one of the most photographed Americans of the nineteenth century. One of the people from whom she requested a card portrait was Edwin De Foe of the Quartermaster's Office in Culpepper. He replied, "I doubt if my picture be of much value to you, but *yours* would be to *me*. You are getting famous Doctor, and will probably one of these days, when some enterprizing individual undertakes to write the history of this rebellion figure very conspicuously." De Foe thought her fame would rest on the work she performed for soldiers' families, but the events of the war were about to unfold in ways no one could yet imagine.[2]

In March, General Thomas directed Mary to Gordon's Mills in northern Georgia, across the state line from Chattanooga. She was to replace the company surgeon who had recently died. For the first time, she wore the uniform of the surgeon with the knowledge that she had an official right to do so. She wanted to emphasize her pride as a woman who had attained this unique achievement: "I let my curls grow while I was in the army so that everybody would know that I was a woman." The Union army headquarters were in the Gordons' home. Mary was assigned sleeping quarters in the large kitchen, along with Gordon, his wife, and several of their children. The officers' accommodations were in another room down the hall. Colonel Daniel McCook, Jr. was the officer in charge. He was an intelligent, compassionate man who had been a law partner of General William Tecumseh Sherman before the war. He and Mary met when she treated the wounded after the Battle of Chickamauga, and they quickly established a good rapport. Captain L. A. Ross was among the soldiers at Gordon's Mills who observed the respect and status that McCook afforded her. Ross remarked in his diary that the two "created a sensation" as they rode into camp together. He thought the doctor "rode her fiery steed with grace and dignity," but noted that most of the soldiers found it an amusing spectacle and an opportunity for scandal-mongering. Ross was inspired to a declaration of women's rights as he intoned, "popular opinion everywhere and the customs of our country are against the advancement and usefulness of the fairer sex" in spite of the fact that their capabilities were unlimited.[3]

McCook's confidence in Mary was demonstrated to the troops when he asked her to don the officer's red sash in order to "revue the videttes" in his absence. She did so, having an orderly ride beside her while the mounted sentries underwent her inspection. "This is the only instance in the war, as far as I know," she proudly asserted, "where a woman made a revue." Not all of the soldiers were impressed with the authority McCook granted Mary. One man from Illinois groused in his diary about being "drilled by Mary Walker." Rumors quickly circulated that she was McCook's mistress or a Confederate spy who had infiltrated the general's good graces. She certainly was not the latter, and it is doubtful she was the former, though there may well have been an attraction. Mary reveled in her new-found power. One day she and McCook sent a joint note to Major Holmes. His regiment housed the brigade's band, and the note read, "Will you be so kind as to send our band up this evening with the string instruments also." The request was written in McCook's hand, but it was signed "Mary Walker, Major and Chief of Staff."[4]

Gordon's Mills did not equal the hellish environment that prevailed at Fredericksburg and Chickamauga. When Mary arrived, most of the patients with life-threatening wounds had been transported out of the area. But her assignment there may have been for reasons beyond her medical skills. McCook suggested that, when she was not attending patients, she go outside the Union lines to tend to the medical needs of the people in the region who were in a dire state after months of battles in and around the Georgia-Tennessee border. Mary knew the assignment was risky, as it often required her to journey several miles away from the security of Gordon's Mills: "It was dangerous going out there, the two officers and two orderlies that accompanied me were armed, and I had two revolvers in my saddle as well." She always carried with her the usual physician's medical kit, which included a scalpel, probes, hemostats and scissors as well as assorted medicines. Although McCook willingly offered her an armed escort whenever he could, there were an increasing number of instances when he could not do so. At one point, Mary was asked to attend to a sick child who resided several miles away in a dangerous part of the country; McCook purportedly determined that she could not have an escort because he could not risk losing any officers when they had so few at headquarters. Mary claimed that she went because, "As they begged so hard for a physician I stated to General McCook that I would go alone and relieve that distress if he would not allow any one to go with me; and here I will say that when I went alone I always removed the revolvers from my saddle." McCook eventually sent two escorts with her, but Mary recognized if she were detained by Confederate soldiers and discovered to be carrying weapons, the situation would go much harder for her. Although she felt the child needed several days' care, her escorts could not be spared from camp for that long. She was not naïve about the dangers faced by a woman traveling alone in enemy territory: "[W]hen I thought of my remaining there alone so far from headquarters where there was but one woman, and that the young mother, the child being . . . between one and two years of age, and four or five men in the house, I felt a little afraid to stay." She left instructions for the child's care and returned to headquarters with her escorts.[5]

Eventually, Mary began to travel more often without her escorts. "The people expressed so much gratitude," she explained, "that I lost all fear of anything being done to myself." There were close calls, however, especially since she wore her blue uniform on these house calls. One hair-raising incident occurred about three miles from headquarters. She was passing an old barn when two Confederate soldiers suddenly appeared and ordered her to halt. After questioning her, they ordered her to drive her wagon into the barn area. The barn was surrounded on three sides by a fence in which "the boards were so close together that one could not see through any of the cracks." She resolved immediately that she would not go into that secluded area with the two men and stalled by saying she needed to reach a patient. After a few minutes, the two men finally allowed her to pass. At headquarters, she told McCook and his officers about the confrontation, describing the leader in detail. The officers jumped to their feet and began to look back and forth at one another. Finally McCook said, "No, it cannot be him," because their suspect had sworn to kill every Yankee who crossed his path. The officers suspected that Mary had been confronted by Champ Ferguson, one of the most notorious, brutal criminals of the war. Years later she saw a picture of the man in a book; "I was so faint with the very thought of how narrowly I had escaped death," she said, "that I could hardly stand up."[6]

The Georgians she encountered had never seen a woman physician or one in a reform dress. On one house call, she determined that the patient was too ill to be left alone, but the only bed the family could offer was in a wing at the back of the house with no access into the house itself, and she requested that the daughter of the family sleep with her so she would not be alone in this isolated location. Unbeknownst to her, the incident created confusion in the family. When she returned a few weeks later and was again required to spend the night, she was informed by the young woman's mother that the daughter would not share her bed. Upon inquiry, Mary learned that neighbors insisted the doctor had to be a man because no woman could know as much as the doctor did. The mother confessed her daughter had made no complaint against Mary, and Mary unbraided her hair to demonstrate she was a woman. The mother gently pulled the long hair. Mary was amused at the woman's abiding skepticism: "[She] said that she had heard they had curus ways of fixing on false hair, still doubted my being a woman, but after a while I convinced her that I was a woman and the daughter slept with me."[7]

As had been the case in Washington, once Mary's efficiency for getting things done was recognized, her assistance was sought for services beyond medicine. One instance involved a woman and her daughter who sought Mary's assistance in traveling to obtain cotton yarn at a nearby mill so they could weave much-needed clothing. Mary knew the dangers of being seen in the area in her Union blue uniform—"they would take my horse away and take me prisoner," she assured the Georgians. But desperation led to creative thinking: the mother suggested that Mary don her daughter's dress and bonnet. Because of the cold, Mary kept her trousers on beneath the skirt, rolled up to keep them out of sight. Confident no one would recognize her in the disguise of a dress, she and the daughter set out. All was well until the return trip. Just as they were ascending a long, steep hill in an isolated area, two Confederate soldiers came riding rapidly toward them. Mary told her companion to give her the reins and whip, apparently intending to try to outrun their pursuers, but the whip slipped from the Georgian's hands. Mary cautioned her it was not safe to get out of the wagon. "I did not dare to get out myself," Mary realized, "because, having on an ordinary long dress, and not having been accustomed to wearing anything of the kind for a great many years before the war commenced, I feared that if I attempted to sight for the purpose of getting the whip I could not do so without having my pants seen, as it certainly would have been dangerous to make the attempt without holding away the dress." This time her fear was not of being taken prisoner but of sexual assault, as they were in an isolated area. As Mary tried to maneuver the wagon up a steep hill and away from the soldiers, the officers rode up behind the wagon and pressed their horses' breasts against the back of the wagon. Once they navigated the hill, one officer rode up next to the wagon on Mary's side and peered down to look at her face. "[B]ut I suppose he thought I was very modest," she noted, "and as I held my head down a little more without seeming to notice his intention to have a better look at my face, he slackened his speed a little, spoke with the other officer, and they then asked what we had got in our wagon." When they learned it was only yarn, they hesitated, then to the women's great relief, finally rode away. It was the last time Mary ever wore a dress and bonnet, but it served her well on that day.[8]

At this point her nemesis, Dr. Cooper, intervened in her life once again. Unwilling to have a woman in the medical corps and furious that his Board's recommendation had been ignored by General Thomas, he took the opportunity to write to the surgeon general, complaining that Mary was "useless, ignorant, trifling, and a consummate bore." He insisted she should never have been given a contract; but his complaints were ignored as the government had other plans. While she did treat a number of general medical cases and occasionally performed surgery for the civilians in the area, the real purpose of her trips outside Union lines while in Georgia was military in nature. General Sherman was preparing for the march on Atlanta in early May, and McCook's request that Mary travel into Confederate territory was in agreement to her request to serve as a spy for the Union army. It was an assignment she willingly undertook. As early as September 1862 she had offered to pass information she gathered in the field to the Union army, as she indicated in a letter to the secretary of war:

> I again offer my services to my country. . . . I refer to my being sent to Richmond under a "flag of truce" for the relief of our sick soldiers and then use the style (of double communication in writing their necessities) that I invented, to give you information as their forces and plans and any important information. No one knows what the style of writing is, except Hon. Mssrs. Cameron Seward and Mr. Allen of the "Secret Service" . . . Any "secret service" that your Hon. Body may wish performed, will find in me one eminently fitted to do it.

"Mr. Allen" was Allen Pinkerton, founder of Pinkerton's National Detective Agency. President Lincoln authorized Pinkerton to establish a Secret Service to gather information about Confederate military activities. That the detective would have sought to engage Mary in the corps of his Secret Service is plausible. In 1860 he had developed Pinkerton's Female Detective Bureau, recognizing that women could sometimes ferret out information to which men might not have access.[9]

The carefully worded written response at the time was simply that her request for "employment in Secret Service" had been referred to Major General Henry

Wager Halleck, General-in-Chief of the army. General Thomas later admitted that he assigned her to the 52nd Ohio Volunteers because she was eager to gather information about Confederate activities. In 1865 the judge advocate general revealed that "at one time [she] gained information that led General Sherman to so modify his strategic operations as to save himself from a serious reverse and obtain success where defeat before seemed to be inevitable." During her pension battles after the war, the government acknowledged that she had undertaken such activities "in accordance with a preconcerted arrangement between her and Federal officers."[10]

The dangers inherent in these actions were extreme and ever-present, and on April 10, 1864, Mary's luck in avoiding detection came to an end. While returning to Gordon's Mills, she encountered Confederate soldiers under the command of General Daniel Harvey Hill and was taken prisoner. There was no denying her affiliation, as she was wearing her blue army uniform. Mary claimed she was only attempting to deliver letters, but the picket guards took her captive at gunpoint. She would not allow them to see her fear, however, and boldly proclaimed she would be glad for the chance to rest her weary limbs. Five days after Mary's capture, General Ulysses S. Grant ordered all women to leave Union battlefield areas. Many women and military leaders ignored the command, but what few knew was that Grant probably feared the exposure of the military's use of a woman spy. Initially, Mary was held for several days at Dallin, Georgia, where Confederate General Joseph E. Johnston's army was bivouacked. From there she was sent to Castle Thunder Prison in Richmond.[11]

Castle Thunder Prison housed political prisoners, spies, deserters, and persons charged with treason. The commandant of nearby Libby Prison asserted that Castle Thunder held "some of the most dangerous prisoners" in the South. Its name was selected by Captain George W. Alexander, the prison commandant, because he wanted a name that reflected the terror a prisoner should feel upon entering the facility; prisoners were described as being "Thunderstruck" when housed there. It lived up to its intended reputation, earning the nickname of the "Southern Bastille." The year before Mary arrived, the Confederate House of Representatives ordered an investigation of Captain Alexander, who was charged with being "harsh, inhuman, tyrannical, and dishonest." He was known to hang prisoners to a beam by their thumbs so their feet barely scraped the floor, and then flog them. His defense was that he was dealing with hardened criminals who required extreme measures, and he was found not guilty. But even Southerners described Castle Thunder as a fearsome place, and the guards were reputed to be brutal in their treatment of the prisoners. A poem about Castle Thunder was published in the *Libby Chronicle*, the prison newspaper, which named General Alexander, Provost General John H. Winder, and other military officers as "of the very meanest stuff." The female ward of this prison was where Mary would spend the next four months of her life. It would demand new levels of strength and courage, especially since one of the first reports she heard upon her arrival at Castle Thunder was that of a young female spy who had been chloroformed, raped, and killed by three prison officers.[12]

The Richmond newspapers delighted in this new subject for ridicule, a "female Yankee surgeon." It was an opportunity for revenge, since Northerners had gloated over the capture of the Southern spy Belle Boyd two years earlier. For four months, the major newspapers in the city made Mary the butt of their jokes and the target of their resentment of the North. In May, when she was walked by guards through the streets to General Winder's office at Libby Prison, she was criticized for her "male attire, which begins to look the worse for wear." Her clothing was undoubtedly in a ruined state, as it was the only clothing she had with her at the time of capture, and the prison was cited more than once for the suffering prisoners endured because of inadequate clothing and bedding. The months of criticism did not alter Mary's assertions of her rights or her Northern alliance. As one Confederate captain noted, she "had tongue enough for a regiment of men." Equally galling to the press were her sympathies with African Americans. The newspapers were not above creating their own fictions about the prisoner; but it was the aspersions cast against her "male attire" that finally elicited a response from Mary. "Simple *justice*," she asserted, "demands correction. I am attired in what is usually called the 'bloomer' or 'reform dress,' which is similar to other ladies' [dresses], with the exception of its being shorter and more physiological than long dresses."[13]

In June, the *Richmond Enquirer* claimed that Mary was "very tired of her captivity in Castle Thunder. She wants to go home, and don't mind if she sinks the Doc in the woman to do so. Sensible female." No doubt she wanted to go home, but the timing of her capture made the possibility of release or exchange more difficult than usual. Both the Union and Confederate armies had accepted the Dix-Hill plan in 1862 that established policies for exchanges of prisoners; but controversies emerged that led the Union to halt the exchange for several months in 1863–64. A few weeks later the *Richmond Examiner* chimed in with one of the longer and most vilifying depictions of her:

> Miss Doctress, Miscegenation, Philosophical Walker, who has so long ensconced herself very quietly in Castle Thunder, has loomed into activity again. Recently she got mad, pitched into several of her room-mates in long clothes, and tore out handsful of auburn hair from the head of one of them. Then she proclaimed secession, and went into another apartment. . . . Her miscegenation suit is getting rusty, and . . . it is said she has a Yankee Major lover among the prisoners at the Libby prison, which is one square below the Castle, and within easy signal range.

The images of a "cat fight" and of Mary as the "miscegenist" seeking "secession" offered a way for the city papers to denigrate her personally and the North in general.[14]

Mary was able to send a few letters during her incarceration. One of the first she sent was to her parents. After her release, she would reveal the hardships of her months of imprisonment, but at this juncture she wanted only to reassure her family. Vesta sent the letter to the *National Republican*, which printed an excerpt from it in late June: "I hope you are not grieving about me because I am a prisoner-of-war. I am living in a three-story brick castle with plenty to eat and a clean bed to sleep in. I have a room-mate, a young lady about 20 years of age, from near Corinth, Miss. I am much happier than I might be in some relations of life, where I might be envied by other ladies. The officers are gentlemanly and kind and it will not be long before I am exchanged." It was far from truthful, but it was a kind letter to send home to parents who were undoubtedly distraught. In reality, rations for prisoners were maggot-filled, water was given only at the permission of guards, and the guards often harassed Mary.[15]

As in many prisons housing enemies and deserters, the food was never adequate. In October 1863 General Winder received complaints from prison commanders that, for the fourth time in recent days, no meat was available. "No force under my command," Winder observed as he argued for immediate attention to their diminished food supplies, "can prove adequate to the control of 13,000 hungry prisoners." Inflation made the cost of feeding thousands of prisoners—as well as soldiers—an unbearable debt for the Confederacy. By the time Mary was imprisoned in Castle Thunder, rations had been severely reduced beyond that which had brought the 1863 complaints. Her diet consisted of limited amounts of cornbread, bacon, and either peas or rice that were used to prepare a soup. Meat was rarely part of the diet by 1864. Further, prisoners were allowed only thirty minutes of exercise in the yard each day, and many prisoners suffered from muscular atrophy. The prison was filthy; Mary's mattress was infested and rats could be heard in the night as they scurried about her room. The air was foul, especially in the hot summer months when she first arrived, and she would often lean out the small window in order to breathe. Somehow she had managed to retain among her possessions a small fan that had an American flag printed on one side. More than one Union prisoner recalled being marched past Castle Thunder on their way to imprisonment in Libby Prison and seeing a small woman at the window, holding the fan so that the flag was turned in their direction. It was a sign of unity and encouragement in the midst of the fears that haunted every new captive.[16]

Finally, on August 12, Mary was part of a prisoner exchange negotiated by the armies of the North and South. Both sides were desperate for physicians, and she was exchanged for a Confederate surgeon from Tennessee. The Richmond newspapers bid her farewell, referring to her as "the miscegenating surgeoness and philosophical bloomer." Her release was reported throughout the United States, and many newspapers also remarked on the fact that she was exchanged for a regular army surgeon. The official notation made in the prisoner lists described her as "The notorious Miss Dr. Mary E. Walker, Surgeoness of the 52nd Ohio Regulars." It would not be the last time she was described as notorious, but it was the proudest. Reports at the time proclaimed that as she left the prison she shouted "Huzzah!" and bowed her farewell to the prison commandants in a manner that "plainly indicated that she had no regrets in leaving." Her health had deteriorated, and she had sustained eye damage due to the lack of healthy food and to the constant presence of gas-burning lamps in the small cell where she was housed. She returned to Washington after her release; ironically, considering all she had endured for the Union army, her contract ended on August 23.[17]

Although "body weak," her spirit was strong. President Lincoln met with Mary to ask about her treatment as a prisoner, and she took the opportunity to express her opinions about the situation in Virginia. Less than two weeks later, she published an account of her imprisonment in the *National Republican*. She chose to write a political satire of her life as a prisoner of war—a "*guest*"—at "Hotel de Castle Thunder." By detailing the scant "bill of fare" that prisoners were given, she emphasized the dire economic conditions of the Confederacy that fed prisoners little and its soldiers barely more, but concluded on the upbeat note that she had now learned her own strength through the experience. "Whoever passes through terrible trials in the vigor of years ought to thank the Hand that suffered the same to be; for every *terrible experience* develops the powers, so that one can calmly say, 'Strike deep, my heart can bear;' so that one can manufacture smiles by the bushel when the heart is breaking; so that, whatever of wrongs or injustice may be met, no glance of the eye can betray aught but a cheerful resignation to 'whatever is.'" Most of her comments about her imprisonment at this time were for the public and reflected either her stoic insistence on diminishing the experience's effects or a graphic rendering of conditions to expose the ruthlessness of her Confederate captors. A few years later, lecturing in London, she would offer a more detailed account of those months, including the fact that at one point in her incarceration she was near starvation.[18]

Mary remained in Washington only for two weeks before heading south again. By September 10, she was in Louisville, Kentucky, where she met with friends from McCook's brigade. Tragically, while Mary was imprisoned, her friend and ally Colonel McCook died from battle wounds. She always remembered him as a kind-hearted, generous man. She briefly considered undertaking a lecture tour of the States, which would have been a highly profitable venture considering the publicity her release had garnered, but she ultimately delayed her career as a lecturer. Instead, she joined the medical personnel in the battlefield who were treating the wounded after the Battle of Atlanta. While caring for the wounded, she wrote to General Sherman. She was no longer satisfied having to negotiate a contract each time she sought to go to the battlefield. She had proved her value as a physician and as a supporter of the Union cause, and now she wanted to be a regular member of the military as were male physicians:

Atlanta Sept. 14, 1864
Gen. Sherman
Sir
  Having acted in various capacities since the Commencement of the rebellion, without a Commission for our Government & three years of Service having Expired—I now must respectfully ask that a Commission be given me

with the rank of Major, & that I be assigned to duty as surgeon of the female prisoners & the female refugees, at Louisville, Ky.

I beg to inform the Gen'l that if there should be a hesitancy, on the ground that no *woman* had ever received *such a Commission*, I have but to remind you that there has not been a Woman who has served Government in such a variety of ways of importance to the great *Cause* which has elicited patriotism that knows no sex.

I still farther beg to inform you, that, I have at various times acted in the Capacity of Extra Assistant Surgeon, for the sick & wounded of our army, with entire satisfaction to my patients & the Surgeons by whom I have been put on duty; & when I have asked the different Surgeons of the U.S.A. for a commission, urging that services that were appreciated by the above mentioned (concerns) could be as well performed with a Commission as without one.

I have been told that "all the reason was because I was a woman" & "female surgeons should confine their practice to their own sex."

I have been informed that the female prisoners mentioned, now number between twenty five & thirty; & that there are over two hundred females & refugee children in Louisville Ky.

I only ask that simple *Justice* be done me as a "Military Necessity."

Most respectfully
Mary E. Walker, M.D.

It was a shrewd request. Having treated wounded soldiers at Indiana Hospital and at the battles of Bull Run, Warrenton, Fredericksburg, Chickamauga, Chattanooga, and now Atlanta, her service record and her skills could not be questioned. If the argument against commissioning her was the usual one for women physicians—that they should only treat their own sex—then her request to be assigned to the female prison countered that argument. Mary also went to see Assistant Adjutant General Edward D. Townsend, seeking payment for her years of service. She now had a large packet of official papers and letters that detailed her work for the Union army. After meeting with her, Townsend contacted General Thomas, asking if there was "anything due the woman and if so what amount for secret service or other services?" Thomas responded, "[H]er services have no doubt been valuable to the Government, and her efforts have been earnest and untiring and have been exerted in a variety of ways." Within two weeks she received $432.36 in back pay—but no commission.[19]

Her argument to Sherman for assignment was successful in part. On September 22, Joseph B. Brown of the Assistant Surgeon General's Office in Louisville wrote to Mary: "In accordance with instructions from *Major General Sherman* Commanding Military Division of Mississippi, *Miss Mary E. Walker, M.D.* will report in person, without delay for duty with female prisoners in this City. By order of the Asst. Surgeon Gen'l." Mary had been so confident that her demands would be met that she was already en route to Louisville. Two days later, the newspapers reported Mary's arrival. For the rest of her life, her every move would be news. She had wanted to be famous, and her accomplishments, her unique personality, and her appearance had cumulatively garnered her that status.[20]

She had barely arrived in Louisville, however, when she sought a twenty-day leave to return to Oswego. Sherman granted her request and offered her permission to apply for an extension if necessary; he knew that her purpose was not personal. The critical election of 1864 was looming, and Mary's goal was to work for Lincoln's reelection and for the Republican Party as it sought to oust the Democratic governor, Horatio Seymour. She applied for and received the extension because, as she noted, the original date "expires *two days before election*. That will give me four days to return to my Post, after working until the *last hour of election day*, which is the 8th of Nov." She dived into this goal with her usual high level of energy and determination. She spoke at a large rally on October 24, detailing her experiences at Castle Thunder Prison. The *Oswego Times* had become increasingly radical under Ira D. Brown's editorship. He supported John C. Frémont's 1861 proclamation calling for the confiscation of Missouri Confederates' property—including slaves; he lamented Lincoln's failure early in the war to accept the idea of African American troops; and he fought against an attempted takeover of the newspaper by conservative Republicans in 1863. Although not without criticism, the *Times* and Oswego County supported Lincoln in the election, giving him 2,500 of the 7,000 votes he received to win the state.[21]

While there were many aspects of the Republicans' ideas that did not appeal to Mary, she embraced the party during the war years because it sided with the abolitionists to the extent of arguing for the end of slavery. It was a cautious alliance for all abolitionist reformers, and one that would not survive the postwar years. Had Frémont remained a Republican candidate against Lincoln, it is likely that Mary would have supported his campaign; she had long been an admirer of his antislavery activism. The antiwar Democratic platform, calling for a ceasefire and negotiations with the South, alienated even those Republicans who had not wanted to support Lincoln. Especially offensive to many was the Democratic candidate George B. McClellan's opposition to the Emancipation Proclamation. Mary's longstanding commitment to abolition was the basis of her support for Lincoln. She spoke at rallies, and when Democrats in the audience attempted to silence her with hisses, the Union soldiers present responded with long, supportive cheers that silenced her opponents. Sherman's timely success at Atlanta gave Lincoln the essential boost he needed, winning with 55 percent of the popular vote.[22]

During the months after her release and while she was in Oswego preparing for the election, Mary maintained a steady correspondence with soldiers and their families who sought her assistance, and with friends she had made while stationed at various locations. Most of the soldiers' letters were filled with the anguish of impoverished men in extremely bad health themselves or worried about the health and sustenance of loved ones at home. Occasionally a prisoner would write her; most of these letters were from deserters who sought to explain their circumstances and ask for her intervention. One soldier she had assisted earlier in the year wrote to her, asserting, "I am endebted to you for my life and I am sure I shall never forget your kind interference on my behalf." Friends maintained contact as well. J. H. Wooll wrote her from Washington, referring to her as "Bell[e] of Libby Castle" and "Heroine of the War of 1864"; he wanted her to return to Washington and sent news of the political scene in Washington—"the assembled political thousands." Susan Hall, who worked at one of the military hospitals in Chattanooga, also wrote to Mary, congratulating her on the appointment to the military prison. "*Who* could object to the *propriety* of your position now?" Hall asked, and hoped that Mary would be given "the rank of *Major*."[23]

After the election Mary returned to Louisville and began her new role as surgeon in charge of the hospital at the Female Military Prison. Mary was not commissioned as a major, but she was again formally contracted as a surgeon, for "at least three months." Her base salary increased to $100 per month and to $113.83 per month with transportation costs "when performing service in the field." Dr. Edward Phelps was the prison's medical director and he and Mary worked well together for the eight months she remained at this post.[24]

The assignment, however, was to be more difficult than she had anticipated. Her patients were Confederate women prisoners held for a variety of reasons; most of the women had children with them as well. Some were long-term criminals; most were there for their actions during the war. All were distraught, angry at being imprisoned, and blamed "the Yankees" for their situation. Mary was successful in helping a few prisoners, including three teenagers for whom she gained an order from Colonel J. H. Hammond for transportation home. She could not help but notice, however, the difference in treatment of these prisoners and her own at Castle Thunder: "They have the best coffee, soup, potatoes fresh beef (over half a pound at each plate) and the very best bread. . . . Could I have had the quality and quantity in a week, while a prisoner in Richmond, that each one of these prisoners consumes in a day, I could not have complained of the 'bill of fare.'"[25]

The women prisoners were no more accepting of a female physician than most Americans of the era. A group of them complained, asking that she be removed. Years later one prisoner recalled "the anomalous creature that was put over us for our sins and I remember . . . wondering what the thing was. The dress was that of a man, but the braided hair and skinny, shrewish features were those of a woman. . . . She wished constantly to dose us, but we had no confidence in her and refused to submit to her experiments." The women did not come to their resentment of Mary solely on their own, however. The former male physician of the prison, Dr. E. O. Brown, had been far more lenient with the prisoners, and he continued to visit and prescribe medicines for the patients, in spite of Mary's many requests that he not do so. Like many male physicians she had encountered in the military, he was sure she must be incompetent. She soon learned that he had told the prisoners to accept only his orders and his prescriptions. But Brown's tactics backfired; when Assistant Surgeon General Wood heard of the situation, Brown's interference was halted at once. This did not, however, change the damage that had been done in terms of Mary's relationship with her patients.[26]

Before her tenure at the prison began, Colonel Hammond had informed General Wood that the prison was "no better than a brothel." Certainly most of the women were not prostitutes, but several of the female prisoners had manipulated a Lieutenant Stephenson; when they complained of Mary's harsh treatment, he reported it to Colonel Coyle. Initially, Coyle accepted Stephenson's accusation. On January 15, 1865, Mary wrote a scathing letter to Coyle. "You have done me a gross injustice in speaking of me as you do when I appealed to you, to sustain me in the right," she began. "I thought you a man of sufficient discretion and judgement to comprehend things as they exist, and then I thought you had sufficient moral courage to pursue a course consistent with an enlightened conscience." If there was any trait Mary inherited from her father, it was speaking out for what she believed was right, regardless of consequences. Mary would not allow her professional reputation to be damaged or tolerate having false information about her own motives offered as fact.[27]

Stephenson blamed her for having the male cooks replaced by females, but Mary insisted the "food question" was just a pretext on his part. If Coyle "had *three* grains of common sence," she asserted, he would recognize that, because the prisoners complained about the food when men were cooks, too. She then gave Coyle a detailed account of the nearly impossible task of trying to maintain order, let alone treat patients, under such conditions, even though she set up a system of rules to establish order. Although Stephenson had thought there was no harm in letting the prisoners sing Rebel songs, she banned them and any other "disloyal talk." She quickly halted the familiarity that had become routine between the female prisoners and male guards, probably the primary source of the tension between the lieutenant and herself. In fact, Colonel Fairleigh had directed her to replace the four male cooks with females to stop such fraternization. There were other problems among the prisoners that led Mary to intervene. She was appalled by the neglect and sometimes outright abuse a few of the prisoners inflicted on their children. One woman, who had suddenly become the caretaker of three of her sister's orphaned children, tried to hang the eldest as a means of scaring her into obedience. Mary threatened to remove children from mothers who continued to neglect or abuse them. It was a hellish environment for everyone. At one point Mary had a prisoner handcuffed for two hours because she cursed at a guard and threatened Mary. She concluded her chiding letter to Coyle with the admonition:

> Give them their filth, unrestrained disloyalty and immorality and it will be satisfactory times with them. I am an eye sore to them, and they want men Cooks again and a man Doctor. They glory in a Lieut that chops open doors and allows them to surround him in the operation. He would not have dared made such an outright idiot of himself if Col Fairleigh had been here. Col Fairleigh has learned my true motives for all that I have done, and appreciates the

trying position I hold, and all my greatest superior officers have confidence in my having done *well* under all circumstances, and that confidence is *merited*.

>With due respect
>Mary E Walker U.S.A.

To Mary's mind, it was not just a question of who was in charge, but even more so of how she was to be treated. Coyle's failure to support her work was an unconscionable breach of her expectations of what was right. Signing herself "Mary E. Walker *U.S.A.*" went beyond a generic sense of location—it represented her outrage at being denied liberty and justice to do her duty for her country. But for anyone to write in such a manner to a lieutenant colonel created a greater stir than the initial complaints from the prisoners. Coyle forwarded the letter to Captain Charles Gould, who in turn forwarded it to Colonel Wood. Had Wood not been a longstanding ally of Mary's and had not Medical Director Phelps been supportive of her throughout her stay in Louisville, the situation could have ended her opportunities to serve in the army as a physician.[28]

There was also an element of sexism in Stephenson's actions against her. As Mary's loyal orderly, Cary Conklin, attested, "Dr. Walker had the entire professional charge of the prisoners and the guard, and was always kind and attentive to both—So much so to the *prisoners*, that some of the union people were very much displeased. The Lieut. commanding the guard seemed to take every opportunity, and study to do whatever he thought would annoy and make the position of the Surgeon in Charge a very trying one," explaining in part why Mary reacted so vehemently. Yet while her suggestion of being appointed to the female prison had been, strategically, an innovative means of returning to contracted service, it did not take into account the psychological consequences for a former prisoner of war on becoming the head of a prisoners' hospital. The quick shift from being a prisoner herself to being in charge of them in the hospital left her with little emotional ability to negotiate the difficult terrain of working with prisoners who denigrated her beloved Union and praised those who had held Mary captive.[29]

While in Louisville, Mary received a letter from Washington. The letterhead had the stamp of the capital city in the corner with "Congress" underneath; its author's name was given only as "Doc." Playful and witty, the letter refers to an indictment in "the high court of friendship" to which Mary was subjected, until a letter from her was finally received. Before receiving her letter, "Doc" was about to settle into a "grave . . . and formal character; dispense stupid wisdom and sensible nonsense. These resolves were no sooner made, than they were broken after reading epistle." It was Mary's use of the word "love" in her letter that enthralled "Doc," who wrote:

> That word in your letter around which revolves so many beautiful sentiments. *That* magic word love set my fancy in flights, to sun gilt cottages, on the slope of romantic hills; lovely companions to share the solitude etc etc.

Oh how happy such a reality will be, for us, when we are married, (excuse my blushes)—when we marry the companions of our choice. How beautifully Shakespeare (that great unfolder, of the mysterious workings of the human heart) speaks of that passion, Love. He says

She loved me, for the dangers I had passed; and I, that she did pity them. How beautifully that would apply in your case were I to reverse the order of the pronouns.

Oh ye muses inspire my old goose quill, that I may sing of love; pour fourty flashes of lightning into my old pen, give it that eloquent passion that love can only dictate;—let it be moved by the hand of time until the clock of eternity runs down;—it could not half express, even in that length of time how I love you-r sex.

Hoping you will not let my California inamort*a* know the expressions of my tenderest philinks toward you.

Subscribe myself—Yours till we meet on the other side

Doc

570 7th St.

Doc's identity remains a mystery.[30]

By March 1865, Mary determined to leave the Louisville prison. She wanted to be back in the field. As she wrote to Dr. Phelps, "Learning that a number of surgeons are being sent to the front, I most respectfully ask to be sent also. It is six months today since I was assigned here, and it has been an untold task to keep this institution in a good condition *morally* & I am weary of the task & would much prefer to be where my services can be appreciated and to do more good *directly* to the Cause." Phelps regretted her departure, but he complied with her request. She was ordered to report to Dr. George E. Cooper, medical director of the Cumberland, in Nashville. In spite of the conflicts that developed, Dr. Phelps staunchly supported her medical practices at the prison: "I bear testimony to the superior talents and acquirements of Dr. Mary E. Walker. . . . While performing her complicated duties at the Female Military Prison in Louisville, she evinced the same active, energetic and persevering spirit which has characterized her in her whole military career." He concluded that she had rendered "even more service to her country than many of our efficient officers, bearing full commissions." As she left Louisville, Phelps assured Mary, "Any thing I can do for you I shall always be glad to." The *Louisville Daily Journal* reported on Mary's departure, praising her for her service: "[W]e believe her government of the institution received the approval of all loyal people, being a surgeon of fine ability and one whose experience well fitted her for the position. Her removal will be deplored by many. To whatever field of duty she may be assigned, we doubt not that she will meet with the success which her splendid talents merit."[31]

Cooper assigned Mary to the directorship of the Refugee House in Clarksville, Tennessee, where she served from April 11 until May 17. It was not the battlefield assignment she wanted, but she acquiesced, explaining, "[A]s there is no prospect of immediate surgical work—I am contented to serve the Government here until called to a more important position." In part this assignment may have been one more attempt by Cooper to keep Mary from practicing in the military as a surgeon, but she was correct that surgical work had lessened significantly. Lee surrendered just two days before Mary's arrival in Clarksville, and the war was dwindling to a close. By the time she undertook the directorship of the Home, many of the refugees had spent four years running from one city to the next, pushed ahead of retreating soldiers and back again as battles shifted, many of them used as pawns by military leaders. Some of the prisoners were filled with rage and contempt, but most were exhausted, defeated, and shell-shocked by the horrors of war. Refugees at Clarksville and Nashville at the time numbered in the thousands, and those staying at the House were among the most destitute of the war, as refugees who had any money paid to rent rooms in boarding houses.[32]

On April 14, as Mary was beginning her new assignment, the country was stunned by the assassination of President Lincoln. If the war itself had not caused enough dissension and animosity to last for generations, the murder of the president sent shock waves across communities North and South that would be remembered for decades to come. The plot had been to kill Lincoln, Vice President Johnson, and Secretary of State Seward, thus destroying the government and swaying the war toward a last-minute Southern retaliation, if not victory. While beautiful elegies such as "When Lilacs Last in the Dooryard Bloom'd" memorialized the President's death, many Northerners reacted with a call for all-out revenge. Soldiers received word on the battlefield within days, and the tragedy invigorated their passionate calls for the destruction of the South. Mary's brother Alvah, Jr. was stationed at Harrison's Landing, Virginia, when he received the news. "I wish the earth had drank the last drop of secession blood," he wrote home to his wife, "for it seems they're not fit to live since they have so cruelly and fiendly murdered our noblehearted and patriotic Abraham."[33]

Mary's reaction was equally volatile and patriotic. On the Sunday after Lincoln's assassination, she attended morning services at the Clarksville Episcopal Church. A flower arrangement on the baptismal font caught her eye—it was made of white Easter lilies with a large red geranium in the center. Believing it was a silent tribute to the Confederacy, she rose from her chair, moved to the front of the church, and placed a blue ribbon on the wreath. Soon thereafter, the rector removed the ribbon and concluded the service. Now assured of the political implications of the flowers, Mary attended the evening services. She placed a small bouquet that was adorned with an American flag, beribboned in crepe, at the front of the church. During the offering, the minister moved the arrangement aside; furious, Mary rose, moved the bouquet back to where she had originally placed it, and returned to her seat. The atmosphere was crackling with tension, but no further incident occurred.[34]

On the 17th of May General Cooper wrote to Mary that "the medical officer in charge can do all the work required of him" and "your services are no longer required in this department." He informed her that she could present herself at his office or that of the eastern surgeon general. The war efforts were ending and one medical officer was probably sufficient to handle the last of the details; but Cooper's opposition to her work as a contract surgeon had haunted Mary for more than a year, and she would not take the easy path and go to the eastern post. Instead, she went to Cooper's office in Nashville to finalize her work. She was ordered to Washington, D.C., and her military service was officially concluded, at her request, on June 15, 1865. She was paid $766.16 for her services at the end of war. She had one moment of celebration before she left the army. In late June she returned to Richmond, to the place of her imprisonment, and wandered through Castle Thunder with a freedom unknown to her during her incarceration. She was even more honored on July 4, 1865, when she was asked to join in the national celebration by reading the Declaration of Independence from the steps of Richmond's Capitol Building—dressed in full surgeon's uniform for the last time. It was a triumphant return.[35]

After Richmond, Mary spent a few weeks in New York City and then returned to Washington. For the remainder of the year, she boarded at a house in which her fellow residents included two generals and their spouses and several members of Congress. She intended to renew her medical practice in the city, but she settled on no other plans for the future. The unfortunate effect of the partial muscular atrophy of her eyes that occurred during her imprisonment was that she would have to curtail her surgery practice and work primarily as a physician. She considered a lecture tour, in which she could regale audiences with her war experiences, and she was determined to renew her active support of women's rights. Like her sister suffragists, she assumed that the support they had given so unceasingly to the Northern cause would be recognized as evidence of their equality and rightful status as voting citizens. Before Mary could make any move toward reshaping her life in the aftermath of war, however, she was reminded of another battle yet to be won. On July 19, Albert Miller wrote to Mary's brother-in-law Lyman Coats: "Can you tell me where Mary is? I have not heard from her or of her in a long time. I think she will yet see that haste does not always lead to the right & regret our separation. I wish also to know if she is in need of any of the comforts or necessities of life. I would willingly assist her at any time, should she need it. After years of trial & sorrow, one is more apt to see the right—I would be pleased to hear from any of her family at any time." They had less than a year before the five-year waiting period for divorce would be completed; if it was finalized, Albert would be legally barred from remarrying for as long as Mary lived. Whatever his motivations, he was involved with several women at this time and had maintained a months-long relationship with Delphine Freeman of Boston.[36]

A much happier letter seeking renewed contact came from Dr. Lydia Sayer Hasbrouck. "Sister Walker," she wrote, "Where in the name of common sense are you to be found? We see your name there there & somewhere—but not one line from you this long time. Now you have done your work in the Army we want you north—We want to go to work in ernest upon the question of woman's right to suffrage & the Dress question. We want to put lecturers into the field & we want you to help us as Sergeant Major to martial our forces . . . in these war times." It was a welcome call to work at which Mary was skilled and which would help to keep her mind off Albert's manipulations. She had not been idle in terms of dress reform, responding to questions about her appearance wherever she had traveled during the war. Although often ridiculed, she also found women who were interested in her ideas about healthy clothing. Early in the year she exchanged letters with Addie Hitchens of Philadelphia who was drawn to the new style of dress but concerned about public reactions. Mary told her that "*talking* a principle is very different from living it." Although most suffragists had abandoned dress reform, Mary was about to enter on a campaign for its acceptance that would last until her death more than forty-five years later.[37]

Mary maintained a medical office in her Washington home at 374 Ninth Street, but she had been absent so often that her patients had dwindled. More to the point, she had been invigorated by the challenges of battlefield doctoring and wanted something equally important to do in the months after the war. Thus she sought a postwar commission as an army surgeon, to serve as a medical inspector in the Freedmen's Bureau in Washington. The Freedmen's Bureau was established to confront the complex problems facing the government in aiding hundreds of thousands of war refugees, newly freed slaves, and impoverished white farmers. A major part of its mission was to insure a basic education for freed slaves and to help them find equitable employment. Women were integral to the success of the Bureau's efforts from its beginnings; Josephine Griffing, an Ohio abolitionist, was instrumental in encouraging President Lincoln's establishment of the Bureau, and many women volunteers went into the South during the war to enact its mission. With her longstanding commitment to abolition and extraordinary record of military service, Mary felt it was exactly the kind of postwar position in which her talents could thrive. But President Johnson had already contended with the outspoken Griffing, who was fired for exposing the government's failure to address African Americans' post-emancipation hardships. The last thing the Bureau and Johnson's administration wanted on staff was another outspoken woman.[38]

Unsuccessful in these efforts, Mary delved into work and activism that embraced her goal of effecting change in women's status. Her return to lecturing created a lifestyle of constant movement—traveling for conventions, lectures, to visit family and friends around the country, to work on behalf of soldiers and nurses, and to attend legislative sessions where petitions of interest to her (and, increasingly, authored by her) were being heard. Although she developed a pattern of spending the months in which the U.S. Congress was in session in Washington and the summer months in Oswego, she never remained at home for long in either location.

Much of her time in these months and for several years to come was devoted to gaining pension benefits for soldiers and wartime nurses. She studied the legislative acts that were passed during the war in relation to nurses. She prepared the argument that, because they had been placed in positions typically held by soldiers, women nurses were entitled to government pensions for their contributions to the war effort. She tracked changes in wages for nurses and hospital matrons and compared them to those of male medical cadets who were contracted by the Army to serve as surgical dressers and ambulance attendants and who were paid the same rate as West Point military cadets. Since congressional and military records were often incomplete during the war years, she corresponded with as many women nurses as she could to gather their written remarks on when and where they served the army, what work they did, and how much if anything they were paid. Researching legislative precedent and then preparing and presenting a petition to the legislature on behalf of women's rights became the hallmark of Mary's activism between 1865 and her death in 1919.[39]

Immediately after the war's conclusion, Mary spent a few weeks in New York City. She liked to tell the story of an acquaintance she made there, "a very fine woman who was in financial straits. I was 'strapped' myself, so I sold my curls and gave her the money." After that initial sacrifice of her curls, she let them grow at various times throughout her life; but even when her hair was long, she tied it into a small bun at the back of her head, never again wearing the long curls she had used to signify she was a woman surgeon on the battlefield.[40]

Perhaps the most important activity she undertook at this time was a form of study that would serve her well for the rest of her life—she attended lectures on the law at Columbian Law School in Washington (later George Washington University School of Law). That training, her own studies of legal texts, and her many friendships with lawyers formed the legal education that allowed her to petition the United States and New York governments on a wide range of women's rights causes. Although Mary never took the bar exam, she served as legal representative for friends and in later years involved herself in several high-profile cases.[41]

In August, Dr. Ann Preston, Dean of the Woman's Medical College of Pennsylvania, wrote to Mary; it had been suggested that Mary be granted an honorary degree from the institution, and Preston wrote to explain the long process involved. Mary had missed Preston when she stopped by the college the week before while in Philadelphia for the Working Men's conference. Preston's interest in Mary was evident: "I regretted very much that I missed [your] call, for I have long wanted to know more of you and one learns more by a 'face to face' interview than by writing." Preston's letter was full of inquiries about Mary's experiences: "Were you regularly commissioned as surgeon in the U.S. Army? What duties were deemed suited to your position and sex? So far as I know you were the only medical woman in the army who was recognized as such." Preston lamented that "the distrust & prejudice of Professional men" kept other women physicians from being contracted by the army. Preston was one of the most revered women physicians in America, so her response to Mary had to be especially pleasing: "I do not know what may be your plans for the future but I trust that a full and happy career may lie before you—A woman who is true to the *great truth* that speaks in her own soul may even now, despite of all opposition, establish herself in the Profession of Medicine & live blessing and blessed in the practice." Preston asked Mary to send her a history of the circumstances that led her into the army and her experiences while on the battlefield. She was especially interested to know Mary's background to better understand what "made you what you are." This may have been the impetus to Mary's detailing some of her war experiences, although she never published an autobiography.[42]

Mary retained many friendships from the years she spent doctoring wounded soldiers in Washington and on the battlefield. One such friend was George W. Morgan of the Treasury Department, who invited Mary to visit him and his wife at their Washington home. Other associates from those years were working to recognize her wartime contributions through formal channels. When Mary sought a postwar commission in the military as a surgeon, President Johnson directed Secretary of War Stanton to pursue the possibility or that of granting an award to a non-commissioned individual; a Washington newspaper reported that his desire to do so was an act of "carrying out the purpose of his predecessor, President Lincoln." Stanton assigned Judge Advocate General Joseph Holt the task of determining the legal issues of doing so. Holt had served as secretary of war prior to Stanton and was the presiding judge at the trial of Lincoln's assassins. His recommendation was conflicted but influential. He concluded there was no precedent for granting Mary a military commission but suggested a balance could be struck by a "commendatory acknowledgment" of her service. As he put it in his twelve-page recommendation, sent in October 1865 to Secretary of War Stanton, what had to be considered was "whether or not . . . her sex is to be deemed an *insuperable* obstacle to her receiving the official recognition." She was informed on November 2 that there was "no law or precedent which would authorize" such recognition.[43]

Holt's letter to Stanton also acknowledged the range of supporters who had come forward on Mary's behalf. Dr. E. H. Stockwell, one of her professors at Syracuse Medical College who now practiced in Cincinnati, Dr. Edward E. Phelps, with whom she had worked in Louisville, and her associate in the capital's wartime hospitals Dr. J. M. MacKenzie wrote on her behalf, attesting to her professional qualifications and her patriotism. Her entire military record was scrutinized; Dr. Green's 1861 letter signifying her "intelligent and judicious" professional work was included, as were military orders from Generals Burnside and Thomas assigning her to medical service in battlefield hospitals. Thomas's 1864 recommendation that she be commissioned as a major was cited. New York political leaders, including Governor Reuben E. Fenton and several state agents who had recommended her for military and government appointment, were also acknowledged. As Holt observed, however, the most extensive support came from Dr. Phelps, who wrote to Senator J. Collamer of Vermont about Mary's qualifications; Collamer

SURGEON, SPY, PRISONER OF WAR

forwarded the laudatory recommendation to Stanton, adding that Phelps' comments "are confirmed by Gens. Sherman & Thomas and by Dr. Wood, Asst. Surg. Gen." Recognizing that the services Mary had rendered were "novel in character," Collamer argued favorably for the award on her behalf.[44]

In spite of the extraordinary number of attestations as to Mary's medical skills from physicians she worked with in the various military hospitals, Holt—who insisted on referring to her as "Miss Walker"—chose to rely on the comments of the Medical Board in Chattanooga which had pronounced her "utterly unqualified." So, too, did Dr. Cooper attempt to block recognition of Mary's service. President Johnson, however, insisted that a determination be made as to any act that would allow him to award her an honorary brevet. This was the common gesture granted military officers for exceptional service, and while it carried no monetary award, it was a promotion in rank that was highly valued within the military and by the general public. Holt wanted no precedent to be set by awarding Mary a brevet, though he acknowledged the level of her service as exceptional in his letter to Stanton:

> It may also be added, that inasmuch as this is—as it is understood—the only instance of an application of this description, it need not be apprehended that—if it be granted—it will be drawn into an inconvenient precedent, or that the Government will again be called upon to testify its appreciation of a case of similar character and merit. Indeed the case of this lady—when her sacrifices, her fearless energy under circumstances of peril, her endurance of hardship and imprisonment at the hands of the enemy and especially her active patriotism and eminent loyalty, are considered—may well be regarded as an almost isolated one in the history of the rebellion; and to signalize and perpetuate it as such would seem to be desirable.

While Holt recommended no formal commission be granted to Mary, he also gave Stanton the leeway to find an alternative means of recognition.[45]

President Johnson persisted. In 1862, the U.S. Congress passed an act permitting a Medal of Honor to be awarded to Union soldiers for special meritorious services, with the president of the United States granted sole discretion as to who should receive such a medal. A congressional act of March 1863 limited the recipients to those who had shown "unusual gallantry in action;" it was the 1863 act that Johnson drew on to recognize Mary's contributions to the war effort.[46]

At some point Mary was given a small gold badge, shaped like a shield, purportedly from a company of Illinois volunteers. It was inscribed, "Mary E. Walker, M.D., Extra Assistant Surgeon, Army of the Potomac, War of 1861," and she wore it proudly. But nothing could equal the honor bestowed upon her on November 11, 1865. On that day, President Andrew Johnson issued the presidential order for the Congressional Medal of Honor to be awarded to Dr. Mary Walker. Commending her "valuable service to the Government," Johnson noted that she "has devoted herself with such patriotic zeal to the sick and wounded soldiers, both in the field and hospitals, to the detriment of her own health, and has also endured hardships as a prisoner of war four months in a Southern prison while acting as a Contract-Surgeon." The Medal immediately became her most prized possession, and she proudly wore it every day for the remainder of her life.[47]

Receiving the decoration made Dr. Mary Walker the most highly honored woman of the Civil War, and the only woman ever to receive the Medal of Honor.

CHAPTER 5

Interlude

At age thirty-three, Mary began her postwar years with energy and enthusiasm but without a clear sense of how to reshape her life. As with most Americans after the war, it seemed impossible to return to the antebellum way of life. Even among women's rights activists who wanted to return to their goals, daily routines were disrupted in ways that could not easily be reestablished. For a woman like Mary who had worked on the battlefield and earned national fame and a Medal of Honor, a return to routine after these unique experiences was nearly impossible. Her first step was to reestablish a medical practice in Washington. Little had changed in terms of attitudes toward women physicians among the general public, and a woman who wore the reform dress and was becoming increasingly outspoken on national issues faced an even greater challenge for acceptance. One means of supplementing her medical income to which she enthusiastically returned was lecturing, working tirelessly in the early months of 1866 for several causes. At the forefront of her endeavors was aiding soldiers who faced a complex bureaucracy in their quest to receive war-related pensions. Letters poured in from veterans. Her years of seeking a commission in the army had given her invaluable skills in negotiating the military structure, and she used those skills to benefit veterans.[1]

Attempting to adjust to their new lives, many veterans wrote to Mary expressing a need to relive moments from the war or to stay connected to a person who knew what horrors had been experienced. Others simply wanted to have contact with the now famous woman physician. One of the most poignant letters came from G. Richmond, who, as Mary noted, was "a very young soldier that was in the rebel army & temporarily confined in *Castle Thunder*." His letter was infused with the need for contact with someone who had experience as a prisoner of war. "I can never forget," he wrote, "how they tried to get you into that Insurection Scrape and what interest I took in you when I first heard of it." Richmond had been incarcerated on the floor below Mary when a ruckus began; one bullet pierced the floor in her room and hit the floor of his room near where he was seated. Repeatedly, he asked her to recall what they had experienced. "[D]o you remember the interest you took in me when I was called down one time and you thought I would be released? and do you remember how I found means to see you once more after I was released? I never forgot any one or any thing."[2]

Many returning soldiers needed to know that someone remembered them and their efforts in such unusual times. "Capt. and Citizen Brockway," as C. B. Brockway of Bloomsburg, Pennsylvania, signed his letter to Mary, exemplified the process of transition from soldier to citizen. He reminisced about the war, the many friends who were "now beneath the sod," and how odd it was to think that he "once wore a sabre." He enclosed a picture of himself so Mary would always remember him and concluded, "The press, had no other reason occurred, would have prevented me from forgetting you. It is with a mixture of curiosity and wonder that I watch your career and wonder where it will end." The enclosure of his carte de visite also suggested the new way in which the popular portraits were being used after the war—to visualize the memory of their extraordinary times together.[3]

People in positions of influence also sought Mary out, including Frank Fuller, vice president of the Northern Pacific Railroad. Fuller wrote to their mutual acquaintance, Jerome Tarbox, insisting that his motive was not "mere curiosity, or a desire to make the acquaintance of a distinguished lady, whom all must delight to honor alike for her loyalty to the cause of her country, her devotion to science and her boldness in striking out a new pathway to honorable distinction for her sex." As Fuller indicated to Lucretia Mott and Anna Dickinson, he believed that "our multitude of ladies who have sought in the elevation of themselves the disenthrallment of their sex, by their own example, from the realm of babyhood and the stature of toys" should settle in New York. He asked to be introduced to Mary because he felt that she "could secure for herself position and wealth, here, in the great city of New York, in the practice of her chosen profession." If he could meet with her, he wrote Tarbox, he was sure he could convince her of the benefits of the move; he assumed that "she has friends who would aid her to successfully establish herself. If she has not, I am sure she would not be without them long." The idea of moving to New York was already a part of Mary's plans, brought about by her ongoing struggles to obtain a divorce.[4]

Through the war years and her many moves from one battlefield to another, Mary never lost sight of the fact that she had to wait five years, until September 1866, to finalize her divorce from Albert. She was stunned, therefore, when she discovered in late 1865 that while she was serving as an army physician, Albert had been granted a rehearing and won a divorce from her, negating her earlier filing. In effect, his action blocked the finalization of their divorce by having the five-year waiting period begin again from the later date, as he claimed she was out of state during the war and thus those years should not count toward the five-year rule. Whatever Albert's motives, Mary was outraged at his action. To have Albert divorce her would forever tarnish her reputation, even though he was the adulterer. She was now forced to make the situation public by filing an act for relief with the New

York State Assembly. On March 15, 1866, Assemblyman Luther I. Burditt introduced "An Act for the relief of Mary E. Miller" before the assembly on her behalf, with a favorable recommendation from the state judiciary committee. It had taken nearly three months of discussions with individual senators for Mary to bring this act to fruition. A woman's character, especially that of an unconventional woman like Dr. Mary Walker, could always be brought into question in such proceedings, so Lyman J. Worden, who had boarded with Mary and Albert in 1856, wrote a letter in support of her claim. He testified, "Dr. Walker always treated Dr. Miller in the most affectionate manner, and took more pains to please him, & assist him, than I have witnessed in wives who had been married as long as she had been." Worden testified that Mary "appeared to have the *entire charge* of the directing of the housekeeping, besides attending to as much professional business as [Albert] did," and he emphasized that Mary was both "a noble, self reliant, business woman, and also an affectionate wife." Her virtue was unquestionable, he attested, "but in speaking of her being called out nights, on professional business; I have heard it remarked that 'if Dr. Walker was insulted, there was no doubt she would use a revolver in her defense.'" A woman physician who made night calls was often seen as inviting assault, and that fear had been used in arguments against allowing women to enter the profession; the depiction of Mary defending her virtue was thus a necessary precaution against the standard arguments about a woman physician's character. Worden also testified that Dr. Miller had long accepted his wife's choice of a reform dress. Perhaps most damning was Worden's observation of Albert's "*mean* manner" immediately after Mary had ordered him out of the house. When Worden entered their home, he learned from Mary that Albert had suggested they remain married and Mary could have the same "privileges" of sexual relations outside marriage. Worden recounted Mary's response: "She said she would never live with a man that was so *vile* as to make such a proposition, to a *wife*, and that people who thought her *so happy* knew little of her *wretchedness*."5

Mary wrote to her parents shortly after the bill was introduced in the senate. She felt that it was proceeding favorably and that she would be able to visit them in Oswego soon. Meanwhile, she directed her parents to forward mail to her in New York. She adamantly charged her family not to respond in any way to Albert: "I wish you would tell Leyman that if that *villan* [sic] writes to him again or *anyone under any pretense whatever*, to forward any such letter to me and not answer, *under any circumstances*. Should he, the vile Miller, ever come around anywhere, don't let him in the house." Her outrage against Albert compelled her to make the situation public through the filing for relief, but it also served as impetus to fight for her independence and her reputation. As the act wended its way through the senate, a Utica newspaper exposed the situation to broader public scrutiny, as Mary had feared would happen. The reporter believed her claim of having obtained a divorce from her husband in 1861, yet he chastised her for seeking special legislation to fight Albert's actions as it "would soon make our divorce laws of no effect in guarding the sanctity of the marital relations." It was precisely the enactment of a precedent for other women that interested Mary, however, as well as the necessity of her own case. The one moment of reprieve in these months came in January when she returned to Washington to attend a congressional ceremony commemorating her receipt of the Medal of Honor; but it would be three more years before she achieved her divorce.[6]

As she gained confidence in negotiating with legislative bodies and built on her experience with government bureaucracy, she turned to another battle that would be an even longer siege before she would gain justice. On May 29, she filed her first appeal to the U.S. Congress in relation to her own pension, based on the damage to her eyesight while imprisoned. That the government no longer had an interest in recognizing her service was part of a larger policy of denying rights to women. Being in New York in May 1866 was an opportune moment for Mary; it allowed her to renew her acquaintance with many of the leaders of the suffrage movement as they organized for new and more complex combat over the right to vote. Much to their surprise, they would have to argue as well that women were citizens of the United States. Having largely set aside their cause during the war in order to support abolition and the Republican Party, suffragists now expected reciprocation in the form of legislation granting the vote to women. Instead, the Fourteenth Amendment, largely drafted by Republicans, conferred citizenship on every *male* born or naturalized in the United States. Intended to grant citizenship and the right to vote to African American men, the gendering of citizenship in the amendment and the refusal to grant women the right to vote was a double betrayal of the suffragists. When Elizabeth Cady Stanton sought support from her old abolitionist friend Wendell Phillips, she was stunned by his reply. It would be unwise at present to "mix the movements," he insisted, because "such mixture would lose for the Negro far more than we should gain for the woman." Stanton's response, like that of many suffragists, was to lash out against black male suffrage. Such responses would tear apart the suffrage movement and delay the goal of suffragists for years. Many reformers agreed with the idea that it was "the Negro's hour"; a smaller number, including Mary, argued that the alliance of rights for men and women of all races—universal suffrage—was the only plan that would work to insure democratic processes in America.[7]

As news spread of the intent of the legislators, Stanton scheduled the Eleventh National Women's Rights Convention for May 1866 in New York City, with the hope that they could change the minds of male abolitionists before the Fourteenth Amendment was ratified. Theodore Tilton, founder of the American Equal Rights Association, noted that the NWRA's convention was scheduled to coincide with the AERA's meeting and suggested to Stanton that the AERA could serve as a coalition group for those seeking the vote for black men and all women. Although Lucretia Mott became president of the AERA and Stanton first vice-president, they quickly learned they were mere figureheads. After the close of the May meetings, Wendell Phillips called for an executive committee meeting in Boston, excluding Mott and Stanton from the decision-making process. At his encouragement, the committee voted to give preference to black male suffrage. It was an endorsement of the gendered Fourteenth Amendment.[8]

In the midst of Mary's personal battles and the collapse of suffragists' hopes, Dr. Lydia Strowbridge invited her to speak at the June National Dress Reform Association conference. Strowbridge told Mary she had followed her actions during the war; having helped to halt the tyranny of the South, she explained, "we much desire your aid in crushing the tyrenny [sic] of Fashion." It was impossible for Mary to make such a commitment while she was immersed in seeing that her divorce act would pass in the state legislature. Unfortunately, the NDRA did not survive the summer. The June convention drew nearly 800 attendees—and a significant number of hecklers—but longstanding tensions between Dr. Lydia Sayer Hasbrouck and Dr. James C. Jackson, the hydropathist and self-proclaimed "father" of the NDRA, emerged. Hasbrouck felt Jackson was monopolizing the discussion at the convention, as he asked to speak more than once and to run some of the policy sessions. That combined with heckling from a small but vocal group of young men made it the least successful of the NDRA's conventions. It might have been less disastrous for the organization had the local newspapers not picked up the dispute. Jackson lit the bonfire with rude public remarks about the mayor's failure to control the crowd, and Hasbrouck fanned the flames by joining seventeen other women in writing a letter to the newspapers criticizing Jackson's behavior at the convention. They made the gendered argument that, as Jackson did not wear a reform dress, he should not presume to understand the issue and that he represented the problem with men interloping into organizations that dealt with issues specific to women.[9]

While the impolitic scene helped bring about the demise of the organization, several other factors worked against its continuance as well. Most important was the fact that Hasbrouck was exhausted and distressed at having been unable to financially maintain *The Sibyl* during the war years. Further, one of the most active officers of the organization and a frequent contributor to *The Sibyl* was Dr. Harriet Austin, Jackson's daughter. These alliances put Austin in the middle of the debate, and her lessening work for the NDRA had an impact. The split in the leadership also affected Mary. In absentia, she had been elected president of the NDRA to replace Hasbrouck. In spite of the demise of the NDRA, Mary remained strongly committed to dress reform, and it continued to be a major focus of health-oriented physicians. Women continued to "live their principles," as Mary put it.[10]

Mary thrived in the active environment of New York City, but on June 5, 1866, a new form of attack on her lifestyle began. Coming out of a millinery store on Canal Street, she was arrested by Officer Patrick H. Pickett of the Eighth Precinct and charged with wearing men's clothing and disturbing the peace. Walking through the streets of the city, she was apt to create a sensation because of her clothing; boys shouted at her, passersby stopped to stare, and it was not unusual to have a small crowd gather around her. At the police station, however, the sergeant in charge immediately released her, insisting it was a trivial complaint that did not warrant arrest. On June 11, Mary was again arrested because of her attire, this time by an Officer Johnson. The arrest received citywide coverage; some of the reports took the usual jabs at her for her clothing, but none supported the arrest. Periodicals that advocated dress reform, such as the Oneida Community's *Circular*, covered the event in detail as well as subsequent charges brought by Mary. The Oneida Community had been an early proponent of reform clothing for women as more practical for the labor necessary to a farming environment; their periodical praised "The Dress Revolution" and referred to Mary's clothing as "sensible" and attractive. They set the stage for their support by reminding the public of her "long service as Assistant Surgeon in our armies during the war, and whose subsequent capture and imprisonment in a rebel prison won for her the deep sympathy of the public." A new ally emerged at this juncture as well: the *New York World* thoroughly covered the story in a balanced manner.[11]

Officer Johnson took Mary to the Essex Market Police Court, charging her with disorderly conduct and appearing in "male costume." The *Circular* described her outfit—"a broadcloth suit, composed of a tight-fitting waist, a short skirt, and loose pantaloons" and a jaunty straw hat "commonly worn in Broadway by ladies"—and insisted that it was little different than the commonly recognized Bloomer outfit. Judge Mansfield agreed with the policeman, however, and held Mary on bail of $300 and an order to keep the peace for one year. A *Circular* reporter insisted that the judge was attempting to force Mary to dress in compliance with his personal ideas about appropriate fashions for women and accused the arresting officer of preferring to wield his authority rather than disperse the "few rowdies" who were harassing Mary.[12]

It became a battle between Mary's version of events and that of the police officer, but it was also an issue of women's rights. Wearing a reform dress was not a criminal offense, only a matter of public opinion. The *Circular*, the *World*, and the *New York Times* all emphasized Mary's good character. The *Times* also noted that she had been "subjected to numerous insults" before being "locked up." Since she did not have enough money with her for the bail, she was "committed to prison in default," but her incarceration lasted only two or three hours until her attorney arrived to post bail. Immediately after news of her arrest circulated, letters from outraged readers began to appear in New York newspapers. One reader wrote to the *Evening Post*: "Last Sunday I attended a fashionable church and there saw that three-fourths of the ladies, in entering the pews, in consequence of their style of dress, made an exposure of their persons that would have made the French dancer blush." Long dresses mop up tobacco juice and all kinds of filth, he observed, and yet are considered the form of propriety. "Why," he asked, "was Mrs. Dr. Walker arrested? Her dress avoided either of these extremes. The Police Commissioners, I trust, will exercise their usual character of fairness by ordering the arrest of any lady whose dress is more objectionable than that worn by Mrs. Dr. Walker." As public opinion swelled, Judge Mansfield reconsidered and within days cancelled the bond. After being released, Mary filed a complaint of improper conduct against Officer Pickett for the first arrest, and a hearing was scheduled for a week later before the police commissioners. Her insistence on forcing the issue was both to argue for the right of choice in women's clothing and to ward off any further arrests. The charge was brought against Pickett and not Johnson because the latter had forthrightly told her why he was arresting her, while the former had duped her, as she revealed at the hearing.[13]

Police Commissioners Acton, Bergen, and Manierre presided at the hearing, held in the Metropolitan Police Court before a large audience. Mary began by testifying that she had long worn this style of clothing and that many female medical students had adopted similar styles. Fashionable female clothing was subject to attracting filth from the streets, she explained, and if a woman wanted to walk to the top of Bunker Hill monument or the Capitol, she could not do so with decency as the wind would blow a hoop skirt so high that the woman's lower body was exposed. The places named for walking were not coincidental, of course, as Mary intended to make this an issue about women's rights through reference to the nation's capital and her own accomplishments at Bunker Hill where she had begun her medical service during the war. She emphasized that she had been coming to the city for several years, always attired in a reform dress, and had been treated with respect and courtesy by the police. "I wish it understood," she declared, "that I wear this style of dress from the purest and the noblest principles and I believe that if there is anything a woman receives from Heaven, it is the right to protect herself morally and with the present style of dress there are circumstances where she cannot do it." She then added her indictment of Officers Pickett and Johnson, asserting, "This country is not so filled with morality that any woman who tries to live a high and noble life should be compelled by a couple of policemen to put on the long dress and live just as they say she should live." Nor did Mary hesitate to recall her associations with the famous: "I was graduated in 1855; have been in the civil and military service; have been treated with consideration by President Lincoln, Chief Justice Chase, and other respectable men, while clothed in this style of dress." Charles S. Spencer, the officer's attorney, interrupted to insist that an oration from Mary was not wanted, but Acton overruled the objection and allowed her to continue. She explained the dangers of current fashionable clothing for women, after which she turned her attention to the specific events leading to her arrest.[14]

Testifying that Pickett asked to see her Medal of Honor and then asked her to go with him, Mary insisted he never indicated an intention to arrest her. The sergeant at the police station further insulted her by asking if she could read and write, to which she sarcastically replied that she did not know a single letter of the alphabet. Only a small crowd gathered, she insisted, and they were in the street initially to observe a balloon ascension, not her. The gathering of spectators created no difficulty for her to leave until she was "annoyed" by a man who wanted to arrest her. She was escorted away from the situation by another policeman and asked to wait in the nearby *New York Times'* offices. Pickett, however, insisted that two hundred people gathered to gawk at Mary and that she resisted arrest. He also claimed that she declared if he arrested her "she would have him broken." While it is hard to imagine the officer truly felt threatened by this petite woman, the comments are not unlike those Mary made in other instances when her fury got the better of her. Although Acton declared early in the proceedings that the hearing had nothing to do with her mode of dress and would focus on the actions of the complainant and the police officer, Spencer insisted on making her clothing the issue. It was a dangerous mistake, he insisted, to assert that a woman could wear any clothing she chose.[15]

Elizabeth Miller, the proprietor of the millinery, and Mary E. Donnelly, the sales clerk who attended Mary, were also called to testify. They supported Mary's assertion that the crowd was not violent and that it was the police officer who twice tried to burst through the door of the shop, inciting the crowd. By then it was nearly six o'clock at night, and Miller asked Mary to remain in the shop. Although Mary insisted she would be fine on her own, Miller asked an officer to escort Mary home. When asked where she lived, Mary replied, "Any place where the Stars and Stripes fly!" The hearing allowed for Mary's wit to come into full play. In one instance, she described her attempt to leave rather than accompany the arresting officer: "While the officer fumbled in his pockets I showed my *Walker* powers and ran down stairs into the counting room, and told them of my adventure." Much laughter supported her witticisms throughout the hearings.[16]

The testimony of Pickett's partner, William B. Moseman, substantiated Mary's account and certainly helped in the verdict. In closing arguments, the defendant's attorney insisted that public peace must be the highest priority and the officer was justified in arresting the complainant if it helped him to disperse the crowd. When Commissioner Acton rendered the committee's decision, he declared that the officer was doing his duty but acknowledged that Mary had a right to wear the reform dress. He cautioned, "If you were creating a disturbance and there was a mob there, he would be justified in removing you." Mary interjected: "Why didn't he let me go my own way? . . . There was a street-car I could have stepped into." Acton refused to be engaged in a debate and turned to Officer Pickett, declaring, "Don't arrest her again, officer. Let her go. She's smart enough to take care of herself." The reprimand to each party concluded the proceedings. The newspaper responses to the commissioners' decision reflected their stance on dress reform and women's rights. The *Nation* criticized the outcome while the *New York Tribune* argued that Mary had the right to wear the dress and should not be harassed for doing so, and the *Circular* insisted it was a vindication of women's right to wear the reform dress. Mary apparently felt the same, as she returned to her usual business without further action. These arrests were only the beginning of a long series of confrontations

INTERLUDE   83

she would have with the New York police over her right to walk about the city in reform clothing.¹⁷

As the summer of 1866 drew to a close, suffragists were planning a number of approaches to insure that the Fourteenth Amendment included women as well as black men. One of the major arguments that began to develop at this time—that in spite of the projected wording of the amendment, the Constitution did not prohibit women from holding office—would evolve in the early 1870s into an argument for women's citizenship *and suffrage* as a constitutional right. Mary supported every endeavor of organized suffrage groups. In August, Elizabeth Cady Stanton changed the scope of the suffrage movement when she nominated herself as an independent candidate for the U.S. House of Representatives from the Eighth District of New York City. Although she was soundly defeated, receiving only twenty-four votes, it was a clarion call that suffragists were not going to accept the suppression of their rights.¹⁸

A new opportunity in Mary's life was about to take her away from the States just as the battles among suffragists split the movement into several separate organizations that were often as much in conflict with one another as with their suffrage opponents. It was, in some ways, a fortuitous moment to be away from the fray. Stanton and Anthony had held the reins of leadership since the 1850s, and they repeatedly abandoned any group that challenged their authority, in a combination of personal and group power building. In 1853, for example, when Mary Vaughan opposed Stanton and Anthony for leadership of the Woman's New York State Temperance Society and Vaughan was elected president, the two women withdrew from the society. In the 1860s, Stanton and Anthony often jockeyed between themselves for dominance. Mary was equally strong in her desire to be a leader, and she would not withdraw from a cause just because she differed with the opinions of the leaders. All three were strong-willed women who had each gained success in her endeavors, and for now they were an extraordinary force for suffrage. But the summer of 1866 was the last time for a year that Mary would set foot on American soil, and she was about to gain international fame on her own.¹⁹

CHAPTER 6

Touring Britain

THE CREATION OF A PUBLIC SELF

In August 1866, Mary received an invitation to attend the Social Science Congress to be held in October in Manchester, England. The trip would give her an opportunity to see the United Kingdom and visit its hospitals, although the cost would be exorbitant. To defray costs, she applied for a position as a ship's surgeon; when that failed, friends pitched in, including D. H. Craig, an Associated Press reporter who supported her desire to visit British hospitals. Leaving a few weeks before the conference, Mary joined Dr. Susannah Way Dodds and her Scottish husband Andrew on board the *Caledonia*. Dodds was a hydropathic physician from St. Louis who believed clothing reform was necessary to the success of suffrage because, through the process of choosing healthful clothing, a woman became "self-reliant, independent, and [able to] determine for herself her political privileges and social status." In Susannah, Mary had a kindred spirit.[1]

It was a rough sea, and Mary's discomfort was exacerbated by being in close quarters with so many smokers. As she wrote her family while onboard ship, "I have been sick enough to feel as disagreeable as possible" and wished all tobacco would be dumped in the Atlantic—a sentiment she apparently expressed often to her fellow passengers. When the ship landed at Liverpool, Mary set out on a boat excursion along the western coast of Scotland to visit several hospitals before the congress convened. Dr. Forsyth, superintendent of the Royal Infirmary of Glasgow, responded warmly to her request to visit the facility and sent a schedule of operations with the invitation to attend any she chose.[2]

From Glasgow she traveled to Manchester for the opening of the Social Science Congress on October 3. Ashley Cooper, Earl of Shaftesbury, presided over the congress; the general theme was "Legislation on Social Subjects." One of the first sessions in which Mary participated was on "The Repression of Crime." In reaction to increases in crime rates, controversial penal servitude acts had been passed in England in 1856 and 1864, and the issue resonated throughout the week-long gathering. After formal presentations, Mary joined Sir Thomas Chambers, M.P.,

Lord Robert Montague, and Sir Eardley Wilmot in discussing the topic of life sentences. She had already formulated strong opinions on capital punishment and argued that the practice was barbaric, un-Christian, and allowed for no recourse if an error was made. As an alternative, she advocated laws to suppress crime and asserted that in capital cases the defendant should be the subject of a physician's consideration as well as of the court's.[3]

Another "Repression of Crime" session focused on the subject of infanticide and was led by Dr. Edwin Lankester, Central Middlesex coroner, who was tracking an increase in infanticide cases in his district. It was an issue of great concern to Mary; she had written on the subject for *The Sibyl* in 1859 when she sought to establish a foundling hospital. She joined the Manchester discussion by arguing that the lack of sympathy from other females led some unwed pregnant women to believe infanticide was their only recourse, an argument that was greeted with applause. Mary's own lecture, "Crinoline," at a session on "Destruction of Life by Overwork," focused on damage to a woman's body from carrying pounds of excess fashionable clothing and was well received as well.[4]

British feminist Barbara Smith Bodichon wrote one of the notable speeches read on the evening of October 8 at a section on suffrage. The woman's suffrage movement was in its embryonic stage in England, and in "Reasons for the Enfranchisement of Women," Bodichon suggested a limited vote for women freeholders and householders. While Mary appreciated the attention to suffrage, she believed its import was diminished because the speech was read by a man. As the session drew to a close, the chairman observed that they had "a distinguished foreigner" in their midst and hoped that her modesty would not prevent her from saying a few words. Mary was an experienced lecturer and believed "modesty" that required woman's silence was only a "sham modesty"; she did not hesitate to speak. With a female monarch, Great Britain should lead the world in granting all women equality, she proclaimed; at present, however, both England and the United States "were most illiberal in their treatment of women." She concluded with a prediction that women would have the franchise in ten years. It was a typical suffrage argument, the kind she had given on many occasions, and although there were some hisses from the audience, many people swarmed around her as she left the stage. On and on the questions came, and with wit and flair, she charmed her audience.[5]

A woman physician was still a unique phenomenon in England. Elizabeth Garrett, Britain's first and only licensed female physician, opened an apothecary for women and children in London only two months before Mary arrived. Tensions about the subject of women physicians were still high, and Mary's success at the congress renewed heated debates on the subject. The *London Globe* concluded that women had been the most notable of the congress's eighteen hundred participants and that Dr. Mary Walker had been "prima donna assoluta"; the elitist and fashion-oriented *Court Journal* surprisingly concurred. While newspapers in the States largely ignored the event, Europe took notice. The *French Economist*, for instance, reported that Mary spoke "clearly and logically on the opportunities for women doctors in civil and military philanthropies." People who were present for the speech wanted further contact with her, and those who did not attend wanted to meet her. Her success led Sheldon Amos of Manchester's Social Science Association, apparently the person who had first invited her to the meeting, to request she participate in a series of soirèes at his chambers in the Temple on Tuesday evenings throughout November and December. The soirèes were "attended by some of the best specimens of the younger members of the legal profession" and entailed "really good conversation on all kinds of topics"; many of the congress's participants, Amos noted, regularly attended. Not only did the Tuesday evenings gratify Mary's love of stimulating conversations, they introduced her to some of the most influential progressive thinkers in England.[6]

One group particularly insistent on a meeting with Mary consisted of "titled and literary women" who wanted to discuss methods for helping British women secure the vote. Although she did not identify this group by name, two possibilities emerge. It was in October 1866 that the Manchester National Society for Woman's Suffrage was founded, and it is possible that they invited Mary to meet with them. More likely it was the Kensington Society, as she had met Dr. Elizabeth Garrett at the Social Science Congress. The society included Garrett, Barbara Bodichon, Emily Davies, and other activists. At the congress, Mary encouraged women to go to the polls and vote, and she was delighted at the rapid progress British suffragists were making in Parliament.[7]

Other Britons sought her acquaintance as well. Some, such as Sarah Cooke, were admirers of her dress reform activities, while others were internationally recognized figures. The American minister Moncure Conway, who read her "excellent address at the S. S. Congress," called on her in London in early November; they discussed their mutual interest in "woman, marriage, dress, and . . . negro equality." Both were supporters of abolition and other reforms that gave them a common basis of interest, though Conway's attachment to his native Virginia left him much more conflicted about the war than Mary had been—indeed, she felt there was only one right position on the war—but they had lively discussions, and they would meet again at the Paris Exposition the following year. George Dornbusch also sought her acquaintance, recognizing in her ideas an alliance with Dr. Trall's school of thought and tagging her as "a sister Vegetarian." Dornbusch had helped organize interest in vegetarianism in London in the 1850s, and Mary became well acquainted with his family over the next few weeks. A particularly pleasing acquaintance she made at Manchester was with Charles and Selena Bracebridge, who were instrumental in introducing her to Florence Nightingale. She and the Bracebridges exchanged a number of letters over the next several months as Mary traveled the country, and they became close friends.[8]

Several British physicians also invited her to visit their facilities and attend operations. In late October, Dr. Holmes Coate, senior surgeon at St. Bartholomew's Hospital, escorted her on a tour of London's Bethlem Hospital for the Insane. Other physicians welcomed her as well. After their initial meeting, Dr.

Waymouth of Middlesex Hospital in London (ironically, the institution that had banned Elizabeth Garrett), sent her a list of operations scheduled for October 31 and invited her to attend, "should Dr Mary be inclined to favour the Hospital with another visit." Mary accepted, startling the all-male student body as they viewed a woman clad in a reform dress escorted through the hospital halls. Waymouth's use of "Dr Mary" suggested the congenial relationship that had developed between the two physicians, but it was also the title by which she would soon be known on an international basis. For the next five decades, her celebrity would be so widespread that newspaper headlines simply referred to her as "Dr Mary."[9]

Other medical men who met with Mary included psychiatrist Dr. Forbes Winslow and several physicians who were active in the Female Medical Society. Winslow was the leading British authority on mental disorders, who would gain even greater fame years later when he became involved in the Jack the Ripper case. His interest in criminal psychology touched a chord with Mary's growing interest in the subject. She also became friends with Dr. Lankester's family and visited the doctor and his wife Gay at their home several times while in the country. During the winter, Mary sought information about having her name added to the British Medical Registry. Dr. Elizabeth Blackwell had done so in 1859 when she visited England, but following Blackwell's admission to the Registry, the General Medical Council enacted rules that allowed them to exclude physicians with foreign medical degrees, at their discretion, which meant no other women were admitted. Mary seems not to have pursued the issue beyond an initial inquiry.[10]

Mary's new friends encouraged her to give a formal lecture while in England, believing her extraordinary life story would attract a large crowd and would help support women's rights and admittance to British medical colleges. St. James Hall in Plymouth opened its doors on November 12, 1866. The hall held three thousand seats, quickly making it a coveted stage for lecturers and performers. Mary was booked for the evening of November 20 for a lecture titled "The Experiences of a Female Physician in College, in Private Practice, and in the Federal Army." The lecture was widely advertised in newspapers and through handbills. It was novel to have a woman physician speaking to the public in England, and one who wore the reform dress was doubly notable. Amelia Bloomer attempted to introduce her reform outfit in England in the early 1850s and was so severely ridiculed that she returned to the States. No one could be sure how Mary would be received; but there was standing room only on the evening of the 20th. The audience included several renowned medical men, a large number of reformers, and an even larger array of people who came out of curiosity. A group of medical students were seated in the galleries, with the intent of disrupting the speech. A year earlier their fellow students had succeeded in banning Elizabeth Garrett from medical lectures, and raucous behavior broke out in the galleries even before Mary appeared on stage.[11]

As the slender figure in a reform outfit stepped onto the stage, a hush fell throughout the hall. She began the most important lecture of her career to date, detailing her youthful interest in medicine, her struggles in medical school, and her early years of practice. She emphasized the importance of dress reform throughout her comments, linking it to health issues but also to an individual's right to live life in her own way. She received sustained applause when she recalled that her first goal as a physician had been to aid the sufferings of the British troops in the Crimea; but when she observed that some Americans told her she should have married a doctor rather than become one, the medical students saw their opportunity and shouts of "Hear! Hear!" followed. Mary stood quietly at the podium until the students' shouts subsided, then commented that some patients thought they should pay less for a woman doctor, but she had a ready reply: "My education has cost me as much as that of my learned brothers has cost them. I have had far greater difficulties to overcome, and if any difference is to be made, it ought to be in favour of the female physician. However . . . I am ready to accept a scale of remuneration equal to that of men." This brought a thorough round of applause. As she continued, the medical students periodically interrupted with outbursts and mocking laughter. At one point she sat down and waited for them to cease. Her audience was not fully receptive to her inclusion throughout the lecture of arguments for dress reform, but when she turned to her unique experiences on the battlefield, she held their full attention. At the end of the lecture, she was rewarded with considerable applause and even some cheers.[12]

Newspapers of all political suasions condemned the actions of the medical students for shaming Britain through their childish pranks and undemocratic attempts to silence Mary. After days of criticism from the public, some medical journals attempted to question whether the disruptions were actually led by medical students, but since the police had arrested one of them, the defensive argument was quickly defeated. In terms of the lecture itself, the newspapers responded with an extraordinary amount of coverage. How they reported on the evening's events depended on their attitudes about a radical woman reformer. The *Court Journal* and the *Medical Times and Gazette*, for instance, lamented Mary's usurpation of male prerogatives by becoming a physician and argued that it was "not womanly to saw off legs and arms, and to operate upon the tibia." Both papers concluded Mary's lecture was a failure. The *Medical Times*' opposition to women physicians also led them to argue that she demonstrated no medical knowledge and to speculate she was only a nurse during the war. Charles Dickens's *All the Year Round* expressed both dismay at a woman doctor and respect for her courage in stepping before the public. The three-page article admonished Mary for abandoning the "M.D." of "My Dear" for "My Doctor," for her "egotism and vanity," and for her "perversion of rare zeal and unflagging energy." But it was equally impossible, the magazine insisted, "to withhold one's admiration for the courage, the perseverance, the self-denial" necessary to achieve all she had. That Mary's appearance was seen as a threat to English class hierarchy was made evident a few months later in an article in *Fraser's Magazine* that addressed recent challenges to marriage laws. If Englishwomen rebelled against marriage, the author warned, a "martyr-spirited heroine . . . who will no more quail from male or female reproof, than Dr. Mary Walker or Dr. Elizabeth Blackwell," will emerge and Englishmen will "find women of the working classes by the hundred and the thousand following the example." Conservative periodicals such as the *Pall Mall Gazette* also denigrated her through sexualization: "The practical way to answer Doctrix Walker would be to make her deliver her lecture, in her peculiar costume, between Power's Greek Slave and the Venus de Medici"—that is, between nude figures.[13]

Newspapers supportive of women's right to speak publicly presented quite a different perspective on the lecture's success. The *Morning Star*, edited by radical activist Justin McCarthy, pronounced, "Dr. Mary E. Walker accomplished a feat last night in St. James's Hall. She cowed . . . as unruly a gallery full of stupid young gentlemen as ever disgraced themselves in a public assembly." Affording her lecture front-page coverage, the *Star* praised Britain's sense of fair play that finally triumphed. The newspaper observed Mary's sensible comments and her ability to dismantle the students' interruptions, and it asserted she received the applause of medical men who were not threatened by a woman physician. The *National Reformer* was even more laudatory in its praise of Mary's endeavor. The reporter, Peter Fox, noted the courage required to stand alone before the barrage of the medical students. Five minutes into her talk, she had charmed her audience with her "intrepid integrity . . . lofty morality . . . her melodious voice, her native spontaneous grace," Fox declared. "It was the Una of Milton's 'Comus' triumphing over the 'rabble rout' which had come to insult and wound her." He noted that her tale of a dying soldier wanting to kiss her was not well received, but she easily recovered, and her "crystalline spirit" and individualism should be praised as highly as that of Ralph Waldo Emerson. When the *Medical Times* report appeared, the *National Reformer* responded with a front-page rebuttal, calling the assertion that Mary's lecture was a failure nothing more than "Arrant bosh!"[14]

The widespread reviews opened the floodgates to lecture bookings for Mary throughout the United Kingdom. Although she was scheduled to return to the States at the end of November, these new possibilities for lecturing expanded what was to have been a six-week visit into a year-long lecture tour. Advocates for numerous causes wanted her to speak at fundraisers, and she developed what would be her most popular and yet at times most controversial lecture, "Dr. Mary E. Walker, Her Capture by the Confederates, and Four Months' Detention as a Prisoner of War." Her encounter with the ruthless Champ Ferguson played a dramatic part in the lecture, as Mary honed her story to attract a broad audience. In these months, she became a skilled lecturer, a businesswoman who knew the ins and outs of booking halls and negotiating fees, and a keen self-promoter.[15]

She was confronted by every kind of promoter, too: genuinely committed reformers, hangers-on, and self-promoters who wanted to gain recognition through association with her. Other admirers sought her out to offer genuine advice. P. F. André, for example, wrote Mary the morning after her lecture with suggestions of how she could improve her presentation. A reporter for the *Commonwealth* and the *National Reformer,* André asserted that the way to repay her "peerless ingenuousness" was to offer her advice. Drop the comments about kissing a dying soldier, he insisted; it suggested naïveté. Spend less time on the "*politics* of the Republican Party and the War. People did not come to hear a political lecture." And especially do not mention that she tore up her "*night shirt*" to use as bandages; virtue demanded that such topics be used solely for a female-only audience. Mary closely studied his suggestions, as they echoed some newspapers' criticism, and some of her subsequent lectures on dress reform were advertised as "For Ladies Only." The kissing episode revealed national differences. It gained such a life of its own in public and private conversations about Mary's lecture that her friends felt compelled to respond in print. One friend sent a copy of Mary's private letter of explanation to the *Pall Mall Gazette,* with a note insisting that, had Mary not been interrupted by the pranksters in the gallery, the story would have been well received. Mary's own explanation read:

> One day while passing through the Washington hospitals, looking for a soldier whose friends at home had requested me to see personally and report his true condition, the low typhous moaning of a young soldier attracted my attention, and, kneeling by his cot, I watched the sufferer a moment. He opened his sunken eyes, and in a pleading tone said, "Let me kiss you—twice, *only* twice!" His eyes looked glazed, his emaciated face had a yellow hue, his lips were parched and full of blisters; and as I hesitated a moment to summon courage to grant so disagreeable a request, a young man, about his own age, told me "he was from the same place, that he was a nice young man, that his only sister had gone as a missionary to Europe just before he enlisted, and he had had no sleep for twenty-four hours. Let him kiss you! His hours on earth are numbered, and he cannot see distinctly; he thinks [you are] his sister; it will comfort him in his last moments, dying away from home, in the glorious cause of *liberty*!" I held my cheek to his lips; he kissed "twice," and while I bathed his face he sank into a quiet slumber and died the next morning.

The image of a woman substituting for a dying soldier's loved one filled the pages of American newspapers and short fiction in these years, but the British audience felt no such attachment to the idea. Consequently, Mary honed the lecture and created others for specialized audiences interested in dress reform, temperance, and women physicians.[16]

Especially important to Mary were the many requests from British reformers who sought support for their causes. Her commitment to the working classes was evidenced in her agreement to participate in a large meeting of the Trades' Demonstration in St. James Hall; she joined members of Parliament and delegates from several reform associations on the platform. But it was her views on women's rights and temperance that drew the greatest number of lecture offers. Dr. James

Edmunds, founder of the Female Medical Society (which trained midwives) and the London Temperance Hospital, sought her aid in promoting women's advancement in the medical profession. He also encouraged her to publish her opinions in the *Victoria Magazine* so her comments could reach a large number of English women. Through Edmunds, Mary met Rev. Charles W. Denison and his wife, Mary Palmer Denison, Americans living in London. Supporters of opening medical colleges to women, the Denisons recognized the ways in which Mary's increasing fame could benefit the cause, and the couple served as her hosts throughout her time in England.[17]

After the success of Mary's St. James lecture, the *London Anglo-American Times* printed the entire Medal of Honor citation, adding, "Her strange adventures, thrilling experiences, important services and marvelous achievements exceed anything that modern romance or fiction has produced. . . . She has been one of the greatest benefactors of her sex and of the human race." Bookings for her lectures soared. In January Dr. Edmunds invited Mary to "a very influential meeting" at which he introduced her to people who could support the society's efforts to establish a women's medical college in London. Yet the more successful she became, the more conservative periodicals vilified her. Part of Edmunds's plan was to help undermine the critics by placing Mary within a circle of influential men who would support her efforts and she theirs. Several women's and feminist periodicals also embraced Mary's efforts. The *Lady's Own Paper* began publication four days after her St. James lecture, and within weeks it gave her front-page coverage. Increasingly she received requests to lecture outside of London as well. The Committee for the Management of the Free Lectures at Fetter Lane Chapel developed a series of lectures designed for the working classes, and they booked her for three dates in early 1867. Negotiating dates became a time-consuming job. She scheduled most of the thirty lectures she gave in London, but she finally hired booking managers to schedule her dates outside the city. Several women, including Ann Cooper and her daughter Ellen, also worked through local organizations to assure their communities had an opportunity to hear Mary. Ann Cooper arranged one of Mary's lectures at the Palace, and Ellen arranged another at the Sydenham Lecture Hall.[18]

Life was not all work, however. Robert Hardwicke, a publisher of biology and medical texts, invited Mary to an evening of "friendly Gossip" in Piccadilly and requested her portrait to add to his significant collection of medical practitioners' portraits. Friends such as Gay Lankester, a Miss Cox, and John Plummer also invited her to attend dances and soirees in their homes. Mary loved to dance, and she accepted such invitations whenever possible, though her schedule was becoming so hectic that she often had to decline. One letter that arrived in January 1867, however, raised a suggestion that greatly appealed to Mary and which she began to develop as a possibility. Edward M. Richards of Ireland, a friend of Dr. Dodds, wanted to come to London to meet Mary. He had followed her career since her days of writing for *The Sibyl* and through the war years. "I always had the greatest wish to be personally acquainted with you," he wrote, "& now since you have done what I supposed no woman could have accomplished viz worn the Reform Dress in London, I am still more desirous of seeing you." He suggested that she remain abroad long enough to attend the Paris Exposition. Dr. Trall was going to exhibit the reform dress at the Exposition, and it was a world stage that greatly appealed to Mary.[19]

In the interim, an event in the States brought her closer to finalizing her divorce. It was the responsibility of Mary and her attorney to prove that Albert had been unfaithful. On January 17, 1867, Nelson Whittlesey filed a report with the New York Supreme Court in the case of *Miller v. Miller*. The State of New York accepted only two forms of evidence of adultery—prostitutes' testimony, or "hotel evidence." The latter necessitated evidence that the accused had shared hotel rooms with a person other than his or her spouse. Whittlesey, who had been on the same lecture circuit as Albert, presented a compendium of hotel evidence against Albert. Even though Mary knew about several instances of Albert's infidelity in the late 1850s, the level of promiscuity revealed by Whittlesey was shocking. He filled three legal-sized pages with details of Albert's affairs. Since the state had a five-year waiting period, these events were considered part of his actions during his married life just as Mary's leaving the state to work for the war cause had been. The report revealed that since the spring of 1862 Albert had engaged in numerous affairs, often with more than one woman at a time. In the summer of 1862 he was arrested for the seduction of Maria Hardy of Marlborough, New Hampshire; Albert admitted to Whittlesey at the time that he had "criminal conduct" with the nineteen-year-old woman who was his patient and who gave birth to a child he fathered. Whittlesey paid more than $500 to settle the matter for Albert. In the fall of 1862, another young woman from Maine also confessed to authorities that Albert Miller was the father of her child. Between 1863 and the present, Whittlesey added, there were several other females with whom Albert was "criminally intimate." He had a longer affair with Delphine Freeman, beginning in late February 1865, and later that year Albert married Freeman. It was not unusual for individuals to remarry before the five-year waiting period was completed, as local record-keeping was imprecise at best and records were rarely exchanged across county lines. Yet Albert's second marriage occurred at the time he had written Mary's brother-in-law, supposedly wanting Mary to reconsider their separation. Although it would take another two years for Mary's divorce to be granted, this document more than assured the authorities that she had a legitimate claim. In that sense, it was a positive turn of events, although the contents of the document were painful reminders of betrayal.[20]

Persevering, Mary immersed herself in the issue of women's advancement in England and the United States. She gave a private lecture in London to several women in which she spoke about her experiences as a physician, gave several lectures for temperance societies, and was lured to the Peel Grove Institute with the assurance that "thousands of working men and their families" would attend. At the same time she was preparing for her second lecture at St. James's Hall. Although it was a benefit for the Bermondsey Poor Schools, medical students turned out in even greater numbers than at her first St. James lecture. As many as one hundred medical students were placed across several sections of the hall; they repeatedly interrupted her, even though the focus was on her imprisonment and not specifically about being a physician. The event became a touchstone of how advocates and opponents would react to her public life. The *British Medical Journal*, in spite of its opposition to women physicians, was appalled at the students' behavior. While it insisted on referring to Mary as "Miss" rather than "Doctor," it condemned the students; not only did they disgrace themselves, the *Journal* insisted, they also inflicted "a public humiliation on the body to which they belong." This time Mary drew attention from the American press as well. Surprisingly, positive comments came from the *National Police Gazette*, a tabloid-style, sensationalistic paper. It asserted the "doctress" was "a woman of grit, and is said to be talented and well-read, and skillful in the practice of the profession she has adopted." It was the mob mentality of the medical students that drew the *Gazette*'s attention, and it reported on the police court hearing many of the students faced as the result of a brawl outside St. James's Hall after the lecture.[21]

The *New York Medical Journal*, which opposed admitting women to the profession, published a scathing three-page attack on Mary for the lecture at St. James's Hall. The article was a collage of quotes from British periodicals, selectively ignoring any positive comments—her appearance, they insisted, "strengthens the opinions of those who hold that women had better not meddle with physic." Under the pretext of finding the British *Medical Press & Circular*'s comments uncouth, the New York journal allowed its extraordinarily salacious comments to conclude their article: "The *Medical Press & Circular*, with a bitterness and intensity of satire surpassed only by its coarseness, styles her the American Medical Nondescript, and suggests as an attractive subject for her public entertainments, 'Why Not? or, Clitoridectomy and Its Uses.'" The *New York Round Table* recognized, however, that male physicians' reactions were "the old story again of opposition to free competition in the labor market." The *Round Table* admired the fact that "Dr. Mary stood bravely to her table" through the medical students' interruption, and hoped in the battle the hecklers were waging against her "it will not be Dr. Mary who will tire first."[22]

In spite of these debates by men of the press, women's desire to consult a woman physician was demonstrated several times when women wrote to her, seeking medical consultations or to talk about the profession. Because Mary was not included in the British Medical Registry, she could not treat patients in England and had to decline such requests by referring the individuals to other physicians. Common and deeply poignant, too, were the many letters she received from women who had been unable to accomplish their dream of becoming a physician. Margaret Kirkwood of Edinburgh, for instance, wanted to practice medicine and wrote to thank Mary for "the open declaration you are giving us of the principles concerning your espousal of the noble profession to which you belong." Kirkwood acknowledged that Mary and other "sister-pioneers have to break down the obnoxious barriers which exist regarding the propriety of training our sex in this splendid field of labor."[23]

In March, while Mary was lecturing at several venues, the *New York Times* aligned her with another woman of the same name who was creating a scandalous reputation for herself. There were three other "Mary Walkers" who gained some level of fame in the nineteenth century, though none on the level of Dr. Mary Walker. Mary S. Walker was a fiction writer whose stories appeared in periodicals for a few years at mid-century and was rarely confused with the doctor. Late in the century, another Mary Walker became an active Spiritualist whom several famous people consulted. But it was the third woman of the same name who created the most complications for the doctor, and by reporting on her activities at the same time as Mary's March lecture at Fetter Lane Chapel, the *Times* implicated Mary's actions as equally improper. The lesser-known Mary Walker purportedly donned male attire, became a barkeeper, and "went to making love to the pretty girls who came after the family beer." She was arrested and incarcerated in 1867, at the height of the Mary's success in Britain, for stealing money from the bar's till. Attacking both women—and by implication questioning Mary's sexual preferences—the *Times* concluded by noting that a young woman who became engaged to the barkeeping Mary Walker "visited her in jail. They are not to be married at present, as woman's rights have not attained to that degree of development." With the *Medical Press & Circular*'s article and now the *Times*'s, Mary's sexuality became an open topic for inquiry and attack, at home and abroad.[24]

Yet the tide-swell of interest in her lectures continued in England into the spring. She was booked for multiple nights in halls that seated several thousand, and continued to offer her services to smaller groups as well. Her friendship with Justin McCarthy was also developing in these months. He and his wife, Charlotte, dined several times with Mary; the two women maintained a steady correspondence during Mary's stay in England, and the McCarthys enthusiastically attended her lectures. Mary recommended Charlotte read John Stuart Mill's *Liberty*, a popular text with women's rights advocates and one that Charlotte found to be "a glorious book." One evening Mary and the McCarthys were joined by Dr. John Chapman, editor of the *Westminster Review*. Several British intellectuals outside the medical profession also sought Mary's acquaintance, including Thomas Arnold, a historian at University College, and, surprisingly, the author Fanny Kortright. Arnold presented an academic paper on Walker, primarily biographical in focus but certainly the first in academia. Kortright became an ardent supporter of Mary's work in spite of the fact that she would soon oppose woman's suffrage.[25]

In late March Mary expanded her lecture circuit to include Edinburgh and Glasgow. She was enchanted by her acquaintances in Scotland, and these visits were long remembered as some of the most enjoyable experiences of her two-year stay in Great Britain. Her booking agent in Scotland, G. W. Muir, arranged more than twenty-five lectures for her over the next few weeks at Carlisle, Glasgow (several times), Edinburgh, Kilmarnock, Dundee, Greenock, Ayr, and Hamilton. By the first week in April, she felt increasingly exhausted, but some appeals she could not forgo, such as the lecture at Albion Hall, which could seat twelve hundred people, for the benefit of the Literary Institute at Barnet. During this time, Mary received a letter from J. Morgan of Regent Street, who had recently met her. He insisted she was "destined to attain a very high position in society. I feel that you will have ere long an introduction to Her Most Gracious Majesty, our poor Widowed queen." There is no public record that an introduction was made, though several people expected it to occur.[26]

Later in the month she had the honor of being invited, as "a great favor" to the sponsor, to participate in a large temperance convention in Finsburg Chapel. Dr. James Edmunds, the Hon. Neal Dow, and other respected personages were joined by Mary on stage. At the same time, however, Mary came under attack by two influential conservative periodicals, the *Spectator* and the *Queen*. The *Spectator* published a letter signed only "Medical Student" that questioned Mary's professional skills, and the *Queen* used the letter as "conclusive evidence" of her lack of medical competency. The *Queen* specialized in domesticity and fashion, especially patterns of Paris fashions which it encouraged British women to emulate. It opposed woman's suffrage and advances in women's education that it claimed would unfit women for roles as wives and mothers. The *Queen* published several negative articles about Mary from her first lecture at St. James Hall, when they described her as representing "everything that woman of sense . . . should avoid" and lacking the mental power to be a good physician. In June the weekly asserted, without naming Mary directly, that American women who were mobbed for wearing bloomers were simply receiving their due punishment. Mary's continuing popularity led the periodical to the vituperative piece that questioned her medical credentials—and they questioned whether she had actually served as a surgeon in the war.[27]

Mary was livid. She sought the legal assistance of David Morgan Thomas of the Temple in London, who counseled her that her sense of the "penance" the *Queen* should be required to make was not sufficient. He informed her he would "deal with *the whole matter* in a manner which will effectually prevent the recurrence of any more impudence in that, or kindred quarters. . . . The time has come when there must be an end of the malicious scribblings of a pack of malevolent boobies whose cowardice is surpassed only by their incompetency." When the editor of the *Queen* received a letter from his solicitor, Thomas insisted, they would have to insert a letter from Mary that answered all of their charges, and "like all cowards, [they shall] tremble, & repent." In the interim, she continued her lecture tour.[28]

In the midst of her hectic schedule, with "quite a run" on tickets for her lectures, Mary received a letter that cheered her greatly. Mrs. E. A. Farmer of Delaware County, Iowa, wrote to inform her that they had established Walker Lodge, I.O.G.T.

in Uniontown, Iowa, "in honor to her whose name it bears." The International Order of Good Templars advocated complete abstinence from alcohol, and the Iowa lodge recognized Mary's ability to carry that message internationally. Not all news was so rewarding. In May, two articles appeared in medical journals that demonstrated the disparate ways in which medical men responded to this woman physician. The *New York Medical Journal*, which had reprinted the "clitoridectomy" comment, published a scathing letter to the editor from Dr. Roberts Bartholow, who had been a member of the Medical Board that attempted to block Mary's appointment as a contract surgeon. Bartholow had a successful practice in Cincinnati and was an ardent opponent of non-allopathic approaches to medicine and of women in the profession. The anonymous letter in the *Spectator* and *Queen* was suspiciously like Bartholow's. His letter was explicitly in response to the coverage the *New York Medical Journal* had given Mary in its January issue, and it was rife with passages that revealed jealousy of the recognition she was receiving in England and disdain for medical women. When Dr. Perin saw Mary, Bartholow claimed, he "was not a little astonished at the apparition [of a woman in "that hybrid costume"], and, I may add . . . indignant that the lives of sick and wounded men should be intrusted to such a medical monstrosity." No phrase about Mary was so often repeated as this line from Bartholow's letter—that she was "a medical monstrosity." Although he insisted he was merely setting the record straight about her abilities, he incorrectly detailed several statements about her background and about military officers involved. Bartholow was an intelligent man, but he was described by some people as "erratic" and unstable in his behavior; ultimately, he was merely an extreme instance of the widespread resistance among medical men to women doctors. To accept Bartholow's assessment of her professional skills would require ignoring the written accounts of her medical abilities from Dr. J. N. Green, Assistant Surgeon General of the United States Robert C. Wood, Dr. J. M. Mackenzie, Dr. E. H. Stockwell, Dr. Preston King, and Dr. Edward E. Phelps, medical director of the Kentucky. All but Stockwell were allopathic physicians. But these were private documents not presented to the public, and as Bartholow understood, a denigrating phrase could be far more powerful than reality.[29]

Mary fought back. In a letter to the editor of the *Spectator*, she detailed the letter's factual errors and cited her medical degrees and the statement from President Johnson that accompanied her Medal of Honor. The prestigious *Lancet* entered the fray by defending Mary's professionalism. Its article was widely reprinted in the States, Jamaica, Europe, and elsewhere. Covering her recent attendance at an operation at Middlesex Hospital, the *Lancet* defined her as a serious medical practitioner and asserted there was "much truth and sound sense in her opinion" that fashionable female clothing was physiologically damaging to women. Still hesitant to recommend the woman physician in general, the *Lancet* concluded, "We may hesitate about the advisability of this lady's example being generally followed by her sex but we cannot fail to respect the earnest purpose which has marked her step in the present instance."[30]

The stress from these charges and her exhausting lecture schedule finally took its toll. Mary began to experience throat problems and at the end of May she had to cancel an appearance because of illness. Good news arrived, however, from David Morgan Thomas. Through several meetings and an ongoing correspondence, Mary and Thomas became friends with shared concerns for reform. He wrote her hurriedly on May 9 from the Court of Chancery that the *Queen* as well as the *Spectator* had been induced to print her letters refuting their erroneous statements.[31]

Meanwhile, Mary maintained ties to her friends at the Female Medical Society in London. Lord Shaftesbury led the society's third annual meeting on May 27, 1867. Although Mary was not on the program, Shaftesbury asked her to speak. *Victoria Magazine* described her comments on women physicians as "graceful, ladylike and effective." Throughout Mary's months in Britain, she never lost sight of the issue of woman's suffrage and often incorporated it explicitly into her lectures. One fortuitous new acquaintance was Harriet Law. A Marxist and secularist, Law was marginalized by mainstream women's rights' groups, but Mary's and Law's interest in suffrage and labor drew them together in 1867. Walker aligned medicine not with privileged elitism but with *labor*—"I *am* a working woman," she often declared. Near the end of Walker's stay in England, she and Law were able to combine their efforts by appearing together on stage. On June 16, 1867, Mary presided at a suffrage meeting at Cleveland Hall in London at which Law spoke on John Stuart Mill's woman's suffrage proposal currently before the House of Commons. Mary followed with a lecture on the role that woman's suffrage would play in the reform of English marriage laws. The speeches were "greeted with thunderous applause."[32]

Mary also continued her commitment to dress reform. Dr. Edmunds and she had attended several medical lectures together, including Edmunds' speech at the London Dialectic Society, and at the Society's June 18 meeting, he invited her to speak before the group on dress reform, hoping to encourage other women to "get into the habit of speaking" publicly. An instantaneous fondness for Mary was a common occurrence among these reformers, and their affection often helped to sustain her against the barbs of her critics. Just as wounded soldiers had fallen in love with her during the war, so too did some reformers—men and women alike—fall in love with Mary in these months. Henrietta Hodges of Newington was one such figure. A women's rights and temperance advocate, Hodges often wrote to Mary, and her letters began to take on the tone of a lover. She called Mary "dearie" and lamented Mary's inevitable return to America. Her only solace, Hodges wrote, was that she could correspond with Mary and hope "to think of your dreaming of me." By early July, the letters became more explicit, as Hodges repeatedly asked Mary to return to Newington for a visit: "I do trust it will not be long . . . before you see us, and My Husband will *always* give *you* up his *half the bed*, but we could only sleep" and signed the letter, "Yours most lovingly, Henrietta Hodges." Mary did not return to Newington, and no correspondence between the women after her return to America is extant.[33]

In July, Mary prepared for her trip to Paris. She did not leave England a wealthy woman, in spite of her nonstop lecturing schedule, having often agreed to speak "for expenses" when it was a cause she strongly supported. But it was an extraordinary experience. The Paris Exposition Universelle was to be Emperor Napoleon III's demonstration to the world of France's superiority, and more than eleven million people attended between its opening on April 1 and conclusion on November 3, 1867. Touring the large exhibit-filled park that surrounded the central hall, Mary could view an English lighthouse, a Tunisian palace, and the United States' one-room schoolhouse. The main exhibit hall, the Palais du Champs de Mars, was an enormous iron and glass structure with a mile-long circumference. The exhibits were divided into ten categories, including industrial products, works of art, and a section on clothing at which her friend Dr. Trall exhibited the hygienic reform dress.[34]

Mary marveled at the displays, but she created a scene herself when she attended the Americans' Fourth of July banquet at the Grand Hotel. The French government was nervous about any large public gathering of Americans because Archduke Maximilian of Austria had been executed two days earlier. Emperor Napoleon III had attempted to establish a puppet empire in Mexico under Maximilian during the Civil War, using the distraction of the war as a means for expanding his empire and influence. Support of Maximilian had been disastrous. Eventually French support troops were pressed by the United States to withdraw; shortly thereafter Maximilian was captured by Mexican President Benito Juarez's forces and executed on June 19, 1867. In Paris on July 2, when the Emperor announced the exposition's prize-winning entries, national anthems were played as each winning country was announced—except "The Star-Spangled Banner." The exposition managers sought to bar the Americans' Fourth of July dinner celebration, but organizers argued it was a private affair. Nearly three hundred prominent U.S. citizens attended. An ardent patriot, Mary's response to the failure to play the American anthem was to wear a sash of stars and stripes to the dinner. In spite of the request from French officials that political commentary be avoided, the night was filled with political tensions. A toast to President Johnson was snubbed by many as was one to the French emperor. Moncure Conway felt it was a very dull evening—until Dr. Mary Walker rose from her chair and walked to the head of the table. She offered a toast to "Our soldiers and sailors," kissed the symbolic flag-sash she was wearing, and quietly returned to her seat. When Mary left the gathering after dinner, she was cheered by a group of French citizens in the courtyard. In his memoirs, Conway recalled that the cheer was an acknowledgment of "Dr. Mary Walker's independence."[35]

She remained in Paris for four weeks and spent much of her time at the hospitals. Her visits to the Surgeries at the Charité and Hôtel Dieu Hospitals were reported as an honor bestowed by her on the French facilities. At the latter hospital, the interns invited Mary to join them at breakfast in their dining hall, and they shared a lively, good-humored exchange in spite of the language difficulties (Mary spoke no French and only one intern spoke English). The young men toasted her health, which delighted her, though she drank water in compliance with her temperance stance. It was one of her fondest memories of Paris, and a refreshing change from the verbal attacks by medical students in England. Only one incident marred her experiences in France. She visited the American Section of the exposition at the end of her tour of the exhibits and was shocked to discover that a photograph of General Robert E. Lee was on display. Insisting it was too soon after the war to display his portrait, she started to tear down the card that flatteringly described Lee. The commissioner-general of the American Department, John Bigelow, pulled her away from the display and explained that it was the decision of the American government to display the portrait. Although not unsympathetic, when she attempted once again to destroy the display, he led her out of the building. To a woman who had been imprisoned by Lee's troops, any attempt to honor the Confederate leader seemed an outrage. In spite of this incident, the remainder of her time in Paris was pleasant. She returned to London in early August.[36]

Mary gave a final lecture in England on August 17. Held at the National Temperance League Rooms, it was titled "Farewell Lecture to the Ladies of London, on Ladies' Reform Dress." George Dornbusch advertised the event for her, sending notices to over forty newspapers and fifty women reformers. The large audience embraced Mary's address, a satisfying conclusion to her year abroad. Afterward she traveled to Glasgow, where she was to depart on the *Hibernia*. As she readied for departure, she wrote a letter to Justin McCarthy at the *Morning Star*: "I must improve this last opportunity to thank the public and the *press* for the many expressions of kindness and attention during my visit in the United Kingdom and Paris. Please say to my numerous friends who have paid me *special* attention, that it was impossible to call upon them all before leaving, but that they are remembered with gratitude and esteem. . . . In a few moments I shall . . . sail for my loved America. I shall leave, feeling, 'not that I love the Kingdom *less*, but my own native land *more*.'" Her year-long stay in Great Britain had been a triumphant success. She remained in contact over the years with several of her new British acquaintances, including Professor Donaldson at Cambridge, with whom she exchanged a series of letters on scientific issues of the day. She returned to the States energized and ready to immerse herself in reform work. Her time abroad served as the impetus to developing a national presence at home. She had learned how to use publicity effectively as a kind of "public diary," writing the details of her life and opinions for public rather than private consumption through essays, interviews, and especially letters to newspaper editors. It was a technique she would use with consummate skill for the rest of her life. Dr. Mary Walker was about to become one of the most widely recognized women in America.[37]

CHAPTER 7

"A Representative Woman"

When Mary returned to the States in September 1867, she was nearing the age of thirty-five, invigorated by her year in Britain, and ready to join the major reform movements in her own country. She made her home primarily in Washington, D.C., but in many ways, America became her home. Washington and New York were the hubs of reform activism in these years, and she was often in movement between the two cities. Over the next five years she traveled across the country and spent time in Connecticut, New York, Pennsylvania, Ohio, Missouri, Kansas, Mississippi, Louisiana, Texas, Maryland, and California on lecture tours and to support various causes.

Reconstruction as both a political policy and a moment of cultural change had stagnated during her absence. Twice Republicans attempted to impeach President Johnson, the second time when he sought to oust Secretary of War Edwin M. Stanton, who was aligned with the Radicals in Congress. Mary knew and respected Stanton, and he was a key supporter for the awarding of her Medal of Honor, yet it had been Johnson who continued to seek a way to acknowledge her extraordinary war service. Thus as she returned home, she found herself in an impossible political quagmire. When Republicans lost the vote on Johnson's impeachment, Mary joined a delegation of congressmen that went to the Executive Mansion to congratulate him. It was an awkward beginning for her change in party affiliations, since she preferred Radical candidates at that moment, but it fit with her sense of duty.[1]

The Southern Democratic successes of 1867 led Republicans to nominate Ulysses S. Grant, a conservative, as their party candidate over Radical candidate Benjamin F. Wade, who was an important supporter of woman's suffrage and well known to Mary. The country was unprepared for the vigorous resistance a growing and vocal group of women instigated when it became evident that the political leaders of both parties envisioned no reconstruction of women's political and social status. Tensions between suffrage activists had also grown in Mary's absence, however—in part because of policy differences, and in part because of personality clashes. For a woman to embark on a public political career in the mid-nineteenth century, she had to be strong, outspoken, determined, and willing to take on new kinds of leadership roles. Not surprisingly, most of the leading activists—including Mary—had strong egos and were often unwilling to accept criticism of their actions.

In October 1867 Anthony and Stanton aligned themselves with George Train, who helped finance the founding of the American Equal Rights Association but who was a blatant racist. Train was running as a Democrat for governor of Kansas, and part of his platform was support of woman's suffrage in opposition to voting rights for African Americans. Train, Stanton, and Anthony toured the state of Kansas, and Train's racial statements ignited a split in the suffrage movement. The press used the alliance to undermine suffrage efforts as well, and it afforded the Republicans an excuse to pull further away from support of the movement. When the AERA's Executive Committee called an emergency meeting in December, Anthony was asked to defend her actions in Kansas and especially her use of the AERA's name without the committee's permission. Her response exposed the status that both she and Stanton felt they had: "I AM the Equal Rights Association," Anthony proclaimed. The passage of the Fourteenth Amendment exacerbated these tensions as suffragists struggled to determine their best avenues of resistance. In spite of the rising tensions, Mary immersed herself in working with the AERA. The old friction between her and Stanton and Anthony over dress reform had never healed, yet together they accomplished important work in these years.[2]

In November 1867, Mary became the first woman to attempt to vote in the state of New York. As she described the experience in Oswego, "I walked up to the ballot-box and was about to cast my ballot when the inspector placed his hand over the box and told me to get out. I protested and told him that I was a property-owner and a taxpayer and had as much right to vote as he did. Another inspector hunted up the law and read it to me," which said only male citizens could vote. Although she was turned away from the poll, her action was in line with the new directions that the suffrage movement was taking in its effort to secure the vote for women.[3]

Unlike many women activists, Mary did not have financial support from a spouse or family money to help fund her activities. She had maintained contact with some of her patients while in England, but she had to reestablish her medical practice in Washington once again. She focused on treating working-class patients and held evening office hours to accommodate patients' work schedules. Some physicians denigrated any colleague who worked with poor patients, insisting it was a sign of incompetence or a misguided sense of duty. It is very likely that Mary's middle-class clientele was small because of her radical appearance and activism. But treating working-class patients was a part of Mary's eclectic philosophy of establishing democratic values in all aspects of life, and she had learned a great deal about labor issues while in England. Eclectics viewed the postwar period as a challenge to medical freedom. With the rise of the allopathic-based AMA, medical examining boards increasingly rejected non-allopaths, "from the motive of pure partisanship" according to eclectics and homeopaths. It was in Mary's home state of New York that the greatest resistance to the AMA's domination was enacted through the establishment of the Eclectic Medical Society in 1863. Shortly thereafter the EMS joined ranks with the Reform Medical Society, which included eclectics and physio-medical practitioners. The united society and the Eclectic Medical College of New York were incorporated in 1865 by the state legislature, setting an example for eclectic physicians and organizations to seek state recognition. Although eclectic physicians would be a key part of medical practice in the United States throughout the century, they were increasingly under attack in the late 1860s. Mary continued to practice eclectic medicine, wrote occasionally on medical treatments, and advanced some of her thinking; but, like most physicians of her generation, she largely held to her training of the 1850s.[4]

Most of the winter of 1867–1868 was spent in Washington, where she renewed old friendships with suffragists whom she had known for over a decade, including Stanton, Stone, Anthony, and Mary Livermore, and developed many new friendships among the extraordinary group of women activists who settled in Washington after the war. One such friendship was with Emily Briggs. Originally from Ohio, Briggs came to Washington in 1861 when her husband was appointed to the position of assistant clerk of the House of Representatives. The Washington political scene quickly attracted her attention, and under the pseudonym of "Olivia," Briggs published a daily column in the *Washington Chronicle* for more than twenty years. The two women shared a fascination with Washington politics, a commitment to woman's suffrage, and keen senses of humor.[5]

Another important, long-term acquaintance was Clara Barton. In addition to their wartime service and advocacy of woman's suffrage, Mary and Barton shared the experience of being highly criticized public figures. Barton's reputation as a "healing angel" was attacked on many sides before her character was redeemed for later generations. Over the years, the two women worked for federal government departments and faced constant harassment from fellow workers. Barton's initial years in the Patent Office, beginning in 1854, were enjoyable and stimulating, but a shift in administrators left her to face a growing animosity from her male colleagues. Each morning as she walked to her desk, rows of fellow workers would spit on her. Similarly for Mary, groups of males would follow her in the streets, call her names, and throw objects or mud at her. Both women were also vilified through rumors published as "facts" in the newspapers. Because she chose not to marry and to work outside the home, Barton was plagued by rumors claiming she was promiscuous, living with a man out of wedlock, or the mother of children with Negroid features. Mary's vilification came from wearing the reform dress—thus she was a "she-man," a "freak," an "anthropoid," and a "hermaphrodite." In reality, Mary and Clara shared keen intellects, a talent for wittiness, and love of political discussions.[6]

Although Barton was never a close friend, Mary developed a lifelong friendship with Dr. Ellen Beard Harman. Their friendship was melded through their commitment to medicine and women's rights, after meeting at the Hygeio-Therapeutic College. Harman lived in Illinois but was often in Washington for various reform activities. She and her husband published *The Reformer* magazine in the late 1850s, and she continued to write as a means of advancing women's rights. Harman was also an officer of the World's Health Association, which consisted primarily of supporters of eclectic medical practices. The WHA included many of Mary's friends, such as Dr. Russell T. Trall, Samuel R. Wells, editor of the *Phrenological Journal*, and Dr. Lydia Stowbridge, who practiced hygenics and dress reform. The WHA thrived during the war years, when Mary was unable to attend most of their conventions, but she and Harman often attended suffrage conventions together in reform dresses. Harman was one of Mary's most vocal supporters at the conventions as well. These friendships helped sustain Mary through the final stages of her divorce and to move beyond her personal sense of loss and failure.[7]

It was also in these years that Mary developed one of her most important friendships—with Belva Lockwood. The friendship was based on their mutual commitment to women's rights and on the ability of each woman to educate the other in ways that advanced their work. Their friendship would suffer strains but would endure until Lockwood's death in 1917. The widowed Belva Bennett McNall and her sixteen-year-old daughter Lura had moved to Washington in February 1866; three years later, she married Ezekiel Lockwood, a dentist and Baptist minister. Her goal in moving to Washington was to be in the midst of the "great political center,—this seething pot—" in order to learn more about how government worked. Few women knew that subject as thoroughly as did Mary, and she willingly shared her knowledge with Lockwood. In turn, as Lockwood sought a law degree, she would advance Mary's legal knowledge. Mary and Belva may have met initially in 1863 when Lockwood moved to Oswego and bought a seminary, the Oswego Female Institute. When Lockwood and her daughter came to Washington, they resided at the Union League Building and opened a private coeducational school. Soon Mary and other activists made Lockwood's rented floor at the Union League Building their locale for political meetings and strategy sessions, with more than a dozen societies meeting there weekly. Belva's intelligence and determination impressed Mary. The two women had much in common: both "exuded ego," came from rural New York, taught school before entering their preferred professions, and were devoted to abolition, suffrage, and temperance. Although Mary was known for wit and love of humor and Lockwood for being rather humorless, they blended their differences as well as their commonalities into a lifelong friendship.[8]

There was another relationship in Mary's life at this time that was more complicated. Stephen R. Harrington, an attorney from Virginia, spent time in Washington on political business for the Republican Party. It is likely he and Mary had known each other since the war, when he was stationed for a time in Washington. By the summer of 1868, their friendship had become much more, as Stephen revealed in a love letter to Mary:

> Mon cer ami.
> "It is Sunday a little after three."—
> What suggestive words.—
> Now, as I read them o'er, memories come welling up as of long ago. Strange, that events scarce four weeks passed should have embeded themselves so deeply in the heart as to claim a peerage with those there enthroned for years,—and so familiarly prompt, hold and guide my thoughts. But away with reflections and *with* realities.
> I am gratified, indeed, with the intelligence brought by the little missive from "Mary at home." It shows what one heroic, determined woman can do, armed by justice alone and opposed by law and public opinion. Am pleased too that your ever busy self seems to be at rest in the quiet of home.
> Myself—well, a restless brain, spirred on by cold, blind ambition, a heart throbing with warmest impulses,—a conflict that of course achieves nothing and unfits me for companionship even to myself. Sometimes I wish I had been born a plodding, practical man. . . . But I was to leave reflection *out* of this letter. Of course I have been "busy as a bee," buzzing round Congress, during the last few days, looking after confirmations and other matters that are always hurried through at the close of a session.—Have "appeared" twice before the public as a speaker on the "great and coming events,"—was "duly appreciated," I presume,—Have looked after the interests of a few clients with considerable success but very small cases. . . .
> I would like to see you *very much* this morning,—from my heart, but what is is written, and my wild wandering thoughts must stay.
> With sincere regards, and memories, kind and perpetual I remain
> Always
> S. R. Harrington

In spite of the closeness evident in his letter, Harrington faded from Mary's life hereafter.[9]

As the winter months advanced, Mary began to plan a lecture tour that she hoped would garner accolades similar to those she received in Britain. But the accolades would be few, especially as the country and the press began to realize that women's demands for equality were not passing enthusiasms. Initially, Mary planned to focus the lectures on her imprisonment at Castle Thunder, a topic that was well received in England and Scotland. She began the tour in Norwich, Hartford, and Willimantic, Connecticut; from there she traveled to New York State, lecturing in Utica, Schenectady, and Amsterdam. She quickly learned that while the lecture on her captivity in Richmond still held some interest, many people wanted to put the war behind them, so she expanded her repertoire. In Schenectady, she spoke on "The Human System," which allowed her to address both physiology and dress reform. The tour was an educational first try at reestablishing herself as a lecturer in the United States. Audiences were attentive and enthusiastic for the most part, and she returned to Washington and her medical practice with the intent of developing new lectures.[10]

Mary's involvement with the founding events of the British suffrage movement was a unique experience among U.S. suffragists, and so in May 1868 she lectured on the state of English woman's suffrage at the Universal Franchise Association's convention in Washington. Josephine Griffing, Belva Lockwood, and Helen White Garrison founded the UFA in 1867 in an effort to stave off the gendering of the pending Fourteenth Amendment. The organization consisted primarily of professional women working in the capital; it was dedicated to the idea that suffrage was a right of citizenship and could not be withheld because of one's sex or race, and thus the UFA welcomed African Americans and men into its ranks (though only women held offices). At the close of the UFA convention, a delegation was organized to meet with the House Judiciary Committee with Mary and Lockwood as its spokeswomen. The response of the members of the Judiciary Committee formed a pattern that would be sustained for many years: they offered sympathy and seemingly supportive comments but concluded that the law forbade women from voting and thus their hands were tied. As the suffragists honed their skills, they would learn which committee members were truly sympathetic and would become more adept at enlisting their support.[11]

At this time most suffrage groups were working in concert. Washington groups such as the UFA joined forces with the AERA and others to market the cause before the public and Congress. Mary joined Stanton, Anthony, Stone, Lockwood, Gage, and their constituents in flooding newspapers and meeting halls with copies of petitions seeking Congress's inclusion of women in its intentions to extend the U.S. suffrage laws through the Fourteenth Amendment. The petitions were concise in their plea—that Congress recognize "the right of voting may be given to women on the same terms as men." The petitions were sent to Benjamin Wade, who would present them to Congress at the end of the year. Working in concert, the suffragists were a formidable force.[12]

In June 1868 Mary presented a lecture at the Union League Hall under the auspices of the UFA. The lecture was titled "Pure Love and Sacred Marriage," but it did not present a conventional attitude toward marriage. She offered variations of the lecture throughout her career; it focused on the need for equal sexual mores between the sexes if marriage as an institution was to survive. Her appearances on behalf of suffrage were gaining an increasingly large public following, and most suffragists recognized the importance of her contributions even if print commentaries were largely critical. One disparaging periodical was the *Eclectic Magazine*.

It was not a medical journal but rather an entertainment magazine published in Richmond; it had been pro-slavery during the war, and its editors had not forgotten Mary's work for the North. They used her as a touchstone for boundaries that the "advanced woman" must not cross and linked her and George Sand as dangerous models for women.[13]

On July 28, 1868, the U.S. Congress ratified the Fourteenth Amendment, granting citizenship to men born or naturalized in the United States. It was a significant advancement of African American men's rights, and it set aside the findings of the Dred Scott case that limited citizenship to white persons only. But the amendment was devastating for women, as its second article referred to "male inhabitants" and "male citizens." It was the first time in U.S. constitutional history that citizenship had been gendered. Just as suffragists had feared, the amendment not only denied women the franchise but citizenship itself. While the passage of the law reinvigorated the woman's suffrage movement, it did not yet bring significant funding to the cause. Suffragists were doubly devastated by their abandonment by several men with whom they had worked for decades in the abolition cause but who had supported the amendment—most notably Gerrit Smith, Wendell Phillips, Frederick Douglass, and Horace Greeley. In the fall of 1868, suffragists in the AERA and the UFA began to advise their members to go to the polls to vote in the presidential election. Going en masse to polling stations on Election Day to insist on their right to vote was the key strategy of the movement at the end of the decade. It effectively encouraged women to work in concert for the vote; it made the issue increasingly public; and it insured newspaper coverage, thereby drawing more women and men to the idea that the time had come for woman suffrage. One of the most effective of these efforts occurred in November 1868 in Vineland, New Jersey, where 172 women, including 4 African American women, marched to the polls. Although banned from depositing their votes in the official ballot box, they symbolically cast their votes in a separate box.[14]

How effective this strategy might have been if it had been maintained will never be known, as suffrage leaders were becoming more and more disenchanted with one another and would soon change tactics. At the end of the year Lucy Stone, her spouse Henry Blackwell, Thomas Wentworth Higginson, and others called a convention to found the New England Woman Suffrage Association. Although they invited Anthony and Stanton to attend, the two women declined since the NEWSA supported the Fourteenth Amendment. Alternatively, Stanton and Anthony held a convention in Washington to express their views. Their tactics alienated many colleagues who had long supported both abolition and equality, including Mary. Their attack on the Republican Party was supported by most suffragists, since the party they so ardently supported during the war refused to reciprocate on behalf of woman's suffrage; but Stanton and Anthony denounced the Fourteenth Amendment in spite of what it had accomplished for African American men. Mary began to view Stanton and Anthony with increasing wariness. Nor did the election of Ulysses S. Grant to the presidency bode well for women suffragists.[15]

On January 2, 1869, Mary's nine-year battle for a divorce came to an end. In a special term of the state supreme court at Utica, New York, the case was finally heard. In November 1867, her attorney B. F. Chapman had filed a motion on Mary's behalf with the New York Supreme Court, asking that Albert's divorce judgment of November 1865 be set aside so Mary could respond to the action. Since she was serving in the army at the time Albert filed, the motion was granted, and the case was sent to a referee, the Hon. Thomas Barlow. His final assessment was fully in Mary's favor, stating "it appears that all the material facts charged in the said complaint are true, and the defendant has been guilty of the several acts of adultery therein charged." The marriage was dissolved. As with the original decree in 1861, it was determined that Mary might remarry "in the same manner as though the said defendant was actually dead." Albert was barred from remarrying until Mary was deceased, as the court was unaware that he had already remarried. When she received her official copy, Mary tucked an old letter from Albert inside the decree and wrote on the outside of the packet: "Divorce & Last Letter of the *Villain*."[16]

In the initial months after her divorce, Mary spoke extensively about the complexities of trying to obtain a divorce, often using her situation to denounce archaic laws and male attitudes toward women ("Most men love women as children love dolls"). But within a year she had stopped commenting on divorce in a personal context and never again spoke publicly of her marriage. Although her name would occasionally be linked with a man or a woman over the coming years, she never established another long-term sexual relationship. She had many friends of both sexes, and thousands of acquaintances; why she chose to remain unattached can only be a matter of speculation. It would have been difficult in the nineteenth century for an extraordinarily independent woman to find a partner who would accept the level of self-reliance she manifested. Susan B. Anthony believed that "single-blessedness" was necessary to the suffrage cause, because spouses and children demanded time and energy. Anthony declared that traveling with her sister activists helped diminish the "all-alone feeling" that sometimes overwhelmed her, though Anthony's preference for single-blessedness was supported by her many romantic alliances with other women. When there was discussion—either publicly or in private letters—that Mary might be involved with a particular man or woman, it was most often presented as an accusation rather than a verifiable fact.[17]

The most common relational incidents connected to Mary over the years were from two types of sources—men proposing to her, and men's accusations that she drew their wives away from their family ties, often with sexual implications. She received several earnest marriage proposals over the years (from war veterans to a President), but she never seriously considered remarrying. Her gender-challenging appearance also made her the subject of much sexual speculation. Men who opposed changing attitudes toward women's roles in society were particularly vitriolic. This combination of responses was evident in a letter Mary received several years after her divorce from an angry California man, A. J. Coyer. Mary lectured in the state and befriended Coyer's wife, Dora. In his letter, Coyer insisted that Mary never again visit his home since she could not forgo her "disposition to meddle with 'family matters' which ought not concern you." Mary met with Dora more than once while A.J. was away and apparently criticized him ("abusing me in my absence in my own house!!"). If the "family matters" included abuse or a domineering husband, Mary would not have hesitated to intervene. Underlying A.J.'s remarks, however, was his claim that during an earlier stay with the family Mary had "gone so far [as] to occupy my bed and sleeping with my wife, a thing which, in consideration of the fact that your sex is questionable was to say the least, imprudent." In these years, Mary still wore long hair; her sex was "questionable" only because she wore the reform outfit. While it was common practice in the mid-nineteenth century for women to sleep together in a platonic manner, Mary may well have been sexually involved with Dora Coyer. Another factor may have forced her to forgo sexual relations after her divorce. Mary was one of the earliest women to discuss the subject of sexually transmitted diseases; as a physician, she would have been far more aware of this side of life than most Americans. Considering the extraordinary level of promiscuity in which Albert had engaged during the four years of their marriage, it is possible that he transmitted a disease to her. The possibility can only be speculation, but as Mary would write in her 1878 book *Unmasked*, it was a very common situation for married women in nineteenth-century America.[18]

Whatever Mary's sexual preferences were, there is no question that in the late 1860s she was perfecting for herself a female-identified life that she began in her youth and which she would maintain until her death. In the late 1870s she would radically alter her appearance in a manner that publicly attested to her desire to undo gender norms. Most nineteenth-century women lived male-identified lives in which patriarchal practices dictated a woman's cultural worth as well as self-worth through her relations to men, her "duties" as a wife and mother, and an economic system that relied on woman's place in the home. While the majority of women accepted their domestic social roles, a growing number were expanding women's professional activities, political involvement, and sense of self-worth, and questioning traditional social structures. Within this group was an even more unusual faction of women who, like Mary, also created environments in opposition to the patriarchal system that dictated nineteenth-century U.S. culture. This meant not only working for women's advancement, but working through women's organizations, with other women, and—rarest of all—without the confines of answering to a male authority. Mary often proclaimed her enjoyment of friendships and intellectual exchanges with men, but believing fully in her self-worth as independent of male approbation, she lived without letting such strictures dominate her independence of thought and action. The many female friendships and organizations that shaped Mary's life were not those of the church or the home—they were those of a profession, of a public life in constant challenge to male-dominated value systems, and of a private life independent of male constraints. Her intellect, actions, and appearance were *lived* challenges to the status quo.[19]

In January 1869, Josephine Griffing, on behalf of the UFA, called for "All associations friendly to Woman's Rights . . . to send delegates from every state" to a convention to be held in Washington on January 21. Coming less than three weeks after her divorce was finalized, Mary found the convention an invigorating moment. The UFA's founding was rooted in the belief that suffrage conventions needed to be held in the nation's capital in order to bring the issue to the legislators' doorstep. It was Grace Greenwood's report on the convention for the *Philadelphia Press* that would be preserved for the *History of Woman's Suffrage*, but the event was widely covered in the press. The gathering offered Mary a chance to convene with sister reformers such as Lucretia Mott, Elizabeth Cady Stanton, Susan B. Anthony, and Lucy Stone. Even more importantly, it was a time to work with old friends—Clara Barton, Josephine Griffing, and Mrs. R. M. Butler of Vineland. The latter reported on what Greenwood called "the gallant band of women" who went to the polls in Vineland in the November elections. Butler also voiced opposition to the separatist tactics that Stanton and Anthony had used, and she echoed Mary's sentiments when she insisted, "As to the question of woman first or the black man first, I mean both together." Greenwood captured the spirit of the day when she defined the role of the various leaders: "while Lucretia Mott may be said to the be the soul of this movement, and Mrs. Stanton the mind, the 'swift, keen intelligence,' Miss Anthony, alert, aggressive, and indefatigable, is its nervous energy—its propulsive force." But Greenwood was conservative in many ways, and she loved "sweet, saintly" women like Mott and Barton rather than Dr. Mary Walker "in her emancipated garments and Eve-like arrangement or disarrangement of hair." Mary had many supporters, but some suffragists did not want to be aligned with a woman who did not represent the "feminine" in a conventional sense. In some ways the attention to Mary's attire in these years confirmed the concerns of activists who had abandoned the reform dress, but as Mary well understood, that attention could also be used to gain a national stage for women's rights.[20]

On the first day of the UFA convention, Mary and Ellen Harman sat in the front section of the hall where their attire was noticeable to most attendees. Mary's turn at the lectern was scheduled for the evening session. Earlier in the day, Stanton spoke angrily about the potential for black men to receive the vote while women were excluded. Clara Barton followed with details about her war work but then declared she did not agree with Stanton; she was willing to have black men receive the vote before her because she was sure they would hold the door open wide for women. Barton concluded with an appeal to the many soldiers she aided during the war to support her now. When Mary spoke to the large audience, she declared that she was proud to have labored and suffered for black men, white men, and women—but she was unwilling to see one more male made a voter until "the whole female population was enfranchised." It was her abiding call for universal rather than individualized suffrage. She had the audience with her throughout this segment of her speech. But as she turned to a discussion of how the law was used against women not only in terms of suffrage but in marriage relations as well, the audience became increasingly uncomfortable. Little had changed in attitudes toward divorce since Stanton's attempt in 1860 to make it a significant part of the women's rights debate. Mary detailed the many ways in which the law had been used against her in the long years of her own divorce proceedings. When a man in the audience called out, "We don't want to hear it," Mary replied, "Well, if you do not want to hear me, your daughter may suffer." As she continued, several opponents of divorce, including Lucretia Mott, attempted to silence her, but she held her ground and completed her comments.[21]

Other controversies arose at the convention, many of which were excluded from Greenwood's flattering report. One major change in Stanton and Anthony's focus was to call for a federal constitutional amendment to ratify female suffrage. Stanton believed that this would be a unifying issue for suffragists. She wrote a note to Lucretia Mott after the first evening of the convention: "At last we shall have a definite, constructive rallying point." Less than three years earlier, Stanton publicly stated while arguing against the Fourteenth Amendment that the Constitution contained "not one word that limits the right of suffrage to any privileged class." Now, however, she and her followers turned to "an amendment wholly our own." Within the next few years, an amendment would indeed become the rallying cry of the soon-to-be-founded National Woman Suffrage Association, but many suffragists did not join the rally and none would become so outspoken in opposition to this new approach as Mary.[22]

The other important issue that Greenwood erased from her reportage was the racially based dispute that emerged. A resolution was put forth on the second evening that declared, "A *man's* government is worse than a *white* man's government; because, as you increase the number of tyrants, you make the condition of the disenfranchised class more hopeless and degraded." Dr. Charles Purvis, the influential African American leader from Philadelphia, criticized the proposed resolution, asserting that women were preventing the African American man from obtaining his rights and calling them "the bitterest enemies of the negro." Mary was outraged at such an assertion. While she was a strong supporter of universal equality, she could also be blind to the privileged status her race afforded her. She demanded of Purvis an explanation of what the women had done against the Negro. Purvis responded that he was astonished at her ignorance. George T. Downing, an African American entrepreneur from Newport, Rhode Island, interjected that women had ordered enslaved men to be bound and burned alive; when Mary demanded to know what the women present at the convention had done against the Negro,

Downing rescinded his assertions by saying that the female conventioneers were an exception. Emily Stanton of Virginia noted that the laws which allowed such barbarities as Downing had cited were not made by women; she called on the black men of Washington who were now citizens to bring that equality to women. Subsequently, Downing presented an alternative version of the resolution that was approved a few weeks earlier by the Central Committee of the National Convention of Colored Men. It asserted that "the privilege of casting a ballot is an individual right, not restricted by color or sex." Although Stanton and Anthony supported the first version, the second version was adopted. The UFA was from its origins for universal suffrage, and its appeal to Mary was rooted in that philosophy, but the heated exchange exposed the fact that racial tensions within the suffrage movement had not abated.[23]

The convention's location in Washington was perhaps the most successful part of its endeavors. Several senators who already supported woman's enfranchisement—Benjamin Wade, George W. Julian of Indiana, Samuel Clarke Pomeroy of Kansas, and Henry Wilson of Massachusetts—now became close working partners with Washington suffragists. Julian presented Congress with the first resolution for a constitutional amendment for woman's suffrage on March 15. Although the resolution did not progress, these months marked a new cooperativeness between a growing group of legislators and women activists. Several suffragists, including Mary, Anthony, Stanton, Griffing, and Mott, remained in Washington after the convention to attend a Universal Peace Society meeting held a few days later. Alfred H. Love founded the UPS in opposition to the Civil War. By the late 1860s, Mary and others who had supported the war were increasingly interested in the idea of peace activism, especially as a number of Northerners were still calling for revenge against Southern states. The UPS was the most radical peace movement in the country. Its initiating idea was that by truly following God's laws the group could return Christianity to its idealized form. Although Lucretia Mott was committed to the UPS's concepts and identified as one of the "perfectionist pacifists," few of the suffrage participants embraced the extremes of this philosophy. They were attracted, however, to the UPS's argument that all people were equal and to its goals of achieving an ideal world through education, reform, and nonviolence. Important to Mary's interest was the UPS's opposition to capital punishment, its acceptance of women as equals in governing the organization, and its encouragement of expressing dissenting views during discussions.[24]

Stanton, Anthony, and Mary were each called upon to speak at the UPS's evening session. Mary asserted that there must be a place where peace began and declared "the place for peace to commence [is] in the home circle." She spoke again of her own situation but also raised the issue of polygamy, claiming no peace could be attained until the practice was abolished and insisting that it was practiced throughout the states, not just in Utah. The issue of polygamy certainly held personal resonance for Mary, since she was still legally married to Albert when he remarried; but polygamy was also part of the broader suffrage arguments. While the anti-polygamy actions of the U.S. government were rooted in debates within Christianity and questions of statehood for Utah, for suffragists it was a question of whether polygamy constituted sanctioned adultery by men, as Mary suggested in her comments. She pursued the idea by writing to Governor Charles Durkee, asking him to send a copy of Utah's marriage laws, and returned to the subject days later when she gave a lecture in Washington on "Love and Marriage."[25]

In addition to attending the peace conference, Washington-based suffragists held a meeting on January 28 to discuss their goals, and Anthony and several other activists remained in the city to attend the session. Led by Belva Lockwood, the meeting focused on what practical steps could be taken in the nation's capital to advance the move toward woman's suffrage. Organizing as the Central Woman's Suffrage Bureau, they debated the best ways to change current laws in order to bring equality to women. The CWSB included several professional women, especially physicians such as Mary, Dr. Susan Edson, Dr. Caroline Winslow, and Dr. Ellen Beard Harman. There was some concern about the relation of the CWSB to the UFA, but as Griffing was in attendance, it was determined that multiple suffrage associations in the capital would be advantageous. Although they appreciated Anthony's presence, they asked her again for an explanation of her alliance with George Francis Train, which she attempted to justify but which was a lingering concern following the disturbingly racialized debate at the UFA convention. Organizational matters were the primary focus of the day's discussion. The use of petitions to Congress was advocated. As Mary observed, however, most women did not yet understand how the vote would affect them. Canvassing to garner petition signatures would be extremely time-consuming if each canvasser had to explain the advantages over and over to individual women. She advocated instead for a meeting at which the advantages would be explained to women and men alike, and for the establishment of a committee to develop organizational plans with the primary goal of educating women to the relation of the ballot and the social system. A petition-signing campaign could follow.[26]

Mary's plan of action was accepted, and meetings for the general public were held over the next two days, followed by another organizational meeting. On the first evening, several men spoke from the audience against woman's suffrage, but Dr. Charles Purvis countered with support. Whatever negotiations had occurred behind the scenes, Purvis's support marked an important moment of bridge-building between white women suffragists and African American men. At the next morning's organizational meeting, plans for canvassing were arranged and several women from around the country who had been in town for the earlier convention offered their support. Anthony did not attend, however, and there was considerable discussion of the course being pursued by the *Revolution*, Stanton and Anthony's year-old suffrage journal. Most of the women present were opposed to its increasing alliance with the Democrats. Although the UFA would be the most powerful of the Washington suffrage groups, the CWSB's efforts came at an important time for the movement.[27]

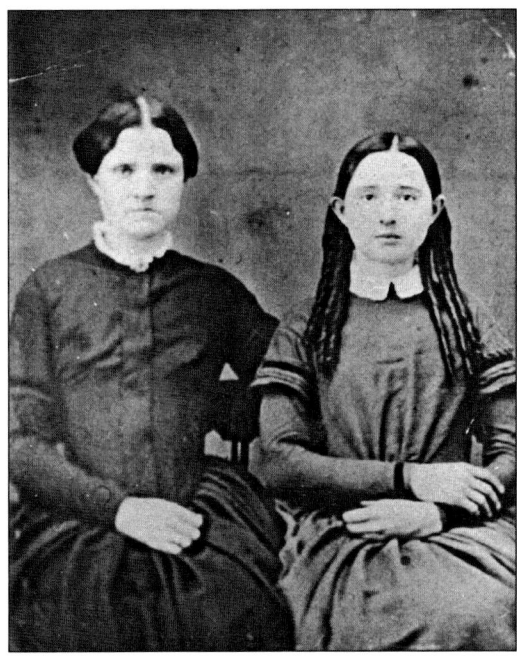

Figure 1. Teenaged Mary and her beloved sister Aurora. Courtesy of Oswego County Historical Society, Oswego, New York.

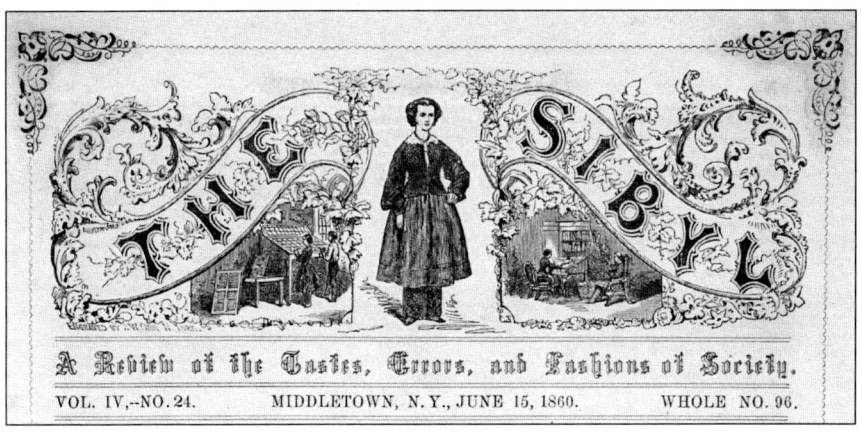

Figure 2. Masthead of *The Sibyl*, where Mary first began her career as a writer in the 1850s. Courtesy of the American Antiquarian Society, Worcester, Massachusetts.

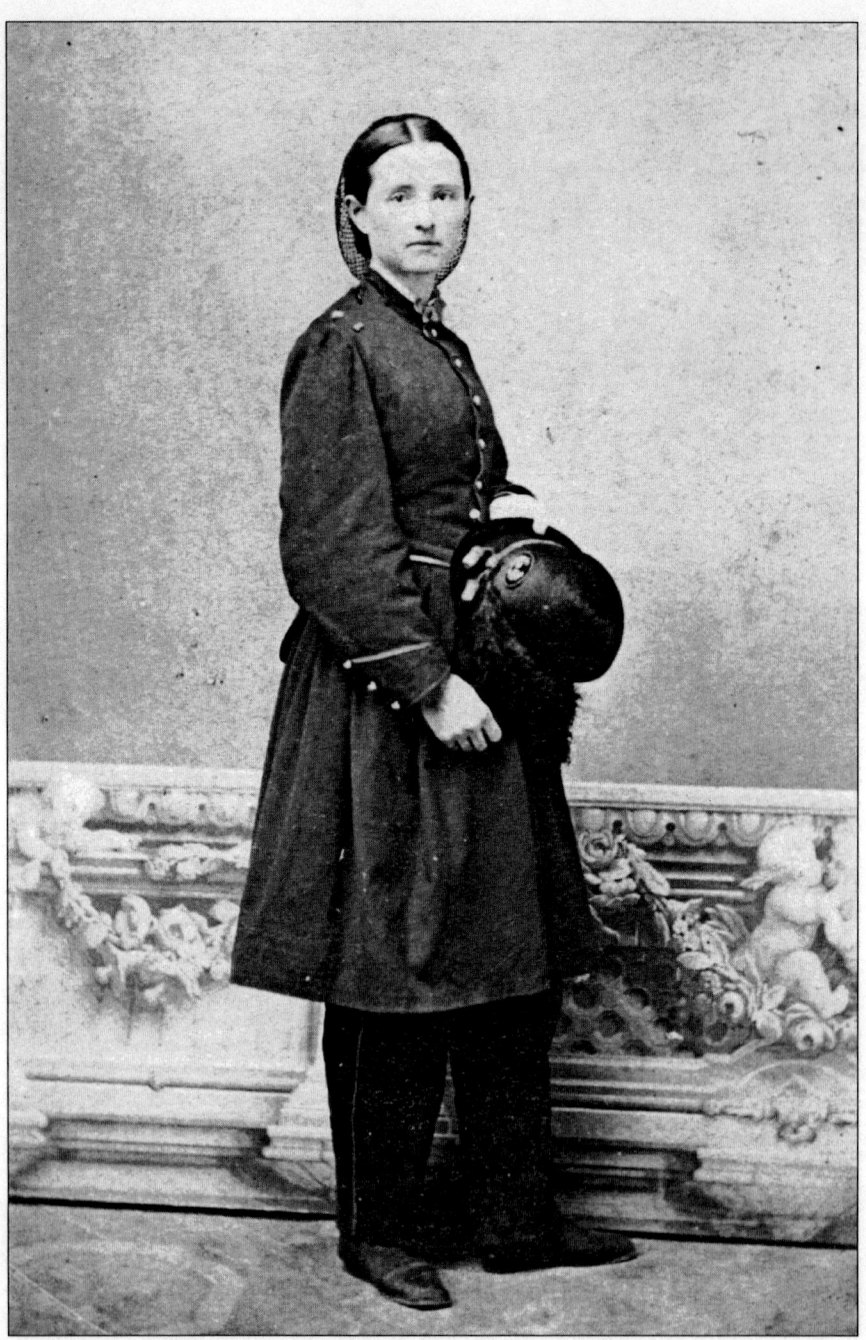

Figure 3. Mary in her Union Army uniform, c. 1864–65. Courtesy of the National Archives and Records Administration, Washington, D.C.

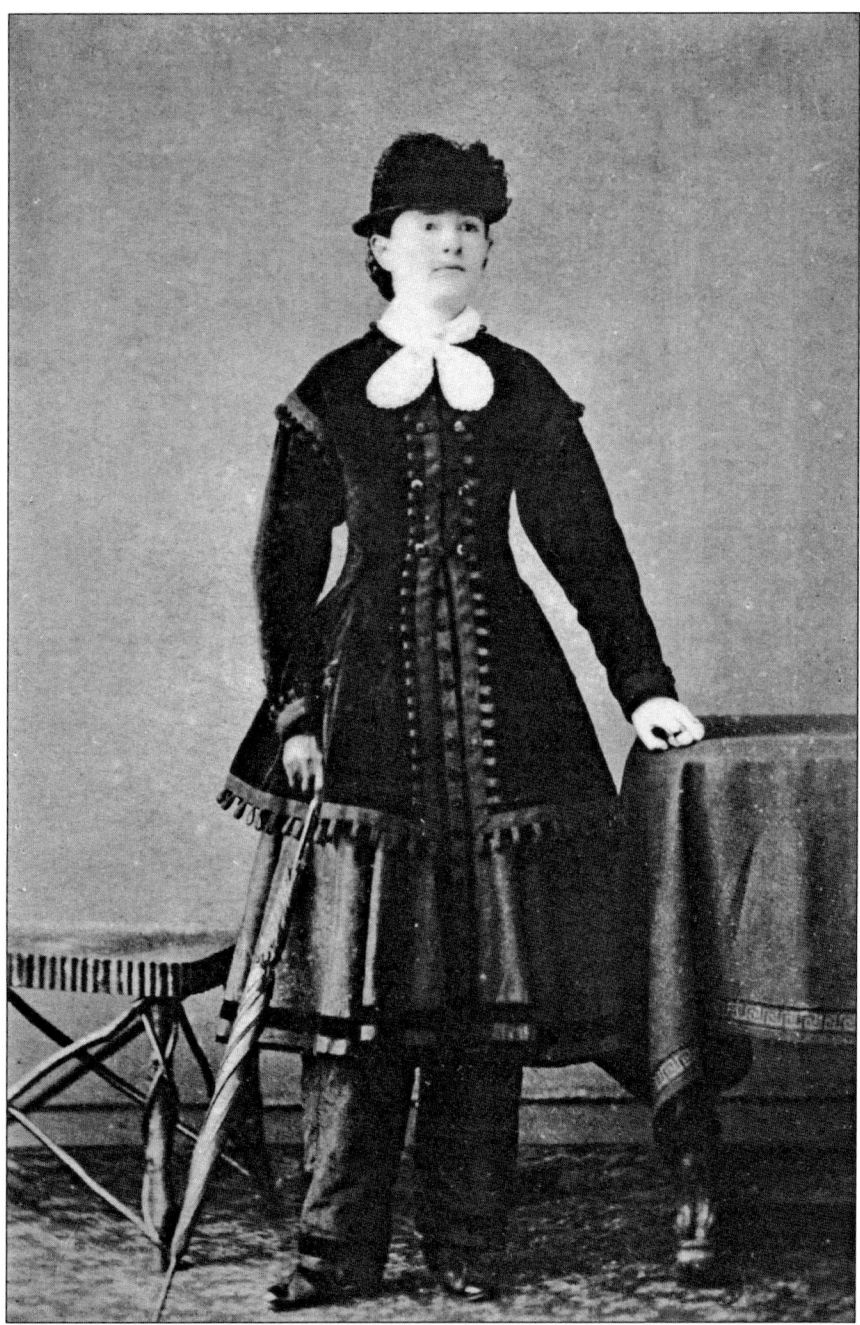

Figure 4. In the late 1860s, Mary continued to wear feminine collars and curled hair. Her Medal of Honor is evident in all photographs for the remainder of her life. Courtesy of Oswego County Historical Society, Oswego, New York.

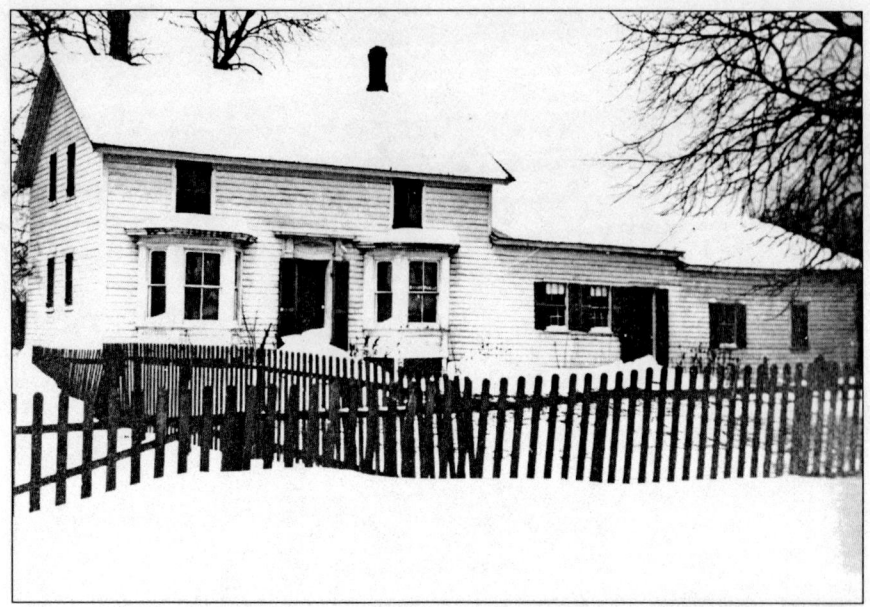

Figure 5. Walker house, Bunker Hill Road, Oswego Town. Courtesy of Oswego County Historical Society, Oswego, New York.

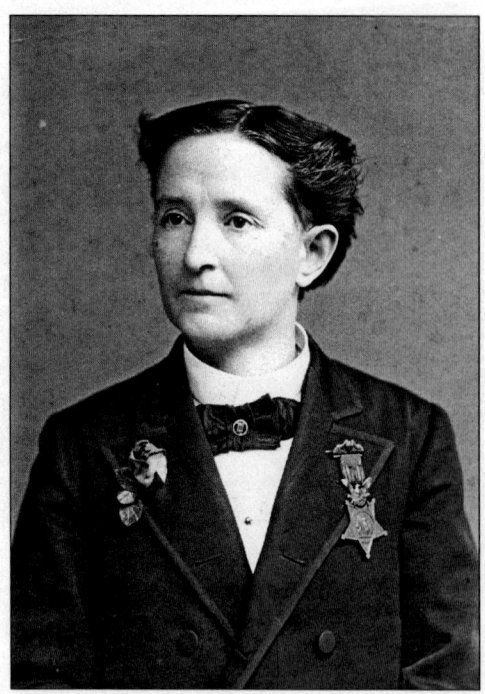

Figure 6. Around 1877, Mary shortened her hair and wore it in the style then popular for men. Courtesy of Drexel University College of Medicine, Philadelphia.

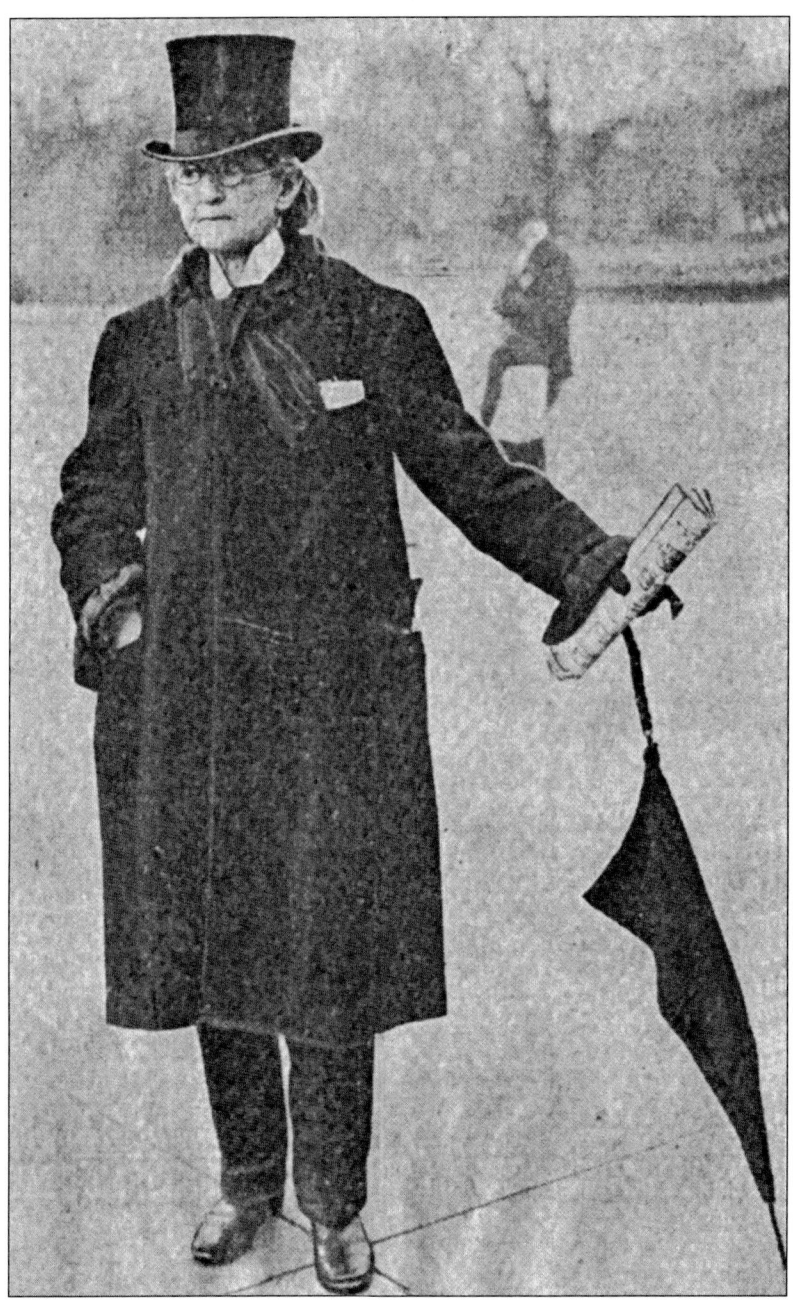

Figure 7. Mary in her famous top hat, c. 1900. Courtesy of Drexel University College of Medicine, Philadelphia.

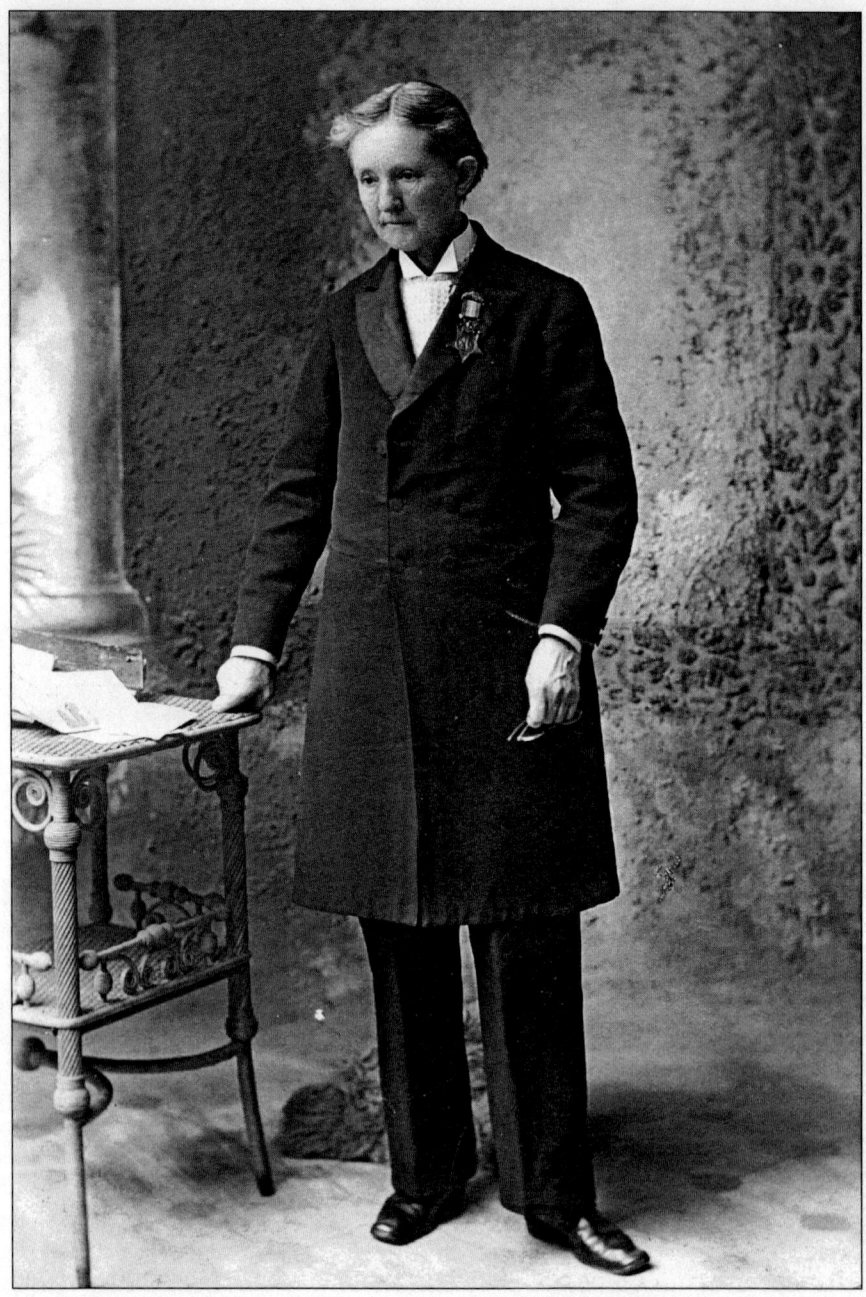

Figure 8. Last-known photograph of Mary, c. 1910s. Courtesy of Oswego County Historical Society.

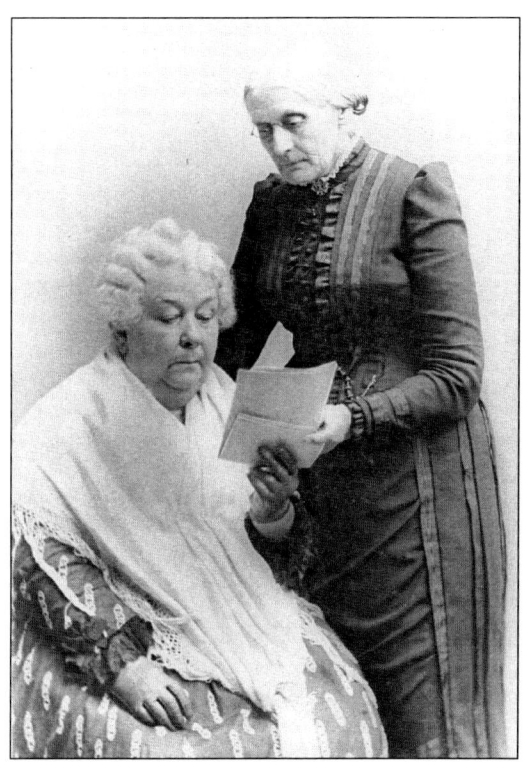

Figure 9. Elizabeth Cady Stanton and Susan B. Anthony, with whom Mary worked closely in the 1860s but differences of opinion about how best to secure suffrage led to a contentious relationship. Courtesy of the Library of Congress.

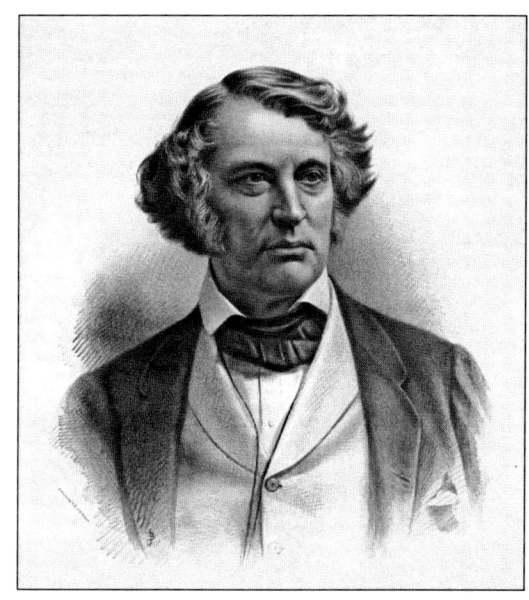

Figure 10. Charles Sumner, to whom Mary refers in all editions of *Crowning Constitutional Argument*. Courtesy of Library of Congress.

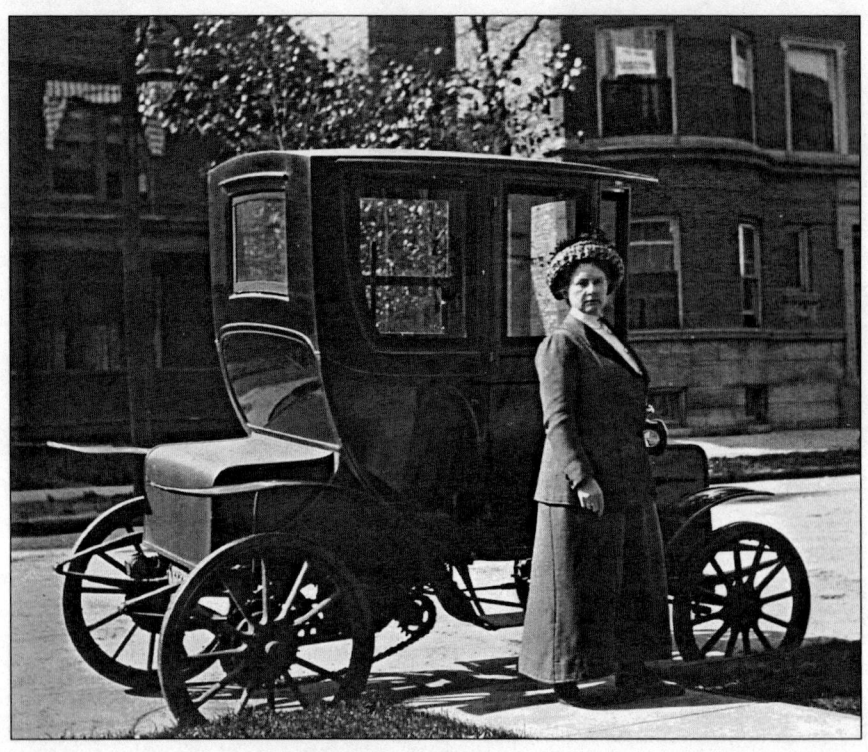

Figure 11. Dr. Bertha Van Hoosen and the electric car in which she drove Mary around Chicago in 1910. Courtesy of Rochester Hills Museum at Van Hoosen Farm.

In February Mary began a new aspect of her writing career—as a newspaper reporter. She applied for a seat in the reporters' gallery of the House of Representatives as a reporter for the *Oswego Times*. Although the request was denied on the grounds that all seats were assigned, she periodically pursued her interests in reporting for the rest of her life. Within weeks, she would surpass the reporters' gallery. In early March, for President Grant's inauguration, finely dressed men and women filled the Senate chamber's gallery. On the floor of the chamber the seats were filled with legislators and dignitaries and—seated near Bishop Wayman of the African Methodist Episcopal Church and Generals Sherman, Farragut, and Thomas—Dr. Mary Walker, the only woman admitted to the floor of the chamber. Perhaps no moment so vividly established Mary's status in Washington.[28]

The suffrage movement was rapidly building momentum in the spring of 1869, and Ohio seemed to be a particularly viable ground for advancing the cause. Mary spoke at a meeting in Cincinnati on April 21, along with Anthony, Stone, Mary Livermore, and others. The large audience responded enthusiastically to the speeches, and the press widely covered the equal rights meeting. Back in Washington, Mary presided over a dress reform convention. She and Dr. Lydia Sayer Hasbrouck were directing their efforts toward reenergizing the dress reform movement. The NDRA had ceased to exist after the battles between Hasbrouck and Dr. James Jackson, but in April the two women physicians reorganized the movement on a national level by aligning it with a broader agenda for women's rights. Founding the Mutual Dress Reform and Equal Rights Association, with Mary as president, they held a convention in New York City on April 28. A strong contingent of women in the United States remained ardent clothing reformers throughout their lives, including Mary's friends Susan P. Fowler and Mary Tillotson. Although a group of "young scamps" hoped to disrupt the convention, Mary's opening speech was "stirring" and "brought down the house," according to the *New York Herald*. When Hasbrouck spoke, she concluded with an attack on President Grant for his negative comments about reform attire. Grant was the object of much ridicule by women's rights activists because of his opposition to all such reforms. Hasbrouck chastised Grant for refusing to meet with Mary because she wore the reform dress and stating he would not meet with her until she came "dressed in garments suitable to her sex." Although the incident was widely reported in the newspapers, Mary rose after Hasbrouck's speech to say that it never occurred—it was another hoax by the press to degrade dress reformers. The young men in the audience became so disruptive at this point that the meeting had to be adjourned, and when the *Herald* reporter filed his story, he shifted tone and joined in the disparagement of the reformers.[29]

Mary called for a continuation of the convention the following night. This time she and Hasbrouck were successful, drawing a large and supportive audience that included the Lockwoods and the philanthropist John O'Donovan. For this occasion, Mary wore a dark green reform outfit with pants, a white shirt, and patent-leather boots. She and Hasbrouck had rethought their strategy overnight, accurately believing that wit rather than anger would win over the crowd. They argued against crinolines, long skirts, and panniers, but included humor along with their medical messages. Mary opened the convention, and Hasbrouck followed with the common procedure of reading letters from absent but supportive luminaries, after which she had the audience howling with laughter as she satirized the misconceptions about the convention that had been reported in the morning's newspapers. Mary did the same, and their ability to laugh off the inaccuracies of the press largely rendered the newspapers' attacks ineffectual. Mary began her lecture by noting she had an apparatus she wished to demonstrate to the audience—if a man could offer her his cane. The pun drew loud laughter from the audience: the cane had long been a symbol of the dress reform movement. She pulled a rather bedraggled skeleton onto the stage (one leg was missing), and her difficulty in getting it to stay in place sent a group of young men into gales of laughter, which she at first assumed was at her expense. Her decision to forgo heated responses momentarily abandoned her, and she remarked that if they did not quiet down she would ask the police to remove them. When an audience member informed her, however, that it was the skeleton drawing the laughter, she joined in, adding that it was "what many women will be like soon if they don't reform their dress," to which the audience responded with approving shouts of "Good, good!" She then completed her lecture on the history and present state of women's dress. The *Herald* reporter in attendance on this day wrote an appreciative account of the evening, noting that Mary presented "some remarkable observations on the hygienic, anatomical, and physiological aspects of the question of dress reform."[30]

In all, the evening was a rousing good time and much more effective than the first night. The convention became national news, with items appearing in papers from Washington, D.C. to Oregon. Over the next few years, dress reform once again became a topic of national debate. More conservative women embraced dress reform as a means of returning to a "plain dress" style, eschewing pants but binding tightness as well, which Mary saw as an important first step toward change. Others advocated a shortened dress, but the true reform dress also gained many followers. A dress reform picnic held in South Newbury, Ohio, in November 1869 attracted three thousand participants in spite of inclement weather. Dress reform sessions at women's congresses began to draw large crowds. Periodicals such as *Arthur's Illustrated Home Magazine* and *Prairie Farmer* embraced the movement, recognizing that women in agriculture often wore pants. The *Oneida Circular* cited Mary's influence as integral to the changing attitude toward the reform dress. Women physicians also became increasingly vocal on the health aspects of the subject. Support for the movement was building to the extent that opponents would lament by the mid-1870s that "dress reform conventions meet everywhere now." In the next few years, with the founding of Wellesley College, the question of women's social roles and dress reform would move into the realm of higher education, and by the last quarter of the century, most women's rights activists would embrace some aspect of dress reform.[31]

In January 1868 Stanton, Anthony, and Parker Pillsbury had published the first edition of the *Revolution*, deciding to publish their own newspaper after Stanton and Anthony broke with their longtime supporter, Horace Greeley, editor of the *New York Tribune*, over the Fourteenth Amendment. Greeley's editorial "A Cry from the Females," in which he mocked female suffragists and asserted woman already "rules the world with the glance of an eye," was the final wedge in their breached association. Publishing their own paper would allow them to advance the movement and control its representation. On May 20, 1869, the *Revolution* announced the founding of a new organization, the National Woman Suffrage Association. Lucy Stone was stunned. In spite of their differences over the upcoming Fifteenth Amendment, Stanton and Anthony had assured Stone that they would work together for the cause. In August, Lucy Stone, Caroline Severance, Thomas Wentworth Higginson, Julia Ward Howe, and George H. Vibbert responded by circulating a call for the establishment of the American Woman Suffrage Association. The AWSA was less radical on several issues, and its focus was on the passage of suffrage laws in individual states rather than nationally. The NWSA, on the other hand, aggressively lobbied the U.S. Congress. Stanton, Anthony, Lockwood, Mary, and many others believed that only an aggressive, nationally focused effort would truly effect change. That level of activism, especially by the tireless Anthony, helped cement the power of the NWSA. Yet the internal conflicts and sometimes outright discord among leaders of the various organizations were now playing out on a national landscape.[32]

A major difference between the NWSA and the AWSA was the reaction to the pending Fifteenth Amendment. Both were opposed to granting black male suffrage to the exclusion of woman's suffrage. The way in which Stanton and Anthony argued for women's inclusion, however, was almost always at the expense of black men and immigrants. They asserted that if women were not included in the amendment, black suffrage should be postponed until the two could be combined. This stance alienated many supporters of the NWSA, including Frederick Douglass and Frances Watkins Harper, both of whom believed that the "Negro's hour" must take precedence over woman's suffrage. The AWSA initially supported the amendment and called for universal suffrage; Harper was one of its founding members. Yet the AWSA leadership was not without its own form of racism. Stone, for instance, spoke of black men's poor qualifications for voting rights, and Henry Blackwell sought support for female suffrage in the South by seeming to offer it as a substitute for black male suffrage. Like most suffragists, Mary was caught in the middle. She believed a national focus was best and yet was deeply uncomfortable with the racial attitudes expressed by the groups' leaders. Both the NWSA and the AWSA made gestures in their formative years to include African American and working-class women, though both soon had a membership that was almost exclusively white. Mary's preference remained with Washington's UFA and CWSB, but she attended both NWSA and AWSA conventions for several years in the belief that working on numerous fronts was best for the cause.[33]

Anti-suffrage journalists thrived in this moment of crisis in the suffrage movement, and they took aim at many of the well-known personages, including Mary. They had been attacking her since her return from England, but their commentaries now took on a new tone of sexually demeaning terminology. She was referred to as being of "a *peculiar* sex" and as an "Amazon," and the *Herald* battered her with diatribes. Privately, however, many war veterans communicated their support. One such man was R. Garner. During the war he requested Mary's carte de visite and now wrote her that the portrait has "been my traveling companion, all the time, Since I left the city of Washington and to day she is kindly over-looking my wardrobe, in my big trunk. . . . I have often been happy, in her presence, in my lonely houses, and hope to enjoy many seasons of pleasure with her, when my soul longs, for the consolations of the beautiful in nature and art." Strangers as well wrote to her, objecting to the attacks and offering their support. Charles Herron of Washington, for instance, wrote that he felt compelled to respond to the "cowardly attacks on you by certain city papers. . . . They would not have been made on any but a lone woman." He concluded his letter by asserting, "You are a representative woman. . . . The self sacrifices you have made will yet receive their proper acknowledgment and you will live when your malingers are dead and forgotten."[34]

Mary now began another phase of her women's rights activism. She felt that her war service warranted consideration for a post with the federal government, and she made a concerted effort in the spring and summer of 1869 to be appointed to a position in one of the government's major departments. She met with Secretary Fish of the State Department; President Grant had recently appointed Daniel Sickles as U.S. minister to Spain, and Mary sought appointment as secretary of legation to Spain under Sickles. The secretary quickly denied her application. Considering her commentary in support of Teresa Sickles during the Sickles-Key divorce case, it was unlikely Daniel would have relished working with Mary. She was rebuffed by Postmaster General Creswell as well when she sought appointment in his department. She was appreciative, therefore, when the Washington correspondent for the *Galveston News* described her as "one of the most remarkable personages now in Washington. . . . [She has] a pleasing countenance, agreeable manners and an inexhaustible fund of conversation." The depictions of her as a "fanatical enthusiast" are untrue, he countered; "There is nothing outré in her personal appearance, and she is highly respected by all who know her." He concluded that some enterprising Southern newspaper ought to secure her as a correspondent because she could "regale their readers . . . with some rich scenes taking place in Washington behind the curtain." The suggestion may well have come from Mary herself.[35]

Many newspapers now referred to her as one of the "major lights" or "the ruling spirit" of the suffrage movement, most often aligning her with Stanton as the primary leaders; thus the *Herald* immediately stepped into the fray and argued vociferously against any government appointment for "this impracticable monstrosity of Bloomerism." The paper contrasted her with Myra Clark Gaines, who was fighting a long and controversial legal battle to recover property in New Orleans that belonged to her deceased husband General Edmund Pendleton Gaines. To the reporter's mind, Gaines was the epitome of "genuine womanhood . . . true to herself and her sex," whereas Mary was going "from department to department in Washington, asking that some poor office-holder may be turned out to starve with his family to accommodate her with a petty clerkship. . . . She talks of her principles, but it is only the hen jumping up on the fence, flapping her wings and attempting to play the rooster in a lusty crow." In fact, Mary supported Gaines's claim, and she and Josephine Griffing attended the trial in aid of Gaines. Ellen Harman wrote in encouragement of Mary's efforts and counseled her to ignore the press's satire: "if a man applied fifty times [for a government position] no mention would be made of it. Well, I hope now you will persevere and squeeze one out of these selfish office-holders."[36]

The press's resistance to Mary's efforts to gain employment with the government continued throughout the summer. At the same time, her arduous traveling and work schedules were playing havoc with what she referred to as her "endurance" abilities, but she refused to curtail her activities. In July, she sought appointment to a clerkship in the Treasury Department, which had been the first government department to recruit women employees. Rumors spread that an auditor in the department had agreed to appoint her to a clerkship, but as the secretary of the treasury refused to sign off on the appointment, the situation was in abeyance. For the present, she abandoned the idea of a government position.[37]

In the meantime, she continued her work on behalf of women's rights in a number of venues. In mid-August, she attended the National Labor Congress in Philadelphia. The turn toward labor by Stanton and Anthony, after both the Republican and Democratic Parties failed to support female suffrage, again brought her into a working relationship with the two women. The workingmen's association was an important group with which suffragists sought alliance, since they engaged in questions of currency, free trade, importation of products from other countries, and the eight-hour work day, which were of vital importance to workingwomen as well. Mary supported Anthony when members of the Typographical Union swayed the congress to refuse Anthony's credentials as a delegate because she helped women typographers organize a union a year earlier. The threat laboring men felt from women's entrance into the field was rooted in the significant increase in women laborers. By 1870, nearly fifteen percent of women worked outside the home; six in ten were servants, a small percentage like Mary were professionals, and the remainder worked in the manufacturing industries. Suffragists recognized the opportunity to recruit this large contingent of women, although many workingwomen viewed middle-class suffragists as already political equals of men and thus not true sisters in the labor cause. Attempting to bridge this gap, Anthony and Mary addressed the committee on female labor, seeking support for woman's suffrage and equal pay for equal work. When the committee proposal went to the congress at large, male delegates removed the reference to female suffrage. The final version of the resolution merely referenced the "duty which should be exercised with pleasure, to guard with vigilant care the delicate and sacred rights of the daughters of toil engaged in various industrial pursuits." Despite this, the two suffragists continued their efforts to be accepted by the congress in the coming months.[38]

Mary's dedication to equal rights, a lingering recollection of the widespread fame she had garnered lecturing in England, and the support of friends combined to encourage her to plan an extended lecture tour, similar to those undertaken at the same time by Stone and Anthony. Originally planned as a trip to Ohio, Missouri, and Kansas, Mary's tour would be extended to include Mississippi, Louisiana, and Texas. It lasted for nine months. On the first leg of the tour, she often joined Anthony, Stone, and other suffragists on the lecture platform as they all crisscrossed the country, promoting state organizations' alliance with the national organizations. The AWSA's first convention on November 24–25 in Cleveland was an effort to draw western suffragists into their ranks. Those in attendance included Abby Kelly Foster, Phebe A. Hanaford, Henry Ward Beecher, Mary Livermore, Frances D. Gage, Antoinette Brown Blackwell, and Amelia Bloomer. At this time Anthony supported Stone's efforts—at least publicly—and, when invited on the first day of the convention to be seated on the stage, she agreed. The alliance of homeopathic medicine with reform causes was also in evidence; the dean and registrar of the Homeopathic College of Cleveland extended an invitation to convention participants to visit the college, emphasizing that in their twenty-year-old institution, "woman . . . has always been equal with man in privilege and honor." It was the goal of Mary's lecture tour to bring a similar message to audiences across the country.[39]

CHAPTER 8

A Crusader's *Hit*

In September 1869, Mary began her most extensive U.S. tour to date. The first stop was Cincinnati, where suffragists from around the country gathered to support the founding of the Ohio State Woman's Suffrage Society. To Mary's surprise, she was blocked by the organizers from speaking because they did not want dress reform associated with suffrage. On the first evening of the convention, however, a woman from Ohio rose to protest Mary's exclusion, noting she "has entertained vast and polite audiences in England before many speakers of today had opened their mouths on the subject of Woman's Rights." The audience agreed, as calls for Dr. Walker rang out around the hall. With no choice but to recognize Mary, the moderator granted her the podium. Mary had no intention of being sidelined to a moment's comment—she announced that she would speak at the next day's meeting. Though the leadership again failed to include her in the second day's schedule, calls from the floor allowed her to speak twice that day. This pattern of exclusion by convention organizers but appreciation by the audience would continue throughout Mary's long career as a suffragist and lecturer. Her longest speech of this gathering supported a resolution Lucy Stone had also advocated—that women, as a class, should be represented in the legislature. She also spoke at length on suffrage, and added her admiration of Ohioans:

> I thank you for having called me out. I believe that there are a great many noble hearts present, and I believe that there are a great many good men in the world. . . . I never have had my feelings more wrought up with gratitude to man than after four months' imprisonment in a rebel prison, I returned to my regiment where I was acting assistant surgeon and found after I had been taken, Ohio men, when the news came to them . . . that Dr. Mary Walker had been taken prisoner . . . great tears rolled down their faces as they said, "She is beyond our power of protection." Never, until the latest hour of my life, can I forget that

moment when my heart welled forth in gratitude to hear that there was so much of nobleness in our great and noble army.

As with so many of Mary's speeches, her comments were equally heartfelt, self-aggrandizing, and skillful in appealing to an audience's pride in their state or town.[1]

From Ohio she traveled to Missouri and Kansas. On October 21, she was pleased to find a good-sized audience in attendance at Fulton, Missouri. While the local press called for her to turn her many talents to a "holier cause," claiming her current actions cast a stigma over all women, they also praised her superior speaking skills. After Fulton, she spent several weeks in the Kansas City region. Her first lecture in the city was sparsely attended, as a driving snow storm kept most people away, but she presented her arguments to the brave few who had come to hear her. Her speech, "Blessed are ye when men shall revile and persecute ye for righteousness sake," asserted that it was erroneous to call the United States a nation of freedom and democracy. She would use variations of this lecture for several years. It encompassed the core themes of her woman's suffrage philosophy: that men's laws perpetuate women's inequality; that women who oppose their own voting rights are ignorant of the conditions under which workingwomen labor; that enfranchising women could help destroy the now-legal sale of alcohol; and that women must not leave change to men but must themselves demand equality. In addition to suffrage lectures, she spoke to full houses in Leroy, Kansas, and elsewhere on "Justice to All" and "Physical Health." But justice to dress reformers was a new idea in Kansas City, and once again Mary was arrested for wearing "male attire," although the charges were quickly dropped.[2]

She lectured statewide in the following weeks, beginning in Topeka and Junction City and extending to Lawrence and Leavenworth. Reports of the success of her lecture tour reached the eastern states. The *New York Tribune* attempted to curtail the impact of her success by asserting that she was advocating a law requiring all men to marry before the age of forty. In spite of such false reports, Mary thoroughly enjoyed her travels. One of the most pleasurable aspects of the lecture tour was the opportunity to meet other women physicians. In Topeka, for instance, she became friends with Dr. Maria DeFord. They continued their friendship via letters over the next several years as Mary focused on the suffrage question and Maria, who lost everything from her practice and her personal belongings in a fire only days after Mary left the state, became an adventurous settler on the Kansas frontier.[3]

The South had always been a "no woman's land" for suffragists; only a few women included Southern states other than Kansas on their itineraries. On this lecture tour, Mary broke that barrier in many ways. Her decision to go beyond the Kansas border into Mississippi, Louisiana, and Texas was instigated by a hoax that cost her much money and time but served as an opening into those elusive Southern venues. While in Leavenworth in December, she received a letter from Mary L. Reed of Port Gibson, Mississippi, who wrote that a group of women in the city had resolved to form a "sisterhood" society to promote women's rights. Realizing they needed links to the North to advance the cause, the Woman's Society sought to entice Mary to Mississippi. A lecture by someone with Mary's "eminent position" in the suffrage movement, Reed flatteringly asserted, would be the necessary impetus to expanding their membership, and they offered her $600 for a lecture. It was an excellent fee, and Mary readily agreed. It was so important to have this opportunity to lecture in the South that she cancelled several speaking engagements and wrote to Reed that she could be there by December 28. "My heart is filled with *more than regard* for the Southern Sisterhood," she exclaimed to Reed, "for you like us, must feel the degredation of all unenfranchised women, in a *professed to be*, Republican country." Mary paid the cost of traveling to Port Gibson, though the expense seemed insignificant in the face of such an opportunity. When she arrived in Port Gibson, however, she discovered that the letter had been a hoax meant to demean her and the suffrage cause. Almost all of the women who traveled on behalf of suffrage were subjected to hoaxes of varying kinds, but it was a costly experience for Mary.[4]

Determined to make the most of the situation, she headed to Vicksburg and Jackson, Mississippi. The Jackson event proved disappointing. She set the entrance fee at $1.25, which limited the audience, but her subject matter was the main block to success. When she arrived at the hall and saw how sparsely it was filled, she cancelled the lecture and refunded the fees, again losing money on the venture. In the midst of this challenging leg of her tour, a surprising attack from an old friend surfaced. Justin McCarthy asserted in several articles that he found Mary's outfit to be "decidedly the most detestable, in an artistic sense, ever yet induced by mortal woman." McCarthy often wrote positively about women's rights activists, including George Sand, but by 1870 he was using Mary as a symbol of extremism in his American publications.[5]

In spite of what had to be painful comments from someone who had been a friend and supporter during her year in England, Mary made no public response. She traveled across Louisiana from late January 1870 through early March, facing considerable resistance. She spoke first in Clinton. The *East Feliciana Patriot* objected to her lack of feminine conventionality and termed her "a specimen of depravity." Mary's lecture was actually successful enough to warrant the scheduling of a second lecture the following evening, but the *Patriot* counseled its readers to forgo attending since Mary had appeared on the streets of Clinton companionably walking with an African American woman. The paper called for every Louisiana community in which she sought to lecture to arrest her for appearing "in disguise." In St. Francisville she was pleased, therefore, to receive a congenial response about booking a lecture hall. Although Charles Furer could not grant her request to use the Social Club Hall on such short notice, he counseled her to book the courthouse, which was "more capacious than the Hall and better adapted for a Lecture room." But the *St. Francisville Democrat* reprinted the *Patriot*'s article on the day of her lecture, limiting the success of the engagement.[6]

Mary intended to travel through Bayou Sara on her way to New Orleans, where she hoped to find better opportunities than she had in the smaller Louisiana cities. At Clinton, she was offered a buggy ride to Bayou Sara by Capt. Thomas P. Jenks. As they rode along, Mary suddenly reached across her escort, grabbed the reins, and pulled the buggy to a halt, having been the first to see the group of bandits that were pointing their guns directly at Jenks and herself. Jenks tried to slip his hand under the buggy seat to retrieve his revolver; one of the highwaymen shouted at him to halt, and Mary quickly pulled his hands upward to indicate he was unarmed. They were forced out of the buggy and behind the high-growing shrubs that grew alongside the road and ordered to throw their money onto the ground. Mary had about sixty dollars with her. As she thought of the long, arduous hours of travel and labor that had gone into earning the money, she clasped a ten-cent piece in her fingers and sarcastically asked the bandits if they wanted that, too. Her challenge brought the threat of a body search and murder if more money was found on her or the captain, so Mary remained silent, if seething, as the highwaymen rifled through their victims' trunks before finally fleeing.[7]

Although the most traumatic, the experience was not the only challenge she faced traveling in the South. She also had to fend off zealous followers who, at times, held quite different values than she. Such was the case with Bradley and Josephine Wightman, directors of an orphans' home for African American children in the Bayou Fiche region. After Mary arrived in New Orleans, she received a letter from the Wightmans announcing that they had met her many years earlier in Rome and explaining that they were directors of an orphanage supported by the Freedmen's Aid Society. While there was some appeal to their request that Mary visit them to see the work they were doing for the nearly one hundred orphans under their care, a second letter from Josephine exposed attitudes disparate with Mary's on the education of freed slaves: "We are . . . teaching the *little darkies ideas* how to *shoot somebody*, and I must say the work requires more patience than *brains*." Mary remained in New Orleans. More pleasing was her renewed contact with D. A. Weber, an African American man she had met in St. Francisville. While in New Orleans, she learned that Weber had been shot, and she wrote to inquire as to his health and invite him to meet with her if he could come to New Orleans. He agreed, writing that he had "entirely recovered from my wound, have also been indicted for Shooting my assailant and *discharged* by order of the Superior court. It is *only* in *free* Louisiana that a man *can* be indicted for protection of his life. I hail with proud emotion the new era which is dawning and trust that when *all* people will have a voice in this government, justice shall not be a one sided affair as it is now." He concluded by noting that "*Our* cause is progressing" in western Louisiana. Weber and Mary were unified in their belief that universal equality was integral to establishing a truly democratic America.[8]

Mary offered a number of lectures while in the city, including "Men's Rights, Women's Wrongs, and Women's Suffrage." This speech was especially successful, and she was asked to repeat it. She discovered in New Orleans as she had elsewhere in the country that, in spite of the many attacks against her in medical journals, individual physicians welcomed her as a colleague. Dr. J. B. Cooper, a surgeon on the police board, and his wife invited Mary to be their houseguest while in the city. In February 1870, while with the Coopers, Mary learned that Congress had ratified the Fifteenth Amendment. Its legal assertion was that the "right of citizens" to vote could not be denied on the basis "of race, color, or previous condition of servitude." Female suffragists tried to take the best possible reading of the language, which did not include the word "male," as the Fourteenth Amendment had. In spite of national support of women's exclusion, Mary was offered the use of the state senate chamber for her first lecture on female suffrage in New Orleans. The large audience included white and black women and men who were part of the intellectual community and several state legislators. Although one newspaper lamented the "evil" of women's rights "invading" the South in the form of Dr. Walker, others acknowledged the lecture was a success.[9]

While lecturing in Algiers, Louisiana, Mary learned that a young woman had been brought before the court and charged with infanticide. Immediately going to the woman's aid, Mary accompanied her to court and assisted her lawyer. She also sent a letter to the editor of a local newspaper after the hearing, admonishing those who denied women equal rights yet were willing to have the intimate details of this young woman's situation presented before an audience filled with men and boys. "A woman has been tried today," she admonished, "but not by a woman judge, not by a woman attorney, not by a woman jury, but all the officials were men in a republican country. What about people being tried by their peers? The woman will be acquitted because there is no evidence to convict her, but the principle is the same." Mary had her own legal challenges to face in New Orleans as well. She was arrested several times for wearing the reform dress; each time she vociferously defended herself before the presiding magistrates. However, when she filed complaints against the officers, Superintendent of Police Cain supported his men and told her that he would have her jailed every time she appeared on the streets of New Orleans. In protest and for her own protection, she made the situation public in a letter to the editor of the *New Orleans Republican*. The action was effective. She returned without continued harassment to her suffrage work, helping to organize the Woman's Rights Association of New Orleans before leaving the state.[10]

From Louisiana, Mary traveled to Houston, Texas. Speaking in the state was risky at this time; few suffragists ventured into Texas. The situation was especially volatile because Victoria Woodhull had recently announced her candidacy for president of the United States. Like Mary, Woodhull's radicalism was drawing concerns among suffrage leaders. The two women held many ideas in common at this time, most notably the belief that the best way to enact woman's suffrage was not through a constitutional amendment but by federal legislation acknowledging women's right to vote as citizens, much as the Enforcement Act of May 31, 1870, would prevent states from discriminating against male voters on the basis of race. Woodhull's political challenge to women's second-rate citizenship in the United

States fueled debates about suffrage as Mary began her Texas lectures. Several men in the state cautioned her about the dangers but supported her efforts. B. F. Luce, a cotton manufacturer from Calvert, reported that he was uncertain how Texans would receive a lecture on women's rights but encouraged her to make the attempt. "I wish you God Speed," he wrote, "and should this great principle, now just beginning to percolate, ever arrive at Maturity, you may justly claim to be its greatest expounder." So, too, did Senator Henry R. Latimer support her right to speak, if somewhat more cautiously. Mary was concerned about violence erupting but also about Latimer's desire to have a sheriff present at her lecture in Austin. He assured her, "The Sheriff is simply discharging his Duty & will patronize the Lecture liberally. I trust you will find my suggestions satisfactory, as I wish to make your visit as pleasant as profitable." The Austin lecture was held at the state capitol, and both lectures drew sizable audiences without violence. Her lecture in San Antonio in mid-May was equally well received and extended for a second night, and she also spoke in Galveston before concluding her tour of the state.[11]

From Texas Mary began her return journey to Washington, stopping only briefly in Indiana and elsewhere along the way. She made little money on the tour, especially after the hoax and the robbery in Louisiana, but she was well satisfied with having advanced her arguments on women's rights to thousands of people in both the North and South. Like all of the touring suffragists, however, she also opened herself to increased public ridicule. Every line of empty space in newspapers and magazines could now be filled with a satirical tidbit at Mary's expense. Her own quick wit often fueled the disparaging reports. For instance, at one suffrage lecture, a young man in the audience interrupted her by shouting out, "Are you the Mary that had a little lamb?" "No," she quickly responded, "but your mother had a little jackass!" The exchange was picked up by newspapers across the country and used to demonstrate the unfeminine behavior of this "male-attired" woman; no criticism was made of the young man's remark. Truthfulness no longer mattered. Story after story appeared in the newspapers, and, as they were published from city to city, they grew in outlandish claims. A few papers did report fairly about Mary's activities, and they often commented favorably on her intelligence and wit. The *Port Jervis Evening Gazette*, for example, reported an incident that occurred while Mary was in Leavenworth, Kansas. Three men called on her, feigning illness. They claimed to have chosen her for their physician because they had heard of her fame. When Mary insisted on being paid five dollars up front from each "patient," the men hemmed and hawed and pretended to search their pockets for money. Through all of their antics,

[t]he silence grew embarrassing to all but the lady, who sat looking like a sphinx. Then one of her visitors got up and went out, then the other went out also. Finally the third got up and ran, without even staying to say good-bye to the doctor or waiting for her to write out the prescription. He did not, however, get away so quickly but what he heard the lady calling after him, "It takes three

smarter men than you to come fooling round me." Her patients having gone, the lady looked round smiling like a saint.[12]

When Mary returned to the East Coast, she was immediately caught up in the political infighting among suffragists. Significant advancements had been made, most notably the enfranchisement of women in Wyoming and Utah, but Susan B. Anthony was forced to end her editorial work for the *Revolution* after George Train stopped funding its publication. The NWSA and the AWSA were competing for members, often holding their conventions on the same dates and in the same cities. On May 14 the AERA had disbanded, transferring its support to the Union Woman Suffrage Society of New York; the next November the Union would merge with the AWSA, effectively leaving the AWSA and NWSA as the most powerful suffrage organizations in the country. The uniting of the groups was not beneficial for African American women, however. In the AERA, they had gained inroads into holding offices; Harriet Purvis and Frances Watkins Harper had membership on the executive committee, and Sojourner Truth and Sarah Remond attended several meetings as guest speakers. The NWSA and the AWSA were run almost exclusively by white women.[13]

Mary gave several lectures in Washington before traveling to Oswego for the remainder of the summer, presenting her popular ninety-minute "Woman Suffrage" lecture to an appreciative audience in her hometown. In the fall she resumed her busy schedule in Washington, working on behalf of suffrage, dress reform, temperance, labor, and general issues of race and gender equality. In spite of her years of appearing in a reform dress, she still had to confront masses of angry men. At one point that fall she was followed by about sixty men and boys who threw bricks, oyster shells, sardine boxes, and wads of wet paper at her; as usual, she continued walking but verbally chastised her abusers. In October she delivered a temperance speech in New York and stopped by the editorial office of Victoria Woodhull and Tennessee Claflin for a short visit before traveling to Ottawa where she lectured on women's rights. Although constantly on the move, she was closely following the developing disagreement between the two suffrage groups, which at the moment centered on an issue about which she held very strong opinions—women's right to divorce. The formation of the AWSA in 1870 was due in part to differences of opinion among suffragists on this topic. The disagreement began before the war, when most suffragists opposed Elizabeth Cady Stanton's efforts to make divorce reform part of the women's equal rights argument. At the 1860 Woman's Rights Convention in New York City, when Stanton raised the issue, the majority of suffragists disagreed with her. Many preferred Stone's view that to discuss divorce would seem to align them with free love, while others believed it hindered current legislative debates about women's property rights and guardianship of their children. As in most of the debates among reformers, personal experiences were behind the differing perspectives. Stone's egalitarian marriage left such issues largely a matter of theory for her whereas Stanton's more conventional marriage and Mary's own status as a divorced woman placed them at the forefront of arguing for change in the divorce laws. In the post-war years, Stone, Lydia Maria Child, and other members of the AWSA continued their stance against linking divorce to the fight for suffrage. Child argued that, while marriage as an institution had been "degraded and polluted by making woman a marketable commodity," it could not be changed without first establishing "equal companionship" between men and women—that is, *after* suffrage had been attained. It was the same argument that was used about dress reform. In Mary's view, such arguments acquiesced to gradual emancipation rather than demanding one's full rights.[14]

In spite of these differences, she attended the AWSA convention in Cleveland on November 22–23, 1870, along with Stone, Isabella Beecher Hooker, her old New York friends Gerrit Smith and Samuel May, Frederick Douglass, Josephine Griffing, and Theodore Tilton. If Mary opposed their stance on divorce, she appreciated the AWSA's commitment to universal suffrage. She joined in the debate at the convention about whether or not the U.S. Constitution granted women the right to vote as citizens. The Fourteenth and Fifteenth Amendments seemed to counter the idea, but Antoinette Brown Blackwell argued that the Constitution did grant women the right. The question began to arise as to whether pursuing a constitutional amendment or going en masse to the polls was the best method for the Association. Mary asserted before the convention attendees "that the fact of women attempting to vote in Washington had done more for woman suffrage than all the Conventions ever held." In opposition to the AWSA's turn toward state laws only, she asserted, "We want a declaratory law . . . passed by the Congress of the United States, giving women the right to vote. This [is] the only way to save an immense amount of labor in the different States." The AWSA would eventually commit to seeking the vote via individual states, and it was the beginning of what would eventually become Mary's split with organized suffrage groups that insisted on abandoning attempts to vote at the polls. A declaratory law would only be enacted, she believed, if women continued to assert their right to vote rather than support a constitutional amendment. A declaratory law would simply acknowledge what their actions proved: they had the right to vote under the Constitution because they were citizens of the United States.[15]

In December, while immersed in suffrage work, Mary also embarked on a plan to found a philanthropic institution for women. Traveling on the steamer *Tonawanda*, she headed for Fernandina in northern Florida with the goal of establishing schools to educate women for nontraditional kinds of work. At the time, there were only two hundred high schools in the United States, and students were disproportionately male. Her vision was to educate Southern women for a new kind of workforce that was only beginning to emerge in 1870. She spent nearly three months in the area but eventually had to forego her plans because of a lack of financial backing. The dream of establishing an institute for women remained a vivid goal for Mary throughout her life, and she would make several similar attempts in the last quarter of the century, culminating in the call for a New Woman Colony in 1895. In an interview by a Savannah reporter on her way to Florida, she proclaimed that before 1876, the nation's centennial, she expected to see Elizabeth Cady Stanton as president of the United States. In spite of their many differences, Mary respected Stanton's intellectual gifts and thought she was the woman who best fitted that position's demands.[16]

There was another issue Mary was advancing at this time as well. At the end of the war, she had begun to work for the establishment of pensions for women who served as nurses, feeling that female nurses were long overdue in their rightful claim to recognition from their government. She had been gathering the names and service information about women in the field for several years, and she turned to that effort in earnest in the early 1870s. Taking her cue from Woodhull's use of the memorial form of a petition, she prepared an initial request for recognition of women's official service during the war. On February 23, 1871, Congressman William Lawrence of Ohio presented her petition to the House of Representatives; it called for land grants and pensions for women who treated wounded soldiers during the war:

> To the Honorable Senate and House of Representatives.
>
> Believing in the right of women citizens to be heard, your memorialist would most respectfully pray the Congress of the United States, to hear the representative of the women who labored for the sick and wounded, during the late war, and grant unto them the same bounties, the same grants of land, and the same pensions, that the United States is giving to the men who served Government as soldiers.
>
> Your memorialist further prays your Honorable Congress to pass an act prohibiting any person or persons from abridging any of the rights of these women citizens in the United States or Territories on account of sex.
>
> She most respectfully submits the following:
>
> ACT FIRST:
>
> All those who left their homes and devoted their time and energies for the relief of sick and wounded soldiers, in our late war, and who were engaged in such service for 90 days, shall be entitled to the same bounty, the same grant of land and if they were permanently injured in health, to a pension for life; the same as the soldiers are receiving from the Government.
>
> ACT SECOND:
>
> The right of the franchise, shall not be denied any of the women citizens of the U.S. or Territories, who labored 90 days, in hospitals for the sick or wounded of the late war.
>
> Respectfully submitted
Mary E. Walker, M.D.

The petition was forwarded to the Committee on Invalid Pensions.[17]

At the same time, Mary was outraged by revelations of the political corruption of the Tweed and Whiskey Rings. It fueled her belief that the government needed women in positions of oversight in order to thwart potential corruption.

With this goal before her, Mary wrote in mid-March to John W. Bell, head of the Department of Justice's General Land Office, requesting an appointment in his department. Although they had not met personally, Bell had followed her career for years, and he was the rare government official who did not reject her request out of hand. Proclaiming that, while her request "deepens and intensifies the admiration I have long felt for you as a woman and a true hearted champion of a good cause, it also strengthens my conviction of the grievous injustice you have suffered"; he praised her "grand soul and noble intellect" and her willingness to speak out on issues that many Americans recognized but few had "the courage to espouse." He lamented that Vinnie Ream could be awarded a $15,000 "pension" (Congress had actually awarded Ream $10,000 for a statue of Lincoln) and Mary none—it should have been $50,000 for Mary, he insisted. More important, and undoubtedly no less appreciated, was his promise to use his influence to attempt to secure a government clerkship for her. It was a carefully crafted letter, offering support but cautioning her about the attitudes she might encounter from fellow clerks should she receive an appointment. His concluding assessment of the short memory of the nation was painfully apparent to Mary. In spite of his position, Bell was unsuccessful in his efforts. Less than six years after the conclusion of the war, many Americans had already forgotten her valiant war efforts.[18]

Suffragists recognized that postwar advances in women's education and in publishing made the written word an increasingly important avenue for reaching wide audiences. The success of John Stuart Mills' *The Subjugation of Women* served as a model for many U.S. suffragists' publications. It exposed what Stanton termed the "hidden depths of woman's degradation." Mary and other leading suffragists would continue to schedule lecture circuits, attend conventions, and go to the polls in an attempt to vote, but essays and books were now an essential part of the suffrage strategy. Mary, who had always loved the written word and had ample experience as a writer, embraced the opportunity to gather her wide-ranging ideas on the major areas in which women's rights needed to be advanced. She drew on her collection of lectures, expanding her ideas as she revised them over the next several months.[19]

Hit was published in the spring of 1871. Her sisters in the dress reform movement immediately recognized the implications of her title—in dress reform circles, "hit" had been a common term used to identify verbal attacks against women who challenged conventional fashions. So, too, was it common among dress reformers to use the idea of a "hit" as the basis for responding to one's critics. Thus, Mary's title acknowledged the many "hits" she had taken in order to live by her principles, and it set the stage for her own assertive responses in the text. She offered several dedications to the book: to her parents, dress reformers, women physicians, and "That Great Sisterhood" of activists. Mary believed that dress reformers had "done more for the universal elevation of woman in the past dozen years, than all others combined" and were "the greatest philanthropists of the age." A full-length portrait of herself in the reform dress graced the book's frontispiece. Her eclectic medical philosophies were evidenced through her dedication to her "Professional Sisters," women physicians "Of whatever School or Pathy." Last, and vitally important to her beliefs and endeavors, was the sisterhood that toiled to establish women's "self-respect and self-reliance" and to "emancipate you from the bondage of all that is oppressive."[20]

Mary included a long preface to the work, in which she challenged those who criticized her for speaking publicly of her own abilities and accomplishments. The theme of the book, she asserted, was marriage, and she insisted she would use "my own language, and express my ideas in my own way." However, because she recognized that "the 'good time coming' has not yet arrived, when an individual can speak of the little personal pronoun *I*, without being gravely charged with the criminal offense of *egotism*," she turned to a well-known phrenologist and friend, Samuel R. Wells of the *Phrenological Journal and Science of Health*, to give a "reading" of Mary Walker's character. Phrenology was enormously popular in this era. Political leaders, suffragists, authors, employers, and many other Americans had phrenological readings done to demonstrate their character and moral nature. By displacing herself and that pesky "I," Mary could present an assessment of herself from a phrenologist that was glowingly flattering and captured her notable vitality. The process both demonstrated her sense of humor and presented her strong sense of self. Wells concluded with a cautionary note: "If you *marry*, select for a companion one who is healthy, intelligent and religiously disposed; one with whom you may be an equal, for you never will consent to play second, nor be held in subjection, but you must have equal rights and privileges in all things. You cannot bear restraint, nor are you inclined to dictate. You simply wish to be free, and to place your accountability between yourself and your Maker, rather than to man." By concluding with this comment by Wells, Mary cleverly revealed the core argument of her text—that a woman must become self-sufficient, develop her own strengths, and follow her own desires in a conscious plan of becoming self-reliant; then, only then, could she enter into a truly equal marriage relationship.[21]

The argument for egalitarian marriage and women's rights in general was presented in *Hit* through eight major avenues of analysis: love and marriage, dress reform, tobacco, temperance, woman's franchise, divorce, labor, and religion. Many of the core arguments of *Hit* were in line with mainstream women's right arguments of the day. A few—such as divorce—placed her in the more radical elements of the movement. It was Mary's experience as a physician that brought a unique flavor to the text. Her years of medical practice afforded her insights into marriage relations and health practices and served as a tableau against which she could enact her political agendas for equality and justice in all aspects of human endeavor. She could argue, for instance, that while the public rendering of marital relations was often idyllic, reality could be quite different: "there is a class of people who *openly*,—and a still larger class who *clandestinely*, live out the belief, that if one is pleased with another, the love element of our being should be exercised without restraint; and such a vast number have so little of Love, and so much of excitability of sexuality, that great wrongs are inflicted on soul and body, to an incalculable extent." In spite of her own marriage experience, she asserted that "[t]rue conjugal companionship is the greatest blessing of which mortal can conceive in this life—to know that there is supreme interest in *one* individual, and that it is reciprocated." It is easy, she suggested, to condemn polygamists and communists for failing to recognize the sanctity of love between two individuals, but their actions "are a thousand fold better than the people outside, who are preaching morality, and practicing the most underhanded and trickish measures, ... cruelly thrusting others out of society, who are victims."[22]

There were two requirements for true love, Mary asserted—respect for and confidence in one another—but both the institutions of law and religion made a mockery of the sanctity of marriage. She offered several progressive ideas in relation to marriage, such as a woman's right to retain her own name. It is "as dear to her as a man's is to him," and "Miss Jane Jones is lost in Mrs. John Smith." If it is so important socially to signify a woman as married, she asked, why is it less so for a man: "why not call a man *Misterer* for the purpose of enlightening the world as to his condition?" She compared U. S. marriage customs with those of other countries, from England to Africa, India, and Turkey; the United States was presented most often as archaic and backwards in its thinking, though the demeaning treatment of women in marriage in all cultures was highlighted. While women's rights arguments often framed marriage as legal slavery for women, Mary's writings were more ardently graphic and filled with research on other cultures, demonstrating both America's barbarity and the universal state of oppression under which women lived.[23]

The subject of divorce was held in abeyance until chapter six. The organizational design of the book revealed an integration of solutions to the many wrongs women faced within the marriage union, the family, and the body politic at large. The initial topic of dress reform posited potential change against the devastating effect of having no legal or physical freedoms in marriage and the consequences of infidelity, tobacco, and alcohol abuse on the marriage relationship. When this picture of woman's condition seemed too bleak to endure, the solution of woman's franchise was introduced. Only then was divorce addressed, for only then could women recognize the rightfulness of ending abuse. Once divorced, the need for an equitable form of labor became clear. Finally, a reformed religious base was proposed as the sustenance of such change. "With woman's enfranchisement," she declared, "comes her unqualified individuality. Without it, just so much, or so little, as men choose to allow her; and that allowance is according to the preconceived opinions, or prejudices, of the men with whom she is related." She examined both the legal concept of women's "dependence" and its implications—if a woman is not an individual in her own right, then everything in her life "depends" on the generosity of a male relative or government representative. The time has already passed, she insisted, when men could "control the *minds* of women successfully, and now the time is almost at hand, when they will be unable to control the *bodies*." Only when women had the vote would marriage laws be made equitable. Her charge to women was powerfully rendered: "Struggle for *political rights*, for it is through such, and such alone, that you will ever obtain *human rights*."[24]

Mary knew that divorce would be the most controversial part of her argument, but she did not come cautiously to the subject. She acknowledged "Whom God hath joined together, let not man put asunder" as the tenet of Christianity that had to be confronted. As with her recognition that "depend" could be used with multiple meanings, she returned to a close rhetorical analysis of this common religious adage against divorce. It was a technique that had served her well since her days of writing for *The Sibyl* when she analyzed a critic's false representations of dress reform in "A Bloomer in the Street." In the instance of "whom God hath joined together," she asserted that she agreed with the premise: "No one can believe more firmly than the writer in the sacredness of the marriage relation." The question, she insisted, is "*whom* God hath joined together, and in *what* joining consists. God's laws are immutable, and if He ever joins two persons together, no man *can* put them asunder." There are marriages in which the couples are truly joined by God, she argued, but far too many marriages are the joining of "purity and impurity" and that combination "cannot harmonize." She used no pronouns in her discussions of the need for divorce. It was not distinctions of sex that created the inequities of marriage—it was laws crafted by men that made women the victims of inharmonious and often brutal marriages. Only men had the ability to live freely and according to their own moral values in a marriage.[25]

Mary poignantly discussed the strange state in which a person finds oneself when trapped in such a marriage without the possibility of divorce:

> To be neither married nor single, and be placed in such a position by the delicate facts of the case, that explanations are out of the question in most instances, is what it is literally impossible for any but the noblest and tenderest to comprehend; and hence the want of sympathy for those who thereafter tread life's path *alone*, imparting happiness to others whose sorrows seem almost unendurable.
>
> To be deprived of a Divorce is like being shut up in a prison because some one attempted to kill you. The wicked one takes his ease and continues his *course*, and you take the slanders, without the power to defend yourself. It is just as honorable to get out of matrimonial trouble *legally*, as to be freed from any other wrong. If it is right to be legally married, it is right to be legally Divorced.[26]

Having established that marriage was not always a morally pure institution and that divorce did not bypass the command to honor God's laws, Mary turned to the question of labor. If women were to be divorced, she recognized, they must also change their attitudes about working outside the home in order to find satisfying means of supporting themselves. The chapter on labor was not strictly linked to divorce. It matters not, she insisted, whether a woman is married, single, or divorced—labor is necessary to happiness for every human being. The public already embraced the idea, she observed; they simply needed to extend it to womanhood as well. She returned to one of her favorite phrases for critics of reform—"the shoddyocracy"—and denounced their patterns of educating Americans to the idea that labor is degrading. To believe that some forms of labor are respectable and others are not "is a part of the chippings of barbarism, that have not yet been hewn off the pillars of civilization. But the axe is already being forged, with edge so keen," she predicted, "that the work will be thoroughly accomplished, long ere the writer shall count her three score years." For all family members to value and participate in some form of labor will strengthen marriage and family relations—and the individual, since "*all* will Labor as a pleasure *and* a profit to *body* and *mind*."[27]

Work constituted the best means to eradicate the archaic thinking of gendered "duties" and "spheres," she argued. Men must embrace the domestic arena as part of their duties and sphere just as women must embrace the public arena as theirs. Further, if everyone engaged in labor, there would be far fewer who had to labor excessively, to the detriment of their health and their intellectual development. She rejected the idea that labor and ignorance go hand in hand: "The great mass of the manual Laborers of our country can comprehend whatever profound reasoning may be brought before them. And who will pretend that the mind that can *understand* is not as great, *naturally*, as the one that can create? . . . I am ashamed of so much of our American boasting, when I look facts in the face, and hear the unsung agonies of thousands of our people, that toil all their lives, and die without owning a little home." In the future, she predicted, "the people of the day will charge the great land-owners, and stock-owners, and *great everybodies*, with selfishness unparalleled" when they learn about the conditions of laborers' lives in mid-nineteenth-century America. "Not one luxurious couch, not one magnificent mirror, not one splendid carpet, not one marble-top table," she proclaimed, "but that, for style and beauty, we owe not only to the *hands*, but to the conceptions of beauty, and the utility of the poor Laborer."[28]

Recognizing that religion was the one field in which women were often allowed to express their own beliefs in a discussion with their spouses, Mary asserted that it was the teachings of Paul that brought most disharmony to the marriage relation. "Any Religion that gives the wife a servile position, is beneath the great plans of Diety. . . . Unless women in all the churches are elevated to their true positions, as companions of men, and not treated in any way as Religious inferiors, the sects that persist in wrongs of this character, will, sooner or later, be swept out of the Religious world." She used this avenue to argue for women to find full voice in all aspects of their lives. The text thereby comes full circle. From her ironic assertions in the preface that the use of "I" could cause such disdain when used by a woman to her final proclamation that only those religions that allow women equal status can survive, she crafted a study of the integrated nature of her work for women's equality as essential to marriage, labor, religion, and the nation. Only with this integration could the United States throw off the last vestiges of barbarism and consider itself a truly civilized nation.[29]

Few periodicals reviewed the publications of suffragists, which was true for *Hit* as well. Its issuance was noted in the *American Literary Gazette and Publishers' Circular*, and the *Albion* printed four lines about it, concluding that it reflected Dr. Walker's "peculiar views." But private letters and diaries indicate the impact such works actually had on women in the country. One young woman from Washington, D.C., who signed her name only as "Winifried," was representative. She wrote to a male cousin, offering her own review of *Hit*: "I must say it is one of the finest Works I have ever read. It treats on Love & Marriage, Dress reform, Tobacco the most degrading habit man ever had because in time will ruin Soul & body, as it generaly leads to every other Vice, Temperance, Womans Franchise, Divorce, Labor & true Piety—it Wholely treats on Virtue, Morality—and the Beauties of Woman & Temperance and I ask as a special favor to speak of this book & get Subscribers, and by Writing the Dr. She will give you all the information wanted. Please do so." For Winifried, Mary achieved her goal of using the written word to increase commitment to the cause of woman's equality.[30]

It had been an extraordinary four years since her return from England. These years set the stage for her vigorous activities in the rest of the decade, which would be some of the most important in suffrage history and in Mary's life.

CHAPTER 9

Women's Rights Unmasked

In April 1871 a reporter for the *Washington Gazette* assumed that, if a woman's political party arose, Mary would be its presidential nominee. Mary proudly identified for the reporter four necessary qualifications for the presidency, which she met; readers would readily have recognized a critique of the abuses of power in President Grant's administration. She had admired Grant during the war and was saddened and then angered to observe what she felt was his moral fall due to alcoholism and political corruption. First, she told the reporter, if elected she would be able to make a fifteen-minute speech "without being held up and prompted." Second, she would entertain dignitaries "without strangling them by the fumes of a cigar puffed in their faces." Third, she would not descend to nepotism in government appointments. Fourth, and especially biting, was her assertion, "I have no taste whatever for gold speculations for robbing the Treasury," a reference to Grant's brother-in-law and the infamous "Black Friday" financial panic of 1869.[1]

In the interview, Mary discussed the major political crises of the day and admonished the administration's plans to annex Santo Domingo. It was the beginning of her fight against U.S. imperialism that would culminate during the Spanish-American War. In this instance, her criticism was more pragmatic than theoretical. How could the government justify spending money on annexation of a country when the United States' own soldiers and "suffering women" had yet to be given their due reparations? Like many opponents of Grant's plan, Mary believed that annexation was less about the proclaimed need for protection from foreign intervention and more about political profiteering. As the next presidential election loomed, the numerous suffrage groups were preparing for a battle they knew would either advance their cause or be a setback of major proportions.[2]

Mary and Belva Lockwood spent the winter of 1870–71 actively planning a suffrage campaign through several venues. Much of their work in these months was done in concert with the CWSB. Its members worked on many fronts: they sponsored a class at the Free National University in which women could study law, pushed for legislation relating to woman's suffrage, and soon would offer their support to the controversial Victoria Woodhull. Members believed that if they could gain the right for women in the nation's capital, they could more easily expand their efforts to the rest of the country. In March 1871 a bill moved through Congress that would deny residents of Washington self-governance. Mary and other members of the CWSB began to argue that the bill should not be thrown out but rather amended to grant all citizens in Washington, including women, the right to vote. A mass meeting in opposition to disenfranchisement for residents of Washington was held on March 17, and a committee was appointed to navigate the bill through Congress. As the meeting ended, participants began to call for Mary to speak. She pointed out to the largely male audience that men in Washington were being confronted with what women had endured their entire lives—disenfranchisement.[3]

When the bill for home rule in the District of Columbia was defeated, petitions were drafted for election officials that called for women to be registered as qualified voters in the districts in which they lived. Mary, the Lockwoods, Sara Jane Spencer, Josephine Griffing, Dr. Caroline Winslow and others orchestrated another march to the Board of Registration. Frederick Douglass joined them in the Marshal's office. With Mary and Belva at the front, the group maneuvered their way through the crowd of surprised male voters who had come to register. A large contingent of suffragists filed into the courtroom in front of the clerk's desk. Signers of the petition included two African American women, Amanda Wall and Mary Anderson, and literary women such as Grace Greenwood and E.D.E.N. Southworth. It read: "We, the undersigned citizens of Washington, believing it to be our solemn duty, a part of the allegiance we owe to our Maker, to our country, and to our homes, to exercise the elective franchise, hereby earnestly petition that our names be registered as qualified in our several districts." Carefully crafted to exert their rights both as citizens—a status denied women under the Fourteenth Amendment—and yet holding to the "feminine" verbiage of "home," the petition was succinct in its demands. Informed that it was illegal for the clerks to register them, Mary and Belva asked that each woman be allowed to complete an application to register so their names would be recorded, and the clerks obliged. Mary made a brief speech while the women filled out their applications:

> Gentlemen: These women have assembled to exercise the right of citizens of a professed-to-be republican country, and if you debar them of the right to register, you but add new proof that this is a tyrannical government, sustained by force and not by justice. As long as you tax women and deprive them of the right of franchise, you but make yourselves tyrants. You imprison women for crimes you have forbidden women to legislate upon.

The effort was a preliminary gesture before appealing to the courts to recognize women's right to vote. Accounts of the event appeared in numerous newspapers over the next month. Most papers refused to print the petition and many reported that Mary had "violently" denounced the registrars or that the clerks had responded with "a very wicked joke" about whether or not the petitioners met the qualification of being male citizens. The false reportage of Mary's violent behavior was the beginning of a decades-long problem. She could become heated in an argument, but stories about her supposed violence—hitting men, boxing a man's ears, punching a man in the face who was smoking a cigar, etc.—became an effective means of diminishing her demands for women's equality by positing them as the ravings of a lunatic woman. In May, Mary attended the NWSA convention, joining Stanton, Anthony, Hooker, and new participant Victoria Woodhull as speakers. Isabella Beecher Hooker gave the opening comments, during which she reaffirmed Mary's and Belva's actions and deprecated the fear some women felt about going to the polls to register. Mary, Lucretia Mott, and others made short speeches in support of various resolutions. It was a successful meeting in which Stanton, Anthony, Hooker, and Mary acted in accord.[4]

The momentum of the April petition drive and the May convention was not to be squandered. Mary and Belva thrived in their work together in these years. They lectured, met with legislators on the suffrage question, and encouraged women to register at the polls in their districts and demand the right to vote. Col. Thomas B. Florence, editor of the *Washington Sunday Gazette*, followed the report on Mary's activities at the registry by inviting her to become a special correspondent for the newspaper. Long having desired to be a journalist, she gladly accepted, and traveled to New York to report on the work of women's rights activists in that state. She would write periodically for the *Sunday Gazette* for the next several years. In late July, she stopped in Oswego to see her family for a short but much-needed rest; while there, Lockwood sent her receipts for the sale of *Hit*. Theirs was a friendship rooted in the drama of causes. Mary sent her articles for the *Washington Sunday Gazette* to Belva so she could deliver them personally to Colonel Florence, and Belva reported on revising her own recent speech into a pamphlet. While Belva acted as an intermediary between Mary and Florence, Mary in turn aided Belva's husband with legal business in New York. The power of this friendship sustained the two women as they worked tirelessly for women's rights and contributed to the broader movement in ways similar to the friendship of Stanton and Anthony.[5]

Mary remained in Central New York through September. She involved herself in the Farmer's Club and Oswego's Agricultural Society, where she gave a well-attended lecture. She traveled nearby for lectures in Fulton and Rome, and in August she participated in one of her favorite annual events, the Oswego Town Fair. The previous summer Mary had offered a prize of "a fine picture" to the woman over age sixteen who had performed the most notable "act that required the greatest amount of moral courage." This year she created an exhibit that displayed the long history of women's contributions to American culture: maps executed by a woman in the 1820s, her grandmother's certificate to teach school from the 1790s, and a 200-year-old warming pan for "women's comfort." She also offered copies of *Hit* for sale. Collecting women's historical artifacts was a hobby Mary pursued throughout her life, and she included one of her own reform outfits in the display to demonstrate the connection between women's history and the present generation. The exhibit, unique in its category, was given a judges' Discretionary Award. Everyone in Mary's family participated in the fair each year. Aurora and her husband Lyman Coats often won awards for canned fruits and best steer, respectively, and Alvah Walker demonstrated his many inventions.[6]

Late in the summer Mary met often with H. C. Stillman, editor of the *Oswego Commercial Advertiser* and a supporter of woman's suffrage and dress reform. By the end of summer they founded a Victoria League in Oswego to support Woodhull's candidacy for the presidency. At the end of September, Belva wrote that one of Mary's articles had appeared in the September 27 *Gazette*, running nearly a full column in length. Belva concluded with a note that she had not sold any additional copies of *Hit* but had given a few copies to relatives. Although *Hit* was not a financial windfall for Mary, it was distributed among suffragists in the States and Europe.[7]

By early October, Mary was back in Washington. The 1872 national convention of the NWSA met on January 10. Mary joined Stanton, Matilda Joslyn Gage, Woodhull, Lockwood, and Hooker as the prominent delegates on the stage. Hooker organized this year's convention, and she presided. While Stanton cautioned about being too enamored of Woodhull, whose radicalism she initially viewed as dangerous, Anthony supported Woodhull's right to speak. The first day of the convention proceeded smoothly. Mary was scheduled to speak in the evening. She began with the assertion that she stood before the audience as a citizen of the United States. She did not agree with Woodhull's call for a revolution to change the Constitution, she remarked. She also countered the racist comments of a man from Rhode Island who had said he supported women's rights because his wife "should have the same rights as the colored man, Irishman, and the heathen Chinee"; they were there to discuss human rights, she insisted. Mary also declared herself to be a friend of the working man and woman, concluding that women would soon have the vote and workers would labor in improved workplace conditions.[8]

The association as a whole was not yet ready to follow Woodhull's ideas, and it endorsed mass efforts for voter registration. Before the convention opened on the second day, the leadership spent the morning presenting their arguments before the Senate Judiciary Committee. Mary led dozens of women to the Senate in support. It was the first major confrontation of the NWSA and the Senate Judiciary Committee. As the women arrived for the scheduled appointment, they were kept waiting and then informed they could not enter. Stanton, Anthony, and Hooker worked the upstairs halls while Mary led a contingent at the chamber doors. When Mary's group was informed they could not enter, she advised her colleagues, "Don't you budge an inch. The women are getting to be a power in the land, and representing, as we do, millions of women, Mr. Trumbull and his committee won't dare to exclude us." After threats of calling the police were ignored by the suffragists, Senator Trumbull acquiesced, and the committee room doors were opened to the women. Hooker, Anthony, Stanton, and Woodhull spoke before the committee. The events of the morning were reported to the convention later in the day, although no mention was made of Mary's efforts to see that NWSA members were allowed into the Senate chambers. Nor was she included as a speaker on the program. Once again audience members began a chant, "Dr. Mary Walker—Dr. Walker!—Walker!" Before Mary could move from her seat onstage to the podium, however, Stanton quickly objected, "Walker is not on the platform, at least not on the programme of speakers. As we pay for the hall we have the right to say who shall speak." It was the wrong tactic to take; her remarks were greeted with laughter from the audience. Anthony stepped forward and suggested they break into groups to discuss raising funds, attempting to shift the discussion, but Mary volunteered to head one of the groups. More laughter followed, as the audience recognized her small victory. The convention closed, however, without Mary being allowed to speak. Ironically, after the convention, Stanton wrote to Lucretia Mott, lamenting the persecution of women who led unconventional lives, naming Wollstonecraft, Fanny Wright, and George Sand. After the convention Hooker also sent Anthony an account of continuing activities: "We have had the usual speeches from Lockwood & Dr Walker all aflame in our first two meetings at Mrs Lockwoods hall—but now we go to our old Committee Room of Agriculture—begun to day—& there will be no further trouble." Suffrage conventions always included controversies, disruptions, and challenges from the audience and among convention leaders. While Mary's relationship with the organization grew more contentious, she was not alone in her tactics or without strong support.[9]

Like hundreds of participants, after the convention Mary pursued the policy of voter registration at local precincts. When Anthony actually succeeded in casting her vote in Rochester, New York, however, she was arrested for the crime of illegally voting. Several women had voted in state elections prior to Anthony's casting of a ballot, but none of them pushed their cases to a trial, as Anthony would do. She rightfully gained extraordinary stature in the movement for going to trial and proclaiming her right to vote. It was a major turning point in the suffrage movement.[10]

After the close of the convention, Mary renewed her efforts on behalf of Civil War nurses, requesting that the U.S. government send her copies of the rolls listing "the names of the women who acted in the capacity of matrons and nurses, and of all the women who were paid by your department for services during the late war." When the auditor for the paymaster general's office responded that it "would require the labor of a clerk for months to examine and prepare such a list as you desire" and thus was not feasible, Mary undertook the arduous task herself. She began by writing to women she knew across the country, asking for details of their military service and the names of other women they knew who had served during the war. Over the next several months, responses poured in. "I was appointed 'Matron' . . . in Judiciary Hospital sometime in the month of April 1861, and served until May, 1865. I only received the small sum of $12 per month for my services there," Mrs. H. E. Speare of Pittsburgh wrote. I was "a volunteer nurse in the Balt° Hospitals during the War . . . as soon as I am able I shall go over myself and get the needed testimony," Sarah J. Carson responded. Julia S. Wheelock recalled that she "gave two years and nine months of gratuitous hospital service during our late war." Mary Gaine supplied a list of twenty-three women she could recall having met while serving as a nurse. On January 24, 1872, Benjamin F. Butler presented Mary's memorial on behalf of "women who labored for the sick and wounded, during the late war" to the House of Representatives. "Believing in the right of women citizens to be heard," Mary's bill asked that women who served for ninety days or more be granted "the same bounties, the same grants of land, and the same pensions, that the United States is giving to the men who served Government as soldiers." There was a second act inserted into the request as well. Mary's lectures since the war's end had often aligned women's right to vote with their service to the country during the war, and the memorial concluded that enfranchisement would not be denied to women who fulfilled the ninety-day service requirement of the first act. Eventually the first act of the bill seeking pensions for women who worked in the military hospitals during the war was granted, though not the right to vote. The women were to receive $20 per month as pensions. It was an achievement that Mary savored throughout her life.[11]

On January 24, Belva and Mary, with a large crowd of supporters, went before the House Judiciary Committee to present a petition for woman's suffrage signed by 35,000 women across the United States. While they were waiting to be admitted to the committee room, Isabella Hooker appeared and insisted that they were acting as renegades and without the NWSA's approval; but as Mary countered, the NWSA had nothing to do with the event. Belva made an eloquent speech as she presented the 240-foot-long document of bound petitions to Representative Butler. The group then moved to the galleries to observe Butler present the documents to the committee. It was a remarkable moment for Mary and Belva, even if it created a greater wedge between them and the NWSA. The interruption of each other's meetings with congressional committees would become commonplace as the various suffrage groups struggled for leadership. In 1881, after Belva had fully joined forces with the NWSA, Stanton and her co-authors of the *History of Woman Suffrage* would praise this document and Lockwood's efforts—and erase from suffrage history the fact that it was a joint effort by Belva and Mary.[12]

Mary also found time during these invigorating days for some lighthearted entertainment. On January 31, she attended a leap year soiree hosted by her friend Professor George T. Sheldon. Mary had a playful side; she loved jokes, and most of all she loved to dance. The evening's dances were titled in keeping with the leap year theme, including the "Grand March—Amazonian" and "Les Lanciers—Leap Year." Subsequent dances included polkas, schottisches, and quadrilles. Mary's dance card was filled by male and female partners for half of the eighteen dances. The evening concluded with a dance called "Galop—Wild Fang," which she danced with a "Little Lady," and the finale, "Quadrille—Line of Battle," with Mr. F. Fothenand. It was an evening of great fun and much-needed revelry after the nonstop campaigns of recent months.[13]

In April, while the NWSA convention in New York was in an uproar over Victoria Woodhull's use of the convention to announce her run for the presidency (with Anthony now fighting Stanton to keep Woodhull off the stage), Mary was fighting another battle. With the success of her efforts on behalf of Civil War nurses, she turned to her own pension case. She had the support of Representative William Lansing of New York, who presented her petition to the U.S. House of Representatives. She sought reimbursement for her unpaid work and for expenses she incurred on behalf of wounded soldiers during her time as a physician in the Washington hospitals and on the battlefield. Lansing asked that Mary be paid $10,000 from the Conscience Fund for her service in the military hospitals. In April, Secretary of War Stanton sent a letter to the Committee on Military Affairs confirming Mary's service. The basis for the claim was that male physicians commissioned as acting assistant surgeons had been granted such funds, and the successful granting of $240 a year in pensions to hospital matrons and nurses left Mary singularly overlooked. Her claim of disability from her months of imprisonment was increasingly relevant; although she would not curtail her day-and-night work schedule, she often had to sit in meetings or convention halls with her eyes closed to rest them. Yet the bill was allowed to die in committee. Over the next thirty years, more than twenty-five bills relating to her pension would be submitted to the House or Senate.[14]

In June, Congress passed a bill awarding a general's widow $10,000 rather than a monthly pension. Outraged again at their refusal to award her a similar amount, especially in light of her military service, Mary immediately set off for the House of Representatives. When the day's business was concluded, she walked onto the House floor and expressed her outrage to various congressmen; she was removed by the doorkeeper. Newspapers across the country reported the incident, with varying perspectives. The *Hartford Courant*, edited by Joseph R. Hawley in the 1860s, had praised Mary's work for woman's suffrage, but under the new editorship of Charles Dudley Warner, it presented a scathing editorial rebuking her actions. She makes her sex "ridiculous," Warner intoned; she is "ludicrous" and "disagreeable." The rage that Mary's actions created in conservative circles was palpable, though a few newspapers referred to her removal as "ungallant and unrepublican treatment." In the midst of this initial battle with Congress on her own behalf, Mary received a letter of appreciation from Alfred Williams, an associate of one of the state's first African American congressmen, Robert C. DeLarge. From the moment DeLarge's term began, he was challenged by Southerners who opposed African Americans in the legislature. Williams referred to charges against him and his associates as false and having been brought about by "political prejudice and partisan hate, as the fact that every man upon the jury was a sworn political enemy, will show." Williams wrote to thank Mary and "your kind lady associates" for the "earnest and kind efforts that you have put forth on our behalf. I was indeed gratified," he added, "to learn from Mr. DeLarge that you had been so persistent in urging and demanding of 'the powers that be,' a proclamation for our emancipation." Williams also expressed his commitment to women's rights. The letter confirmed Mary's belief that the best fight was for universal suffrage.[15]

As the fall of 1872 brought presidential politics to the forefront of national discussions, suffragists struggled to find an appropriate candidate to support. Mary felt that Horace Greeley was a better choice than Grant and his corrupt administration, and she began to campaign on Greeley's behalf. To support him was not an easy choice, since he had abandoned female suffrage, but Mary joined many other Americans in believing he would make real efforts at Reconstruction, and with less violence against African Americans than the current administration had allowed. Suffragists split on the issue: Stanton endorsed Grant, in spite of her attacks only a year earlier against people who did so. Later and with considerable reluctance, Anthony also endorsed Grant, noting it was only because she preferred to "see Beelzebub president than Greeley." On Election Day, hundreds of women in Washington and across the country marched to the polls in an attempt to vote, some singing a revised version of the Civil War song "We Are Coming, Uncle Sam, with 15 Million More." With Grant's reelection, Mary's frustration with the American political scene increased; but the glory of women marching to the polls remained the ideal of her subsequent political action.[16]

Following the differences between Mary and Stanton and Anthony during the elections, interactions at the 1873 convention were more contentious than ever. Beginning on January 16, the convention drew a large crowd that included Mary, Anthony, Stanton, Gage, Lockwood, author Lillie Devereux Blake, and Sara Jane Andrews Spencer. Anthony assumed, not without warrant, that she would be the center of attention at the convention because of her arrest at the polls the previous fall. When she arrived, many members were overjoyed, as they feared she would be in jail for her act of voting. Anthony did not want Mary or anyone else drawing attention away from her agenda for the convention. One major issue set before members was the proposal to form a stock company for a woman's national newspaper. The short-lived *Woman's Campaign* published two special issues about the goals of the paper, which included arguing for women's legal equality and "a more equitable division of the products of labor between the laborer and capitalist." When Anthony, Stanton, Gage, and others met at the National Hotel on January 18 and 19 to write the report of the convention, a dispute arose between Anthony and Stanton about how to represent Mary's role in the report: "Mrs Stanton would not allow Dr. Walker's name to be mentioned in it—I protested but to no purpose—it is precisely the Lucy Stone Boston way," Anthony wrote in her diary.[17]

From the leadership's perspective, it did not help that the first day of the convention was one of the most sparsely attended in recent years. Further, as a resident of Washington, Mary knew many of the local reporters and newspaper editors, and capital newspapers often reported favorably on her activities. The *National Republican* began its coverage of the convention by noting that Mary "had fallen into disgrace with the *ton* leaders of the suffrage movement" but applauded her independence. Unlike Mary, Lockwood was a scheduled speaker at the convention, as she was increasingly moving into line with the NWSA's goals. Mary remained quietly seated on the stage throughout the first day of the convention, but on the second day she stepped up to the podium. Many women not on convention programs used this tactic—Sojourner Truth was one of the earliest—but Mary's yearly use of the tactic was galling to the convention organizers. As she moved to the podium, Anthony hesitated but then introduced her. Rather than turning immediately to the issue of suffrage, Mary made a personal statement. She traced her work for the movement in the States and in England and asserted that because of her international prominence the leaders of the NWSA were trying to ignore her, but she would not be ignored. Further, instead of celebrating Anthony's act of voting, Mary observed that to do so she had to accept the New York law that required swearing to be a male citizen in order to vote. Such actions were stultifying, Mary insisted, and she refused to do so when she attempted to vote in Oswego years earlier. She admonished Anthony, Stanton, and Stone for abandoning dress reform, and for the NWSA's attempt to silence her at the last convention. *She* had not been "cowardly"—she endured numerous arrests for her clothing choice, and she endured disdain because of her courage in continuing to support dress reform and for expressing her own ideas about suffrage. Finally Mary turned to suffrage, discussing women's constitutional rights. She criticized the NWSA's insistence on lamenting the "negro amendments" to the Constitution. Throughout her speech bursts of applause came from the audience, as did some hissing. She concluded by praising her own efforts during the war and, surely knowing it would offend Stanton and Anthony, offered a eulogy to the recently deceased Horace Greeley.[18]

In March Stanton, still furious with Mary for her comments at the convention, presented herself in a letter to Martha Coffin Wright as a martyr: "I want your opinion of conventions . . . I am so tired of them. . . . I endured untold crucifixion at Washington. I suppose as I sat there I looked patient & submissive but I could have boxed that Mary Walkers ears with a vengeance." Undoubtedly her anger was exacerbated by Mary's publication of the *Crowning Constitutional Argument* immediately before the convention. In some ways, *Crowning* was Mary's most important work because her adherence to the beliefs expressed in the broadside dictated the path she took for the remainder of her life as well as her relationships with other suffragists, the press, Congress, and friends. She had thoroughly studied the Constitution and would often claim that she knew the document better than most congressmen. Addressed to the U.S. Senate and House of Representatives, *Crowning* began by referring to herself as a "Women's Representative," exposing both the gendered exclusivity of Congress and her place in the movement. While the NWSA was turning its efforts toward a Sixteenth Amendment that would grant women the vote, Mary's argument was rooted in the belief that the Constitution already included women's enfranchisement and that Congress simply needed to acknowledge that point; thus to seek a Constitutional amendment was to deny women's rightful citizenship. This was the argument that Stanton had made only a year earlier, as had Belva Lockwood, Dr. Caroline B. Winslow, and Dr. Susan A. Edson in their 1871 memorial to Congress, *The Right of Women to Vote*. Many of these texts raised topics included in Mary's document: women had the right to vote in colonial New Jersey, women's enfranchisement was due on the basis of natural rights, and the Constitution did not deny women the vote nor grant enfranchisement solely to men. The difference between Mary and the NWSA was not the goal but the means of achieving it. *Crowning* returned to the point that members of Congress are "*sworn to support*" the Constitution and to deny women the vote was a failure to meet their sworn duties to the nation. Anthony's arrest and trial limited many women's willingness to pursue registration agendas; combined with the new amendments, it forged the NWSA's shift to a constitutional amendment.[19]

Before she had the broadside printed for distribution, Mary gave copies to associates she had known since the early days of her involvement in the abolition movement: Senator Charles Sumner and Chief Justice Salmon P. Chase. Both men praised the document. According to Mary, Sumner exclaimed upon reading *Crowning*, "I am astonished at such an argument being brought to me! I am astonished that a woman's brain has seen the Constitution in its true light as no jurist has ever seen it! Dr. Walker, your Crowning Constitutional Argument will open the door through which all women will walk through and vote!" Sumner asserted as early as 1866 that women would gain the vote "whenever the women in any considerable proportion insist that [the question] shall be settled." The *Crowning Constitutional Argument* would be reprinted at least eight times between its first publication and its final printing in 1916, often with lengthy revisions but maintaining the core of its arguments.[20]

Crowning was presented to Congress on January 15, 1873—the day before the NWSA convention opened—and it received considerable coverage in the newspapers. Mary continued for several years to attend NWSA conventions, but she always worked through other venues as well, and now she focused on efforts in Washington that were spearheaded by the UFA and other local suffrage groups. She was sustained by friends across the country, such as Dr. Preston Day, who was enthusiastically in support of the arguments she presented in *Crowning*. He sent copies to friends and offered Mary sound advice as to the long road on which she was setting out: "*Begin at the beginning*: apply your powers to the voters *en masse*. The Republican Party will probably deny you; the 'Liberals' are sure to reject you; the politicians will wait for the *voters* to push them on. *Ergo*, a long and tedious process of agitation and teaching—not at Washington—but *amid the homes of the people*. This is what I see ahead." He offered encouragement by calling her the "Coming Woman" and "the one who is going to be the next President of the U.S.A.!" Susan B. Anthony was also an astute political activist, and soon after *Crowning* was published, she used donations from suffragists to publish the transcript of her trial. With ten thousand copies circulated throughout the United States, her text overshadowed Mary's—and it placed Anthony as the premier representative of suffrage activism in America.[21]

Mary took Preston's encouragement to heart and undertook a short lecture tour. She also returned to writing at this time, an increasingly important avenue for expressing her medical and reform opinions. Medicine and reform were inseparable to her way of thinking, as demonstrated in an essay on "Smallpox and Dress" she published in the *National Republican* in January 1873. The capital was besieged by cases of smallpox that winter, and physicians were providing hundreds of vaccinations daily in an effort to squelch the outbreak. She argued that a change in people's clothing was necessary to help eradicate the epidemic. "'[F]umigating street cars, filling outside burial cases with chloride of lime, hoisting yellow flags, and enlarging smallpox hospitals'" had done little to slow the disease. Drawing on the medical profession's attention to Benjamin Franklin's experiments with "the difference in the absorbing qualities of light and heat by clothing of different colors," she articulated the need for the public to wear "fine, closely woven fabrics," preferably white in color because they absorbed heat, odors, and "effluvia from without" less readily than did coarse, darker colored fabrics. Infants and laboring men who were typically dressed in dark flannels were particularly susceptible, she argued. Onions should not be eaten, although they could be cut and placed each day in the yards where smallpox cases had been detected because they so readily absorbed air-borne poisons. She also recommended carrying bits of camphor gum as an easily transportable disinfectant, part of her focus on sanitary conditions to help abate the disease's spread. Such remedies were commonly advocated by eclectic and homeopathic physicians of this era, and Mary's successes with non-allopathic treatments of disease were sometimes published in homeopathic medical journals.[22]

Mary was back in Washington in time to attend a historic event involving Belva Lockwood. On March 3, Lockwood's long struggle for equal rights as a lawyer was confirmed by her admission to practice before the Supreme Court, the first woman in the United States to gain the right. Mary attended the ceremony, cheering her friend's accomplishment. From there she turned again to pursuing payment for her services in the army, although with little success. One positive event amidst this disheartening process was a letter of support written by Mary's former orderly, Cary Conklin, of whom she had been very fond. He sent an affidavit to the Committee on Military Affairs on her behalf, detailing her professionalism and his pride in being her orderly. Wisely not waiting for her own pension to be approved, however, Mary decided once again to pursue a government position, with the support of Francis E. Spinner, treasurer of the United States. Spinner had been treasurer through the Lincoln, Johnson, and Grant administrations and thus knew Mary's work during and after the war. As the spring advanced, she felt increasingly hopeful of finding full-time employment. If she could work as a clerk at the Treasury, she could still hold office hours for her patients in the evening and somehow she would find time to write and lecture. When the process seemed to stall, she went directly to President Grant's office, but he refused to see her. In response, Mary began to appear at the White House on a daily basis. Still she was pushed aside. To make her point, she decided to become a very public thorn in Grant's side. She bought a gas stove and camped out in the East Room, cooking her meals on the small stove. Nineteenth-century Americans viewed the White House as the property of the people and believed every American should be able to make himself or herself at home there, but Mary's gesture was more "at home" than ever expected. As the *Washington Chronicle* reported, "Grant has since that trying time been frequently heard to say that the campaign before Richmond, on the James, was nothing to the manner in which Dr. Mary drew her parallels and lines of circumvallation, and issued proclamations announcing that she intended to fight it out on that line if it took all summer. Grant at last surrendered." His offer of a truce was tainted. He exacted a promise from Mary never to camp out in the building again; only then did he tell her that gaining a position in the government was contingent on her wearing a conventional dress. Of course Mary refused; yet she had given her promise and she never again camped in the White House lobby.[23]

Finally, after numerous visits with Secretary of the Treasury W. A. Richardson, Mary was appointed to a clerkship at the Treasury with an annual salary of $1,200. She was sworn in and eagerly reported to the Treasury, only to be blocked by the doorkeepers. Unable to gain access, she began a process of appearing punctually at the office each day, even though she was turned away without fail. As the *Chronicle* noted, "with her profound legal knowledge she well knew that Uncle Sam sooner or later would have to foot the bill." Although she occasionally left the city, she would continue most days to appear at the Treasury Department in the morning, only to be turned away. After more than a year of this pattern, she filed a petition with Congress seeking $900 compensation for the government's failure to pay her. She had been appointed to a clerkship and she had appeared for work each day, she argued; it was not her fault that she was barred from doing her work. The solicitor general of the Treasury wrote a statement agreeing that Mary had been unconscionably mistreated and deserved both back pay and the clerkship, but she received neither immediately. The salary would eventually be paid, but it would be 1882 before she was appointed to a government clerkship and it would not be in the Treasury.[24]

In July she made a short trip to Baltimore, only to be arrested for appearing on the streets in "men's clothing." Her attire in these years was that of a reform *dress*—she typically wore "pantaloons," a frock coat with a skirt that reached below the knees, and a "stylish Mackinaw hat." She still wore her hair in curls or coiled into a bun and could hardly be described as looking like a man, but any form of pants was considered men's attire. Police Officer Ross arrested Mary in her hotel and locked the door to her room, imprisoning her. After her repeated demands, he finally unlocked the door. She immediately filed a complaint asking that he be dismissed from the force; when the Baltimore police commissioners convened to consider the charges, however, they dismissed her complaint. In spite of her arrest, Mary offered a scheduled lecture on the evening of July 24. In "Women's Dress and Men's Rights" she argued for woman's right to choose her own taste in clothing.[25]

She continued periodically to write essays for the *Washington Sunday Gazette*, and her article "Moral Statues" appeared on July 20, 1873. It was undoubtedly a means of releasing some of her frustrations over the way her goals had been thwarted, and letters from friends and acquaintances in response to the article helped as well. B. M. Reese of the national cemetery in Annapolis sent a letter praising her as "a powerfull writer and a deep thinker. But," he added, "the great trouble with you Mary is, You are not popular with those who sit in high places. . . . there is truth in all you assert—but who cares to hear truth from that little nondescript Dr Mary Walker. But don't get discouraged Mary tell the truth and shame the Devil,—no matter what shape he assumes—and no matter if it makes some of our would be rulers squirm at what they term your audacity." But Reese could not forgo adding a postscript: "This is a free Country, and of course you have a right to dress as you please, but it would please me and many others to see you doff them funny looking coat & breeches." Attacks against her reform clothing began to appear again in the newspapers. To add to her troubles, the fall brought news that her application for a pension had been denied.[26]

In the face of these disappointments, Mary used the final months of 1873 to reenergize herself and did not attend the January 1874 NWSA convention. Yet she was still disparaged by Stanton and Anthony, who told reporters at the beginning of the convention that they would get a lot done if Dr. Mary Walker and dress reformer Dr. Hannah Tyler Wilcox stayed away. The *Washington Chronicle* began its coverage of the convention with their assertion, adding, "Just why these two women should be ostracized by the pioneers of this onward movement is unknown." Instead, Mary appeared at a National Sanitary Convention where health and hygiene concerns were discussed. But an event occurred in early January that reaffirmed the righteousness of her long battle with the government. On January 5, 1874, Mary was granted a pension for her military service based on the damage to her eyes while she was a prisoner of war. The pension was $8.50 per month. It was an important acknowledgment and a step forward in her battle for recognition, though the amount of the pension paled in comparison to that awarded to male contract physicians and to nurses.[27]

Her elation at having her military service officially recognized was squelched, however, by a personal attack rendered against her in early February. There were growing tensions between herself and Belva Lockwood over how best to work for suffrage, but their years of friendship had as yet sustained them through their differences, including Lockwood's continuing preference for conventional feminine attire. In February, however, Lockwood's niece by marriage, Lella Crum Gardner, published a scathing attack against Mary: "There stalks about our city unmolested by the police a curious compound of flesh and blood which has the appearance of being 'neither man nor beast,' but altogether ghoul. It is clad in pants cut like a man's, and a half-fitting basquine with a skirt reaching to the knee; a head of short curls is surmounted by a woman's hat. The wearer of the promiscuous dress is called Dr. Mary Walker." Gardner questioned Mary's medical degree, disparaged her claim to be "a *suffering* woman, but tak[ing] no stock in Miss Anthony," and concluded that while she may have a mission, "people have failed to see fruits of her good work." Lockwood's response is unknown, but the friendship was bruised, and it would be many years before the two women fully reconciled.[28]

Wave after wave of setbacks seemed to come in 1874. Mary's request for an increase in her pension, in spite of strong support from the surgeon general and others, was denied. Far more painful was the death of her old acquaintance Charles Sumner in March. His had been an important voice of support for the *Crowning Constitutional Argument* and he was a leader Mary had deeply admired. His death was a crushing blow to the African American community as well. As Sumner lay dying, a group of African Americans surrounded the house, and several black women kept a vigil in the parlor, where Mary joined them. Her action of solidarity was later criticized by the author Gail Hamilton, however, and the criticism was reprinted widely. Hamilton focused on what she viewed as the impropriety of Mary being the only white woman in the parlor.[29]

Perhaps as an outlet for her frustrations on so many fronts, Mary became immersed in the details of the Charley Ross kidnapping in the fall of 1874. The entire country was absorbed by the first case of a kidnapping for ransom. Two men had abducted four-year-old Charley Ross from a street near his home where he was playing. Drawing on her belief that physicians were best educated to understand criminal psychology, Mary began to follow the case and offered lectures on it and criminality in general. Questions about the kidnapping surfaced, but as Charley was not found and his kidnappers remained unidentified, the news story and Mary's involvement with the case waned. It was a tragic event, but the chance to immerse herself in something in which she felt she was helping others was rejuvenating.[30]

In January 1875 she chose to attend the NWSA convention. Unfortunately, Stanton and Anthony had been feuding for nearly three years, though they maintained a public face of congeniality. Anthony resented Stanton's failure to support her during her voting rights trial, and Stanton resented Anthony's ongoing support of Victoria Woodhull. Anthony also seethed over Stanton's greater popularity, when she was the one who managed the day-to-day work of the NWSA; the organization would not have survived without Anthony's unfaltering commitment, as Stanton had attended only five of fifteen NWSA conventions between 1870 and 1879. These tensions exacerbated the conflicts between the two women and Mary. Predictably, the women's differences exploded on the stage, especially as Mary continued her pattern of refusing to be silenced. After Carrie Burnham spoke at the evening session, Mary walked to the podium. Stanton quickly turned to the audience and asked whether Mary should speak or they should follow the program. With the voice votes seeming about equal, Mary started again to speak. The tensions were further exacerbated, however, when Stanton referred to Mary as "Mrs. Walker." "That's not my name," Mary chided; rather than acknowledge Mary as "Dr. Walker," Stanton continued to ask for a vote. Mary asserted that she had not attended the previous year's convention because Anthony had insulted her at the 1873 convention. Furious, Anthony called for another vote, and with a clear majority voting to follow the program, Mary returned to her seat. Many members were unhappy with the refusal to let Mary speak, however, and at the end of the next day's session, Stanton attempted to explain what had happened with "Mrs. Walker," as she continued to call Mary. Under pressure, Stanton reported that Mary would yet have the privilege of addressing the convention.[31]

When Mary spoke, she questioned the character of "some of the ladies on the platform." Anthony knew this comment was directed largely toward herself and asked the audience if they wanted to hear personal attacks. Such a remark opened the door for Mary to ask if the personal abuse against her the previous day was acceptable. Anthony stepped back, and Mary presented a short speech, concluding with a resolution calling for Congress to pass an act defining proper attire for women. Stanton wanted no vote on dress reform and reminded Mary that the committee on resolutions was the proper place for such ideas to be presented. Pandemonium broke out in the hall as some members supported Stanton and some Mary. Anthony finally called the convention to a close until 2 o'clock in the afternoon. During the recess, the leaders on stage gathered together and disparaged Mary, some going so far as to suggest she belonged in a lunatic asylum. They finally left the stage—only to have Mary move to the podium where she read the *Crowning Constitutional Argument*, noting that when she first presented *Crowning* to the convention in 1873, it was omitted from the convention's annual report. Most of the audience members remained in the hall to listen to Mary's speech. After the recess, Stanton announced that all future resolutions and documents must go to the proper committees, and then turned to other business.[32]

During the reading of *Crowning*, Mary uncharacteristically stumbled over a few words, for which she apologized, saying she was not as young as she used to be and that she had difficulty with her eyes. Her eyesight was a constant irritant, but she was undoubtedly shaken by the day's events. Earlier in the day she admitted that she was deeply hurt by the treatment she received from Anthony and Stanton. At the close of the convention, Anthony wrote to Isabella Hooker to give her the details of the seventh Washington convention. It was "a perfect jam of people," she recounts, "with no *single man on the platform*—save the old gent [Ezekiel Lockwood], at whose appearance the *crowd*—the *curiosity* seekers—seemed quite as much amused, as at the artistic presentation of *Dr. Mary E. Walker*—both of whom seemed careful to come on late & to get the most conspicuous seat on platform—." Anthony went so far as to term the small cadre that she saw as the leadership of woman's suffrage in the nation—herself, Stanton, Gage, Brown, and a few others—as "the *elect* . . . who *have* the *helm* of our good *national craft* in hand." Anthony's and Mary's personal animosity threatened to override their commitment to the suffrage cause, but they remained incapable of negotiating a truce.[33]

Mary loved nothing more than to be before the public, espousing her opinions, and after the convention she decided to return to more active lecturing and writing. While most of her writing was focused on political issues of the day, she retained her great love of literature, and her lectures and articles were peppered with literary references. She began at this time to consider how to combine her interest in literature with the need to find a source of income to supplement her small medical practice. Thus on February 28, she published a call for "the well-to-do and appreciative" members of society to help fund a writers' retreat at Watkins Glen, New York. Mary would serve as director of the retreat. Lamenting that "people of brains are not only seldom rich but often actual sufferers for the necessities of life," she presented a romanticized vision of the starving artist: "The sweetest poems, the most thrilling stories, the brightest gems from the deepest recesses of the heart, often come to light in garrets where the comfortable grates in bitter cold days are only things of fancy, portrayed with hands so chilled that the pen at last falls from the grasp, and the refreshing drink from some cool, shady bower is written of in all its deliciousness while the writer is actually suffering in that garret home for a cup of cold water to slake a thirst that the tepid water of the hydrant fails to do." Putting the question in terms of national standing, she reminded her readers that England generously offered pensions to artists, thus it was the least that Americans could do to send subscriptions in support of the writers' colony. She found a reasonably priced house in Watkins Glen with sufficient acreage and a good spring on the premises, conveniently located near a railroad line. It was, she assured her potential patrons, "a lovely and inspiring place both for soul and body." But as with many of her attempts to found an institution, she was unable to attract financial backers to make the plan feasible.[34]

In the fall Mary began a lecture tour to California. She lectured to large audiences along the way, making Ogden a major stop both en route and on her return. She spoke on dress reform in San Francisco, Oakland, Santa Rosa, and elsewhere around the state, explaining that women's clothing unfit them for business and that men would not survive one week under "the terrible tyranny" of women's heavy clothing. Women were bound under "dressical slavery" because they were not educated to the physiological realities of female anatomy. She also connected contemporary fashion to class hierarchies: the wealthy wear these abominable styles and the middle and lower classes believe they must emulate their supposed betters. She concluded the lecture with advice to parents on how to dress children to prepare them for better lives as adults. One day during her travels around the city, Mary was onboard a steamer nearing the Walnut Grove landing when a drunken man knocked a young woman, Katy Barrett, overboard. After Barrett was pulled out of the water, Mary tended to her for two hours, finally bringing her to consciousness. Barrett's injuries were serious, and Mary continued to treat her in the coming days. While in San Francisco, she also had another portrait taken. She was forty-two years old and feeling healthier than she had for some time. It became one of the most popular of her portraits, as she stood erect, with one arm slightly resting on a Greek pillar. It is the last known picture of Mary before she radically altered her appearance two years later.[35]

She needed the strength of conviction in these months. In October, the Supreme Court upheld *Minor v. Happersett*, which argued that the Constitution did not equate citizenship and the right to vote. Particularly offensive was the court's equation of women with children and criminals—all could be denied the right to vote by state legislatures. The ruling fueled the NWSA's insistence that fighting for change in legislatures state by state would be too slow a process and thus a constitutional amendment was the only reasonable course. For many suffragists the decision was the death knell for mass registration efforts, but Mary believed that the most efficient and just way to proceed was to argue against the decision and retain the conjunction of voting and citizenship.[36]

She remained in California through the winter of 1875–1876. Being in California conveniently precluded attending the annual NWSA convention, but more importantly, it gave her an opportunity to experiment with several speeches she was revising. On January 6, she presented "Pure Love and Sacred Marriage" for a female-only audience, and the next night "Woman" for a male-only audience. She had presented versions of "Pure Love" for nearly ten years, and the theme was integrated into *Hit*. The second lecture was the beginning of a series of more forceful ideas Mary was presenting on how men should view women and on the social problems occurring because of male promiscuity. She was planning a second book, and the lecture circuit allowed her to hear responses to her ideas before she published the book. As a physician, Mary was trained to address concepts of sexuality, and her years of practice resulted in an even greater education in the subject. When criticism of her subject matter arose, a rather surprising supporter surfaced: Julia Ward Howe. Although Howe was a member of the AWSA, she was not as conservative on issues of sexuality as most women in the nineteenth century, and her poetry was frankly erotic. The *Atlanta Constitution* published a brief item on January 13 in which Howe defended Mary as "a good, true woman."[37]

When Mary returned to the East Coast, she immersed herself in preparations for the Centennial Exposition of 1876 to be held in Philadelphia. She joined with several women's groups who intended to mark the anniversary with public demands for woman's suffrage, and this preparation drew her to Philadelphia often throughout the year. There she found a publisher for her controversial second book, and she met several influential people, some of whom would become lifelong allies. She quickly became a recognized celebrity in the city as she was seen strolling the streets with Elizabeth Gillespie, organizer of the Centennial Tea Party to demonstrate women's lack of equality in America; George W. Child, editor of the *Public Ledger*; influential businessmen such as A. J. Drexel and John Welsh, president of the Central Board of Finance; the poet Walt Whitman; and political leaders, including Mayor William Stockley. But the Centennial was Susan B. Anthony's shining moment. A public demonstration was critical at this juncture in the suffrage cause, which many felt had stagnated in recent years, and Anthony offered the needed boost to reenergize its forces. After the Declaration of Independence was read in Independence Hall, Anthony marched up to the stage—in spite of being excluded from the program—and presented the speaker, Senator Thomas Ferry, with the Women's Declaration of Independence. She then joined other women outside in reading their alternative declaration.[38]

In the fall, as Mary organized a lecture tour in New York State with provocatively titled speeches such as "Who Dare?" she closely tracked the presidential political scene as it unfolded in Washington. At this time her longtime ally the *National Republican*, under new editorship, began to publish demeaning commentaries about her. All suffragists were facing the problem of political party alliances, and increasingly they would move toward support of the Democratic Party as it began to agree with the call for woman's enfranchisement. If the national political parties faced a contentious battle, Mary was about to do the same at the annual NWSA convention. It was in many ways a repeat of the 1875 convention, and reports that deemed the incidents unseemly were accurate. The convention as a whole descended into a series of lamentations. Much commentary at the convention was tinged with a note of hopelessness. With the presidential election still festering and the arduous labor for women's rights showing few results in spite of the Philadelphia demonstration, the toll of years of endeavor was showing. Although Stanton and Anthony were healing their differences, new tensions were arising between the original leaders of the NWSA and the next generation of suffragists. The leaders perpetuated the idea of their aged status. When they disagreed with younger women, they sometimes referred to them as "babies," and the younger women often failed to respect the decades of labor these women had already contributed to the cause. The younger members wanted to try new avenues of fighting for the vote, some of which were viable and others naïve, but their suggestions were often set aside with the tired assertion that such ideas had been tried in the past and failed.[39]

Through it all Mary remained seated quietly on the platform with Stanton, Anthony, Matilda Josyln Gage, Lillie Devereux Blake, Phoebe Couzens, Belva Lockwood, and others. After several curtailed debates, the convention turned to its resolutions. The call to work for a constitutional amendment was passed, and Phoebe Couzens stepped to the podium for her scheduled speech. Wanting to offer her usual counter to the constitutional amendment, Mary rose from her seat and declared she had a resolution to offer. Instantly, the audience erupted into shouts of "Couzens" on the one hand and of "Walker" on the other. Anthony called for the police to be brought in to arrest Mary, which caused the room to explode with agitated debates about the propriety of such an action against a sister suffragist. When the police arrived, Mary returned to her seat but exclaimed as she sat down, "You are not working for the cause, but for yourselves." This incident had a long-lasting effect on Mary. It was one thing to be arrested by police on city streets, but to have Anthony call for her arrest as a means of silencing her was beyond the pale. She was still writing about it as late as 1907 in a revision of *Crowning*. As always, Mary could have handled the situation more diplomatically, as could have Stanton, Anthony, and Blake.[40]

After the convention, Mary continued her efforts on behalf of suffrage. She submitted memorials to Congress, lectured across the country, gave interviews in which she espoused her support of suffrage, and published numerous texts on women's rights. One petition she submitted to the House in January was later published in the suffrage section of the multi-volume *Great Debates in American History*. But she was now fighting both for and within the woman's suffrage movement.[41]

In early February 1877, Mary turned her attention to presidential politics. The fall voting had resulted in one of the most complicated crises in presidential election history. Mary had supported Governor Samuel J. Tilden of New York, a Democrat, over Rutherford B. Hayes, the Republican candidate. It was a difficult choice for many people as they believed a Democratic win would usher in the end of Reconstruction, yet it would also end the Republican hold on the presidency that had lasted for a quarter of a century. The Republicans' abandonment of suffragists led to Mary's disenchantment with the party and the belief that much of their abolitionist zeal had simply been political expediency. Further, she had known Tilden for many years. His election would have given her unprecedented access to the president of the United States and very possibly the government appointment she had been seeking. She stumped tirelessly for Tilden and was devastated by the electoral process that resulted. Although Tilden won the popular vote by nearly 300,000 votes, the Electoral College favored Hayes by one vote. The compromise that emerged included a specially appointed electoral committee of eight Republicans and seven Democrats to consider disputed electoral votes—and the results were 8–7 in favor of Hayes in every instance. The behind-the-scenes negotiations by Hayes's team had the most devastating effects—the promised overthrow of Republican control in South Carolina and Louisiana, which meant the rapid disenfranchisement of black men in those states.[42]

Negotiations dragged on, and Hayes would not be inaugurated until March. While the negotiations developed, Mary wrote Hayes on behalf "of the women of our common country." Because Congress had failed to pass a bill acknowledging women's right to vote, she reminded him, "we could not exercise the potent '*influence*' of the ballot in the last Presidential election, neither are we called upon to sit in decision with the '*fifteen*' in the complexities regarding the Chief Magistrate of the Nation." It was not only women's fate that concerned Mary. Her outrage grew on the page as she asserted that Hayes had to know his claim to fear for the interest of African Americans under a Tilden presidency "was groundless"; indeed his attacks against Tilden were "unkind, unjust, and unmanly." She prophesied that it was not too late for Hayes to recover "the dome of fame" and righteousness that would "better the conditions of the anxious millions that your party have placed where they are," namely, he could withdraw his challenges to votes for Tilden and halt his attempt to usurp the presidency.[43]

When a call was made by Tilden's camp for Hayes's opponents to assemble in Washington on March 7 to block the inauguration, Mary attended. George W. Julian, a reform-minded Democrat, and others offered speeches. Mary had known Julian for over a decade; he tried to aid suffragists in 1868 by having the term "male" removed from legislation on enfranchisement. Although the anti-Hayes group accomplished little, they did succeed in publicly denouncing the electoral commission. By the end of the month, Mary was involved in another protest, this time a personal one. She had gone to the Treasury building to see the secretary, when the doorkeeper, Walter R. Baker, ordered her to leave the building. Mary exclaimed that she was a citizen of the United States and had a right to sit in the anteroom. Baker threatened to "put her out," so Mary gathered her papers and began to leave. Suddenly Baker took hold of her wrist with one hand, put his other around her waist, and began propelling her out of the building. Outraged, Mary called loudly for the secretary and everyone in the building to see how a citizen of the United States was being treated. She went immediately to the police court and filed charges against Baker. On March 23, Baker appeared before the police court in Washington. He asserted that the previous Secretary of the Treasury Morrill had ordered him to keep Mary out of the building. After Mary recounted the events of her ouster, the court agreed that her rights had been violated and that she ought to be respected in the same manner as all citizens. It was also promised that Baker would appear in court when the case was called.[44]

The *New York Sun* broke the story on the front page of its Washington special and initially reported the incident without bias, but subsequent accounts by that paper and others were dramatized in order to make Mary appear in the worst light. The *Hartford Courant* reported that Mary yelled "go to hell" when Baker asked her to leave; they also said it was a janitor who removed her, thus making it appear that she was the trash being thrown out. Rather than let Baker be brought before a court of law, Treasury Secretary John Sherman stepped in. He sent Mary a letter two days later indicating he had ordered the superintendent of the Treasury building to admit her to all the facilities of the building, but he patronizingly added, "I shall trust to your good sense not to abuse a right which I fully concede to you." Mary responded with a letter thanking him for acknowledging her "citizenship rights," the basis of her argument for women's constitutional right to vote, but she felt a private reconciliation was insufficient. The *Sun* altered its position when Mary sent them a long letter detailing frauds she claimed were taking place in the Treasury Department. They published Mary's lengthy letter and supporting documents in full. After countering the misrepresentations of her behavior and defining it as "in accordance with the purest and most refined womanhood," she wrote that while waiting to see U.S. Treasurer Wyman she inadvertently learned of the fraud by overhearing a conversation between Wyman and his clerk about payments of several hundred thousand dollars. She termed it the "Assistant Secretary of Treasury Conant Ring," thus comparing it to the recent Tweed and Whiskey Rings of corruption. Mary asserted that her knowledge of the corruption was the real reason she was forced out of the building. By creating a scene and then lying about her behavior, they hoped to discredit her in the eyes of Secretary Sherman so he would not believe her charges. The *New York Times* lambasted her for the letter, linking her to Democratic Party values and mocking her as a "(so-called) female." Ironically, by devoting a two-column editorial to her letter, the *Times* gave her claims a far wider audience than they ever would have had in the *Sun*.[45]

Newspapers with Republican sympathies or opposed to women's rights responded by fabricating episodes in which "Dr. Mary" was "on the 'Rampage.'" She was once again figured as an angry, insane woman who might burst into violence at any moment. The satiric *Puck* began to run items about her in almost every issue. Their account of the Treasury building incident had Mary pulling a gun on the doorkeeper, kicking him in the shins, and yelling "murder." But a poet identified only as "Patti" turned the focus onto the excessive actions of government officials as the truly outrageous acts:

The Washington Scare

It is over now, the terror's past,
Those valiant men breathe free at last.
But for a time Hayes' heart was sad,
And Sherman said 't would drive him mad.
So the Cabinet met and talked it up,
And all agreed 'twas a bitter cup,
While Schurz became so down in the mouth,
He vowed it was worse than the "Solid South."
But they faced the worst, these bold statesmen,
And like the Ancient Council of Ten,
Plotted darkly, for there was need,
Since here was a dreadful foe—
Just one *small woman* in bloomers.

Through five stanzas, the poem satirized the statesmen's suppression of Mary and her removal from the Treasury, concluding each stanza with "one *small woman* in bloomers."[46]

With renewed vigor, Mary traveled to New York City in May to attend the spring NWSA convention. In spite of the press corps' frequent disparagement, Mary could at times also manipulate them into serving her own purposes. By inviting reporters to a private lecture the evening before the convention opened, she used them to publicize her ideas, which she knew she would have trouble doing at the convention the next day. Her lecture focused on "The Reform in Women's Dress," but she began informally with what she called "a nice little talk" to set the record straight. She bemusedly noted that Sam Tilden had never proposed to her, as had been reported. Further, she declared, "I don't hate all men by any means. I want to be with them all I can." With the fallacies about her relations with the opposite sex clarified, she began her lecture. On the walls were hung plates and diagrams depicting the deformities caused by conventional fashions. Not one word about the leaders of the NWSA passed her lips. She thereby had her say, which was covered widely by the newspapers the next day, just as the convention began. As she rightly guessed, she was not allowed to speak at the convention.[47]

She did try. Lillie Devereux Blake blocked her way, however, and insisted that she was not welcome at the convention. As Blake anticipated, a reporter for the *World* who was standing nearby detailed the incident in the next day's paper. He clearly admired Blake's "grace and proprieties," "lithe figure," and "tight-fitting dress." His seeming admiration of Blake quickly passed, however. He observed that her actions, with threats of calling the police, resulted in a very cold shoulder being given to Mary by other participants, even though Mary "attempted to converse pleasantly on political and social topics with those about"; as a consequence, Blake came off badly, especially as she complained that Mary was "crazy." The ostracism led to several papers admonishing the NWSA for its exclusionary practices. The *World's* headlines proclaimed the first day to be "a trifling meeting in which Dr. Mary Walker was not allowed to assist," and the *New York Herald*, in an article titled "Woman's Wrongs," belittled the leadership as having used "characteristically feminine" means to "drive this lady from their midst." The manipulation of the press by Mary, Blake, and other suffragists garnered no long-lasting benefits. Infighting allowed the press to report the battles within the movement and to sublimate the suffragists' platforms to the end of articles about the convention, if they were included at all.[48]

The summer brought a reprieve from contentious political maneuverings, and Mary again turned her attention to lecturing and her practice. She continued to travel periodically to Philadelphia for the Exposition. On the 2nd of July, reports of a strange event occurred. Someone went so far as to send out cards of invitation to Mary's wedding to an unnamed "distinguished gentleman of Washington." She wrote a letter to local newspapers denying the news and explaining that it was an attempt to embarrass the man by saying she had refused him. More important was the fact that during this year, Mary donned a more tailored style of clothing. Instead of an overcoat that flared at the bottom like a skirt, she now wore a straight overcoat and straight-legged pants. She also cut her hair in a style popular with men in this era. She sat for a portrait in 1878, painted by A. P. Hubell, and had several photographs taken of herself with her new appearance; it was a change that Mary wanted visually preserved. It was quickly reported that she had donned "fully male" clothing; thus the joke of the wedding invitations was that a man had been refused by another "man." The attacks on her sexual identity grew exponentially. Mary described her radical change in appearance in her usual terminology of a healthy style for an active woman, and she continued to insist that she did not wear men's clothing. But this was more than just a seasonable change of style. Previously she wore long curls, frilly neck ties, and flowers in her hair. These feminine signifiers were now shunned as she dramatically embodied a recoding of gender identity. Although she would occasionally let her hair grow a little longer, she never again wore curls, and she maintained this gender-challenging style of clothing for the rest of her life.[49]

In the fall, good news arrived. Mary's claim for $900 in back pay for appearing for work every day at the Treasury Department was granted. Some newspaper accounts blamed Mary's banishment from the office on other female clerks for protesting against her reform clothing, but she knew that the situation was much more complicated. Solicitor Raynor's notice said that he based his analysis on whether or not Mary had "any just claim for redress upon the Treasury Department"; he found that she was justified in her complaint, as special requirements were arbitrarily set for her that had no basis in government provisions. While it would take more than a year and another House bill before she would finally be paid, Mary was so certain of winning the suit that a month earlier she entered into a legal contract with her father regarding the family property and home in Oswego. The quit-claim deed, signed November 3, 1877, granted Mary rights to the estate for $1,000 with the stipulation that she would give one-half of her income toward her mother's support after her father's death. Owning this property would become central to Mary's plans to found women-oriented institutions over the next few decades.[50]

During the winter, Mary resettled from 919 Seventh Street, N.W., to 1014 F Street, only blocks from Belva Lockwood's home, the local courts, and the U.S. Law Library. It was to be a richly productive year of work. On January 1, 1878, Mary's second book, *Unmasked, or the Science of Immorality*, was published. Although the writing was credited only as "By a Woman Physician," her authorship was soon known since she carried copies with her and sold them with the acknowledgment that she was the author. The book was less an advice book than social analysis, and her decade-long commitment to the emerging field of social science was evident in the book's content and structure. In the same year, Dr. Elizabeth Blackwell published *Counsel to Parents on the Moral Education of their Children* in London. Considered very frank, it was quite sedate in comparison with *Unmasked*. Blackwell did caution against young men's solicitation of prostitutes, but she only remarked in passing on the consequences for women. The major difference in the women physicians' texts, however, was Blackwell's emphasis on the racial superiority of "Anglo-Saxons." Her argument insisted that maintaining the "purity of the race" was central to moral education, and her advocacy of early marriage was to support "the production of a strong race." Mary did not subscribe to the emerging eugenics race theories, and she had a quite different agenda in mind when she wrote *Unmasked*. She intended to expose the double standard in marriage in very explicit terms and then to suggest ways to eradicate this moral disparity.[51]

Although within a decade the shift to a much greater frankness about sexuality would begin to emerge, in the 1870s such discussions were still shocking. Mary believed an open discussion of human sexuality and morality was the best route to enacting change; thus she proclaimed in the opening pages of *Unmasked*, "Knowledge must ever be the basic principle upon which the purest morals are founded." The concept was ingrained in her identity as an eclectic physician trained in theories of interrogation. The book's central theme was that men had become complacent about their devolving moral standards; thus she intended to shine a light on this degeneration in order to help men find their way back to "the right path" of morality, a path that was equivalent to their expectations for female morality. Mary knew the dangers of making the kinds of controversial arguments that shaped *Unmasked*. Anna Dickinson's extraordinarily successful lecturing career was largely ended by her decision to lecture frankly on "Social Evil," and Susan B. Anthony attempted similar lectures in 1874 but quickly returned to "Bread and the Ballot" as her focus—and neither woman had gone as far as Mary in her forthright discussions of sexuality. Yet she was especially pleased that the book "was obnoxious to Mr. Comstock" and proudly proclaimed she had written it to defy him. Anthony Comstock was the self-proclaimed Special Agent for the Suppression of Vice and the man who, in later years, would make the distribution of birth control information through the U.S. mail illegal. His puritanical beliefs included the idea that woman's place was only in the home.[52]

Unmasked established six categories of male codes of morality. At the top was "the code of a pure life, where no sexual wrongs to him or to a woman have ever existed." Few men live up to this code, Mary insisted; if they did, "so much contention, strife, rapes, seductions and murders" would be eliminated from American society. The second code was held by men who "sow wild oats" and then marry "a pure girl," priding themselves on being one of the very best of men. The middling codes of morality included men who discreetly had affairs while married and those who boasted of their multiple extramarital conquests, with no regard for the women they seduced and sometimes impregnated. In the fifth category were men who visit houses of prostitution yet think of themselves as moral because they did not seduce the women or invade other men's families. At the bottom of the scale were sexual predators who were "constantly on the alert for victims." These men had no boundaries: "Rapes are committed by them and even small girls are victims." (In later sections, she discussed sexual predators of young boys as well.) With this exposé as the opening caveat of *Unmasked*, Mary turned to an extended argument advising men how they could abandon their own debasement and that of their female victims. The first step was to rein in sensual motives in favor of reason; doing so, Mary asserted, would naturally lead to an understanding that "the true position of women is always one of equality with [men] in all the relations of life." Sexual excess created a state of constant unrest, but when men used reason to establish their moral standards, not only love and respect for women emerged but equally so their own "peaceful satisfied condition of both body and mind."[53]

The text as a whole was graphic in its articulation of sexual intercourse, anatomy, and bodily functions. At times it descended into archaic myths and yet at other times captured the advances in medicine's attitudes toward and knowledge of human sexuality. Chapters were devoted to "Hymens" and "Seminal Weakness" and to discussions of masturbation, menstruation, and other aspects of bodily knowledge. Perhaps most surprising was the chapter on hermaphrodites—a groundbreaking text, as no woman physician had written openly on the subject of hermaphroditism prior to the publication of *Unmasked*. Mary approached the subject with a certain level of sympathy, but she also claimed that hermaphroditism was a product of licentious antenatal conditions. Having had patients who were hermaphrodites, she based her claims on observations of their histories, and her interest in relating these histories was to assert that "[h]ermaphrodites are but legitimate results of abuse of either or both soul and body. No woman's body *can* be abused without a suffering of soul, and *vice versa*." In labeling hermaphroditism as "this strange freak of nature," Mary presented the dilemma of her analysis: as a medical professional, she could objectively describe the physical conditions, but as a woman activist outraged at the common occurrence of sexual abuse in marriages, she drew conclusions on a social rather than medical basis and used the denigrating phrase "freak of nature" common among physicians in these years—a term that had often been used against her.[54]

The purpose of the chapter was to admonish men into changing their moral behavior: "Men will be better when the true principles of social life are fully *unmasked*." The chapter on hermaphrodites came early in the text. The issue of greatest concern in *Unmasked* was the transmission of venereal diseases to the wives, mistresses, and children of profligate men, and Mary cited statistics that one-fourth of infants who die before age one suffered from "some syphilitic taint." Her concern with the medical and social problems of sexually transmitted diseases emerged during the Civil War, when all battlefield physicians learned to confront the issue. During the war, the proliferation of syphilis among the troops reached such epidemic proportions that at one point General Rosencrans ordered the removal of all prostitutes from Nashville and other areas. Much attention in *Unmasked* was given to barrenness as a result of syphilis, and the longest chapter in the text was that on "The Social Evil" of prostitution. Men could not write properly on this subject, Mary insisted, because they continued to believe that women's passions were not as strong as men's. In reality, she asserted, the path that often leads to prostitution for women begins with curiosity about sexuality and their "natural instincts." Woman's menstrual cycle was designed to have monthly intensifications of sexual excitement "that every month gives new power to vaginal nerves"; thus women's passions were at times greater than men's. One need only examine women's willingness to undertake "all the risks of passing through the agonies of abortions" to understand the strength of their desire. "We must take human nature as we find it," she insisted, "and then try to make the world better by lessons of history, observation and experience." Most women were saved by relying on "moral sentiments," not by a lack of sexual desire. In asserting the reality of women's sexuality, Mary denied men the premier avenue through which they excused their promiscuity. If the majority of women were capable of rising above their passions to live moral lives, so, too, were men.[55]

For those on the other end of the scale of human behavior, Mary showed little mercy. "The only just way to deal with a man guilty of rape," she asserted, "is to *castrate* him." A prison sentence would not change his habits, and he would continue to symbolize for young boys that physical force was the means of ruling over women. She also insisted on the legitimacy of the concept of marital rape and went so far as to claim that it was the basis for the majority of births. One solution she offered against rape for married and single women was dress reform. Current forms of dress for women debilitated their bodies and, in physical misery, lessened their mental strength, thus leaving them vulnerable to rape, she asserted. Mary was never satisfied with merely pointing out social problems. She advocated that women learn the power of fighting a rapist by aiming for the attacker's scrotum. Such knowledge was woman's "power of protection"—an assertion that challenged the conventional idea of man as woman's protector. "Men will never have just laws," she intoned, "until women physicians are the great councils of the nation." The text included illustrations of her own design of a reform dress, and she offered testimonials on the correlations between dress and social evil. Letters from men and women physicians, concurring with her opinions, were printed in the text, as were letters from dress reformers and their supporters such as Mary Tillotson, William Lloyd Garrison, and Lucretia Mott.[56]

Unmasked concluded with a chapter on "The Language of the Nerves." Mary's goal was to have convention shift from the male to the female as initiator of sexual intercourse: "If men were better informed in regard to women," that is, to the construction and sensitivity of the vaginal nerves, "they would understand how it is for their own physical and mental interest to respond to a wife's call, as the ruling power in all relations." Indeed, the "whole question of the essential part is settled by *woman always having supreme control of her person.*" It was her hope, she concluded, that "through this little volume" women would live under better conditions in the future. If this should occur, she could then "feel that [my] earthly life has been one of noble effort." It was Mary's most thorough argument for a woman's right to control her own body and for men to make active efforts to improve their moral character.[57]

Mary attended the annual NWSA convention in January 1878. It began, however, with a women's prayer meeting, presided over by Isabella Hooker, at which a large contingency were anti-suffragists. Thus, when Hooker opened the floor to anyone who wished to express her sentiments, she was immediately challenged by a regular disrupter, Mrs. Frank Churchill, who charged Hooker with holding a political rather than prayer meeting. Churchill claimed the NWSA was preaching Woodhull's free love and that the passage of the Fourteenth and Fifteenth Amendments had enfranchised African American women while she, a working-class woman, struggled and sacrificed to survive. Pandemonium ensued. Hooker and Dr. Clemence Lozier attempted to calm the crowd, but Lozier's frustrated claim that Churchill was insane and should be removed reignited the chaos. Finally, a chant arose demanding Mary take the podium. Hooker, Lozier, and the other scheduled speakers resisted, creating even more vehement calls for "Dr. Mary." The stage was now a mass of bodies arguing about how best to control the situation. Mary rose from her seat, walked to the podium, and when she was blocked by Hooker and others, pulled up a chair, stood on it so her head at least could be seen above the others, and gave a speech on women's rights in which she called on African American women to vote in the next presidential election because they were enfranchised by the Fifteenth Amendment. Hooker, Stanton, and others finally left the stage, and the morning session ended shortly thereafter. In spite of this event, the rest of the convention proceeded without major incident.[58]

On January 16, 1878, Mary and her friend Mary Tillotson were joined by Mrs. Napoleon Cromwell of Alabama at a hearing before the House Judiciary Committee. The women urged Congress to move in favor of women's enfranchisement and to recognize that the Constitution already included women as citizens. There was no objection this year from the NWSA leadership when Mary and others worked separately on behalf of female suffrage. On January 28, Mary and Sara Jane Andrews Spencer were granted a hearing before the House Subcommittee on Territories, during which they argued against a bill that proposed disenfranchising the women of Utah. Spencer, like several other NWSA members, remained friends with Mary in spite of her challenges to the organization. The purpose of the bill that concerned them was purportedly to suppress polygamy, but as Mary and Sara argued, it would only suppress women and have no impact on the practice of polygamy. They had a carefully orchestrated plan of protest: Mary argued that Congress should not interfere with polygamy because it was, from a psychological standpoint, superior to monogamy. Although it was a social evil, it was a more enlightened phase than that of monogamy. Spencer then argued that it was audacious for the members of Congress to disenfranchise polygamists when so many of the politicians were "practical polygamists." The latter was a charge that Mary had also made in her discussions of male promiscuity. The backlash was swift. Days later, when Mary's bill requesting an increase in her pension was presented to the House Committee on Invalid Pensions by Representative Haywood Yancey Riddle (D-Tennessee), it was tabled. It was the briefest report to date, simply saying that an increase would be a special act specific to her and that such increases should only be made by general laws applicable to everyone. The decision conveniently ignored the fact that Mary's pension rate was unique in the system—far less than any male contract physician received and less than half of what female nurses received. Again, newspapers reveled in her loss. The Marion, Ohio, *Daily Star* went so far as to joke that her tailor had sewn her pants the wrong way, with stripes going round the leg, and she was arrested "as an escaped convict," implying her demands for equality were criminal. Although she applied annually, it would be twenty years before she would be granted a pension increase.[59]

Mary moved on to another issue that was about to shock the American public. She decided to apply for a position as an officer with the Washington, D.C. police force. As she explained in an interview with a *Washington Post* reporter, she was disgusted with the treatment she and other dress reformers received at the hands of policemen. She was so well known in Washington that she was never arrested there, but many policemen turned a blind eye to the abuse she and other reformers endured. She was often insulted in public by boys who yelled for her to "Take off your pants" or "Pull down your vest." To stop such abuse, she applied to the force. The petition read:

> *To the Honorable Board of Commissioners of Metropolitan Police of Washington:*
> GENTLEMEN: I hereby make application to be appointed a special policewoman on the Police force of this city. I claim that I am the only woman in the United States that is qualified to hold such a position, as I am the only one who ever held a commission in the United States Army, having been honorably discharged as a contract Surgeon in the regular Army at the close of the war.
> MARY E. WALKER, M.D.

The Board informed her she could speak on the issue at their March 7 meeting. That morning, she published a long letter in the *Washington Post* detailing her qualifications for the position. She asserted that women in the capital "demand that I be a Policeman, upon the ground that they have a right to have 'a protector' that fully comprehends the importance of woman's necessities." She offered to hold a dual role—women's protector and police surgeon of the District of Columbia. As the latter, she would offer free medical service to policemen and their families, and she argued that it was the duty of the government to serve police officers by providing a police surgeon. She sympathized with the financial strains of policemen and their families and argued that their wives and daughters would be healthier if they wore the reform dress. With young thugs' attacks on the increase and their apparent freedom "to insult women old enough to be their mothers and grandmothers," the need for a woman police officer was urgent. She concluded her argument by condemning the Washington press corps for its role in "these outrages" and called on them "to make the *amende honorable*."[60]

That evening Mary spoke before the Board of Metropolitan Police Commissioners. She made her arguments, recommended that they all read *Unmasked*, and concluded with the offer of free medical services for the police: "Think of it sincerely, gentlemen, and I trust you will grant my request." They did not; but she had exposed their failure to curtail the harassment from men and young boys. The combination of her application and the publication of *Unmasked* resulted in a continuing backlash—from the press and soon from the police and the sensational but extremely popular *National Police Gazette*. Press releases increased their sexualized attacks against her. The *Washington Post* ran a poem, "When Mary Walker is Policeman," in which she was depicted attacking a young boy who had thrown mud on her. The poem ended with the victory of the boy who tears her clothes half off of her. "Stay, Muse," the poem's last line read, "this is too much!"—not the boy's action, but the naked body of Mary Walker. It was the beginning of a years-long open season on Mary by the press, describing her as partially naked and her body as too horrible to contemplate. The *New York Times* shockingly declared, "We must have both men and women, and we must resist any attempt to combine the two sexes in one person, as Dr. Walker has attempted to do. *Her trousers must be taken from her*—where and how is, of course, a matter of detail—and, henceforth, clad in the garments of her native sex, the refeminized Dr. Mary Walker will no longer *tyrannize over men* with her lofty claims to exercise the joint and several rights of men and women." It was a blatant call for violence against Mary's person, and it was not the only such call to be published. The *Burlington Hawk Eye* looked forward to the time when "some man will just haul off and give her the most he-awful old kick." Persons committing acts of violence became the heroes of the anti-suffragist and anti-dress reform newspapers' commentaries.[61]

For the first time in her life, Mary became seriously ill and was hospitalized for several days, after which she left Washington to stay with her Aunts Mary and Vashti Walker who lived in Greenwich, Massachusetts. Their home had long been a place of refuge for her, as she visited them most summers. By early June she recovered, but it was the beginning of several serious illnesses, almost all linked to exhaustion, that would beset her in middle age. It was then that the most blatant response to her application came from the police. They made it publicly known that they were considering suppressing the sale of *Unmasked* on the charge that it constituted "broad vulgarity." Mary wrote a note to Samuel Tilden asking to meet with him, apparently to seek legal counsel if the police pursued the suppression of her book; but the danger passed with no formal action taken against her.[62]

Before returning to Washington, Mary attended a Spiritualist camp meeting at Lake Pleasant, Massachusetts, where male speakers denounced Old Testament Christianity in favor of "the Human Divine." Spiritualism continued to attract a large following, with nearly five thousand people attending this sixth annual gathering. Mary's interest in Spiritualism included the desire to communicate with her deceased sister, Luna. At this meeting, the president of the association denied her and several others the right to speak, so she gathered a large crowd around her at the end of the formal meeting and made her comments there. She was also vocal on what she felt was a questionable moral atmosphere at the camp and spoke in favor of "a pure and holy life." Mary's critics rarely understood the high moral standards she set for herself and for the nation. Living a "pure life" was a major aspect of her personal creed, and she believed the way to achieve that standard included personal integrity and working for justice for all citizens.[63]

CHAPTER 10

The Courtroom, the Legislature, Party Politics

In the fall of 1878, Mary was forty-six years old and thriving in her activism as she worked to advance numerous causes, participated in Washington suffrage organizations, and lectured throughout the country. She was well known in the halls of Congress, and she focused her writing on petitions, pamphlets, and letters to newspaper editors. In mid-November Mary undertook a short lecture circuit that began in Connecticut, where she spoke in favor of dress reform, suffrage, and greenbacks (paper money). She supported the maintaining of paper money as opposed to a specie-based monetary system because the latter held the danger of allowing the government to limit the value of wage labor. Keeping greenbacks in circulation, many believed, would aid both small businesses and farmers.[1]

While in Connecticut, Mary visited an old friend, Dr. Lucretia Bradley Hubbell, and she wrote again to Samuel Tilden. "I have been among the New England hills for some time gathering strength, and preaching as well as practicing," she related, but quickly moved to the purpose of her letter: "I need legal counsel that is of the highest order, and hope you will advise me without a *retainer*." In spite of her concerns, opponents were never successful in suppressing *Unmasked*. In late November she left Connecticut to continue her lecture circuit into New York State. Once again, police harassment confronted her in New York City. On December 5, Patrolman Lawrence Flannery stopped her, demanding to know if she was a man or a woman and what business she had in the city. Mary aggressively asserted her right to walk in the city without being harassed, but she was arrested and "dragged through the streets" to the police station. When asked her name by the sergeant, she defiantly replied, "Dr. Mary Walker, American citizen, and old enough to take care of myself," upon which she was taken to headquarters and escorted into Superintendent George Walling's office. Mary knew the law and emphasized that she had committed no crime and therefore had been illegally arrested. She also insisted on bringing charges against Flannery. The usual process played out:

Walling agreed that she had committed no crime and dropped the charges, but her suit against Flannery was also dismissed.[2]

By January 1879, Mary was back in Washington. She continued to house her medical office in her rooms at 1014 F Street, N.W. and ran a large-print notice of her practice in the city directory. Along with her medical practice, a new aspect of Mary's political activism began this year when she became immersed in a criminal case—the Charley Ross kidnapping, which initially attracted her attention in 1874. At the time, Pinkerton Detective Agency sought leads by distributing a flyer across the Northeast and mid-Atlantic states. Profiting from the situation became widespread. A song, "Bring Back Our Darling," quickly appeared with sheet music available for sale, and several books were published on the topic. A police informant told Superintendent Walling, who was heading the investigation, that his brother William Mosher was a known burglar who had once proposed a similar plan. He believed that William had an accomplice, Joseph Douglas, and noted that Mosher's sister was married to a policeman, William Westervelt. Walling brought Westervelt into the case and secretly watched to see if he was involved, as Westervelt's searches always ended with a failure to trace Mosher and Douglas. Charley's father, Christian Ross, began to receive messages that indicated the kidnappers were in New York City. When the father finally decided to meet the kidnappers' demands, against police advice, all communication from the abductors stopped.[3]

In December 1874, Mosher and Douglas attempted to burgle a Long Island home and were shot by the homeowner. Mosher died instantly, and Douglas purportedly confessed that they had kidnapped Charley but only Mosher knew where the child was, and Charley was never recovered. The police then turned their attention to Westervelt; in spite of little evidence, he was convicted on conspiracy charges. But the events surrounding the child's disappearance did not end. Publications of true crime stories thrived, and in 1876 Christian Ross published *The Father's Story of Charley Ross*. By 1878 the story was waning, when Ross published a reprint of his book and gave lectures on the case in Boston. Suddenly the story was front-page news again, and Mary's involvement was part of the attraction.[4]

The *Boston Globe* printed a tantalizing front-page story about Mary's theories, and newspapers throughout the nation reprinted the account. Mary observed that the case was lucrative for many people who had published articles and books on the subject—including Charley's father. She asserted that the child had not been kidnapped and that his parents knew where he was from the beginning, a charge that had been made by a number of people since Charley's disappearance. It was a fraud perpetrated for monetary gain, she insisted, noting that the Rosses were impoverished when Charley was supposedly kidnapped, but with the money donated from sympathetic people around the world, they were now comfortably situated. Like hundreds of others, she claimed to have seen Charley, but she added details of his whereabouts for the past five years. The most newsworthy aspect of her charges was that there were telegrams naming the child that could be tracked to the various locales where Charley had been hidden. The

National Police Gazette was critical of her efforts but noted that "beyond circumstantial evidence and the dying declaration of Douglass [sic], there was little proof that he and Mosher stole the child." In spite of Mary's assertions, Charley was never located.

As a physician, Mary was interested in the psychology of the criminal. Drawing on her medical experience and legal training, she believed that physicians were the best interpreters of whether or not a criminal was insane—a position she asserted as early as 1866 when she attended the Manchester Social Science Congress—and it was a topic she would pursue through many legal cases over the next several years. To educate herself further in criminal legal procedures, she began attending the District's criminal court sessions. Carrying a large portfolio, she took copious notes on the proceedings.[5]

In addition to her medical interest in criminality, Mary continued to be a recognized presence in the political circles of the capital. She frequently petitioned the legislature for women's rights and her own pension, and in one case argued for women to compose at least half of the jury when a woman was the defendant. She was vocal in opposition to political corruption, but her vocality was challenged when she carried it into the Senate galleries. One such incident occurred at a session in which Senator Zebulon Baird Vance of North Carolina spoke and she tapped her umbrella upon the floor. Instantly, a doorkeeper was sent to the gallery to remove her. When Mary refused to leave, he called two of his colleagues and a police officer to help remove her. By this point, no one was paying attention to the speeches on the floor. Mary braced herself in a defensive position and refused to move from her seat. Rather than use force, the officer remained next to her throughout the remainder of Vance's speech; she did not thump her umbrella again, nor did she leave until the Senate adjourned. Newspapers across the country reported authorities had "wilted" when confronted with Mary's determination. The incident continued to attract attention throughout the summer. Most commentators embraced the attempt to remove Mary, but the *National Citizen and Ballot-Box*, a newspaper edited by Matilda Joslyn Gage, came to her defense. Although a longstanding member of the NWSA, Gage was far more radical in her approach to women's rights than Stanton or Anthony. Gage's goal for the *National Citizen and Ballot-Box* was that "[w]omen of every class, condition, rank and name will find this paper their friend," and she held firm to the democratic spirit of the publication when she supported Mary. As Gage recognized, the issue was not Mary's tapping of an umbrella but her unconventionality: "If Dr. Mary Walker or any woman is to be arrested for wearing male attire, why not arrest the Supreme Court of the United States when they appear in their big-sleeved, voluminous black satin gowns? What is sauce for the goose should be sauce for the gander also." The attempt to oust Mary from the Senate gallery was followed by another rebuff in relation to her petition for an increase in her pension. Commissioner of Pensions J. A. Bentley denied her claim, asserting that only a limited amount of money was available for adjusting pensions granted before 1879 and that "some delay may occur in the settlement of your claim." As for so many deserving participants in the war, the delay would stretch to decades.[6]

In these months Mary also outlined a series of articles she was planning to write: "Why 'Unmasked' Appeared"; "American Homes: Wife & Mother Royalty"; "The Marriage Question," which would address Mormonism; "Laws of Heredity," including attention to women's dress; "Black Vomit & Mahogany Corpses," on the causes of yellow fever; "The Near Future," addressing the country's political outlook; "Moral Purity," to which she appended, "Vice rules its little hour, / Virtue late and long"; and "King Tobacco." Not all of the topics would become articles but the issues were integrated into many of her lectures.[7]

Spending at least part of the summer in Oswego was an annual reprieve for Mary from political life in the nation's capital. Summer activities were lively in the area, from meetings of The Old Settlers Society and the Oswego Town Farmers' Club to the county fair, traveling lecturers, and discussions sponsored by the Farmers' Agricultural and Horticultural Society. Her Oswego Town home was often filled with visitors, including working-class women whom she brought to the farm for a healthful respite from their labors and many aging Civil War veterans who still held Mary in high regard. One of Mary's neighbors, Ella M. Carrier, often met the visiting veterans: "all spoke very highly of her and her life in war time, of her kindness to the sick and quite a number told us they considered she saved their lives or limbs." One of Mary's greatest joys was to offer a speech each year to acclaim American independence. As R. S. Ould, owner of the local clothing store from which Mary purchased most of her clothes, recalled, "No Fourth of July was complete without a speech by her." These summer respites always energized Mary; but while she was out of town this summer, the *Washington Post* ran a scurrilous attack on *Unmasked*. The *Post* supported the editor of the liberal *Truth Seeker* who had been prosecuted and imprisoned by Anthony Comstock on charges of distributing obscene material; although the *Post* referred to Comstock as "a bigot, even if an honest man," they turned to contemplating why Comstock had not prosecuted Mary for similar charges. *Unmasked* was, the paper intoned, the "most revoltingly obscene and disgusting book we have seen for a long time" and lamented that it was still being sold by Mary in public places throughout the city.[8]

When Mary returned to Washington, she attended the National Labor Party's convention, and spent the fall and winter engaged in suffrage activities and the ongoing battle for an increase in her pension. She would struggle financially for the remainder of her life; a small pension increase or a lump sum payment would have made a significant difference, but it became increasingly evident that the failure to attend to her petitions was politically motivated. She spent months attempting to negotiate through Congress a bill for an increase; in spite of support from several congressmen, her efforts were unsuccessful. Just as she was again immersing herself in reform work, devastating news arrived: Mary's father had died, after struggling throughout the spring with pneumonia, on April 9, 1880, his eighty-second birthday. He had been one of the most important supporters of his youngest daughter's unconventional life. A local newspaper described him in terms he would have appreciated: "a kind neighbor, a generous friend and a christian citizen." The funeral was held on April 11 at the family home and was attended by a large number of friends and neighbors. Mary's brother Alvah Jr. read a tribute to his father, noting that he did so "without the knowledge or consent of my friends or any other person, and consequently hold no one responsible for what I may say." Alvah Jr. was a difficult man, often at odds with other family members, but his remarks were not offensive. Though he expressed his own ardent agnosticism, he fairly detailed his father's nontraditional faith as a member of the Methodist church yet a nonbeliever in a literal sense of hell. When Alvah Jr. noted that his father had "in him a disposition to except and advocate, regardless of all creeds, regardless of all issues, whatever (in his judgment) was right and true" and that he "was determined to maintain his individuality, a synopsis of which, would fill volumes with interesting reading, and he never allowed another to do his thinking . . . and no popularity or unpopularity, could deter him from expressing that thought regardless of consequences," he unwittingly depicted his youngest sister as well. Mary had learned her father's creed, shaped it to her own needs, and lived her life accordingly—regardless of consequences.[9]

In addition to the loss Mary felt at her father's death, she was frustrated with the progress of women's rights. Suffragists in general were facing increased criticism. An anti-suffrage group, the Remonstrants, was particularly vocal, and political commentaries and cartoons unsparingly satirized suffragists. The attacks did not curtail die-hard suffragists' determination, but it made their efforts considerably more difficult and frightened away many potential participants. While continuing the battle, Mary turned to a new endeavor. She appeared before the House District Committee on June 3 to argue on behalf of the establishment of a home for "friendless women and children." She succeeded in establishing a temporary refuge of this kind during the war, but in spite of many months of urging passage of a bill in favor of the institution by Mary and others, the government declined to act. Tired and melancholy, Mary decided to spend the late summer in her beloved White Mountains and by August was on her way to Lake Pleasant. Her return trip to Washington demonstrated the difference between the ranting, confrontational woman depicted so often in newspaper accounts and the real-life woman who was politically astute and adept at winning over her opponents through charm and intelligence. On the train back to Washington in September, a few male passengers began to taunt her about her style of dress and, seeing that smoking was anathema to her, filled the railcar with tobacco smoke. But when it was discovered she was *the* Dr. Mary Walker, she was asked to speak. It was the only inroad she needed. She quickly gained their attention discussing the laws of health related to her attire and her medical reasons for opposition to tobacco smoking. An account of the train incident was reported in the press, with the following assessment: "Miss Dr.

Walker is a lady of refinement and taste, modest and unassuming, possessed of a tender and sympathetic spirit; a patriot, philanthropist and friend" and that "[a]t Washington, her acquaintance is extremely large. She is recognized and respected in every Department of State." She invited some of the train's passengers to board at the Hillman House Hotel where she was staying and offered them a tour of the city that included an introduction to the vice president of the United States. To complete the enjoyable day, she hosted an evening party with entertainment that included readings and recitations in which Crypti Palmoni, Washington's popular lawyer-turned-elocutionist, participated. The evening was a great success, and the railcar critics left as converts to the merits of Dr. Mary Walker.[10]

A difficult family task was required of Mary that fall: she filed a pension claim for her brother. Described as Alvah Jr.'s "dearest friend," Mary claimed that he was non compos mentis, relating to sunstroke he suffered during the war. The claim was rejected by the Pension Office with the notation that his work habits, appearance, and "mental eccentricities" were little different than before the war. Any change was attributed to advancing age. Mary may have felt that the benefits of such a claim would aid her brother, but it enraged Alvah Jr. Within a few months, he challenged Mary's inheritance from their father's will. The property agreement made with her parents years earlier had been filed with the county court, and all other property, according to Alvah Sr.'s will, was divided equally between the surviving children upon the death of his wife. Alvah Jr., who lived next door to the family home, contested the will, on the basis that he owned the barn on Mary's property. The court and other family members recognized the intent of their parents, and she retained ownership.[11]

As the November presidential elections neared, Mary's attention turned to national politics. Although she still eyed all party politics with caution, she hoped for a Democratic win. The election was widely viewed as a referendum on the Republicans' failure to meet the promise of Reconstruction. Winfield Hancock, the former Civil War general renowned for his actions at Gettysburg, was the Democrats' nominee against Republican James Garfield. Since Mary still believed the best way for women to gain the vote was to appear at polls and demand their rights, she traveled to Oswego and presented herself once again at the polling station on Election Day. When she was told that she did not meet the necessary voting qualification of being a male citizen, she replied mockingly, "I am a fe-male citizen and therefore a male citizen," but she was turned away. Although Mary had not supported the new Republican President James Garfield and his running mate Chester Arthur, her life would soon be intricately intertwined with theirs.[12]

The new year brought an unwelcome reminder of Mary's strained relationship with her brother. He appeared to be the source for a story that circulated in newspapers claiming that Mary refused to support their eighty-three-year-old mother and that Mary was insane. When Mary purchased her parents' home, it was with the stipulation that she would help support her mother and allow her to continue living in the homestead if her father died. She and her mother had always been close, and she welcomed the arrangement; but since Mary lived in Washington most of the year and Vesta's health was declining, Vesta had moved in with Alvah Jr. By making the issue public, he gave her critics more fodder, so it was pleasing to her when the *New York Times* published a surprisingly positive note about her in a front-page article shortly thereafter. Remarking that she had been a "familiar figure in the corridors of the Capitol for several years," the *Times* added, "Dr. Mary Walker is a quiet person in manner and appearance, and it is not easy to recognize in her the subject of the many sensational sketches and descriptions which have been given to the public by those who seem to have found her an interesting study."[13]

In spite of the *Times*' cautionary note about the need for fair representation of Mary's activities, the *National Police Gazette* began a sustained attack on women physicians in general and Dr. Mary Walker specifically. Women physicians were most often depicted in the pages of the *Gazette* as abortionists; nearly one hundred articles on the subject of abortion appeared in the periodical in these years, and the *Gazette* became the champion of the self-proclaimed moralist Anthony Comstock. The *Gazette* argued that a woman submitted herself to bodily dangers when she became a physician. Several articles and full-page illustrations appeared about women physicians who were attacked or murdered; usually the women were reported to have been out on a call at night and thus were charged with making themselves vulnerable. But it was Mary in her gender-challenging attire who struck a particularly volatile nerve with the *Gazette*. For more than two decades, they published items about her and made fantastic stretches of imagination to connect her to any form of what they considered aberrant female behavior. Because Mary chose to dress in pants rather than a skirt, her body became an accepted object of public scrutiny and mockery, with depictions of her as a hybrid male-female. The most common tactic of the *Gazette* was to use her name in criminal cases that had no relation to her. One illustration of a crime, for example, was set in a tavern with a dead, nearly nude man on the floor, a knife in his chest out of which blood was oozing; a young woman—dressed in pants—sat with legs spread apart on a beer keg, holding up a mug of beer while several approving young men joined in the toast. The case had nothing to do with Mary, but the caption read, "The Masquerade of Death. How a Wrecker's Daughter Avenged an Insult and Set Up as a Rival of Dr. Mary Walker with the Proceeds, at Currituck, N.C." In another illustration, a disrobed young woman was depicted as fleeing "a peculiar situation" and holding only a burlap bag to cover her naked body. Although the event again had no relation to Mary, the illustration was titled "Beating Dr. Mary Walker," suggesting only nudity exceeded the impropriety of Mary's attire and again reflecting critics' imagining of her nude body.[14]

For the *National Police Gazette*, as for other periodicals, there was a double bind inherent in this tactic. The emphasis on her physical body conveniently diverted attention from her politics, but it also presented paradoxical assertions concerning her sexuality. She was masculinized and "desexed" on the one hand, and yet the attention to her supposed nude body also sexualized her female body in a promiscuous manner. It was purportedly Mary's choice of attire that gave the periodicals the opportunity to sexualize her, but her radical assertions about the human body and about human sexuality in *Unmasked* undoubtedly played a significant role in their casting her as a public pariah. Because of her threat to such masculine-identified institutions as the police, her body also became a target for their anxieties. Not only was she aligned with the spread-legged, beer-drinking female murderer from North Carolina, but she was subsequently depicted as sexually aggressive or as usurping masculine rights in items that questioned her sex, such as, "It is said that Dr. Mary Walker is anxious to receive the appointment as minister to the Isle of Man." A year later they reported on her visit with the president, depicting her as the only woman hobnobbing with male political leaders; such a visit, of course, had nothing to do with the paper's focus on criminal activity, but to the *Gazette*, a crime had definitely been committed against both femininity and masculinity.[15]

It was one thing to be castigated by a rag such as the *Gazette*, but it was a much more painful experience to have the *History of Woman Suffrage*, written primarily by Elizabeth Cady Stanton, Susan B. Anthony, and Matilda Joslyn Gage, deny Mary's contributions to the cause. The first two of the *History*'s six volumes appeared in 1881, covering the years 1848 to 1878. It was an amazing text in many ways, as it captured minute details covering decades of suffragists' activism; but as Mary, Lucy Stone, and others soon learned, it was also an extremely biased document that sublimated or erased activists who did not adhere to the party-line of the NWSA. Stone at least had been invited to offer her version of the AWSA's activities; she declined, feeling the time for such a history was premature. Mary and many others were given no forewarning about their own depiction in the pages of the *History*. By the *History*'s account of events, Mary had never been on the stage at a convention, never participated in lecture tours, never been an active part of the suffrage cause, and never published books or pamphlets on the subject. In the more than 1,700 pages that constituted the two volumes, she was sublimated to only a footnote and one or two brief mentions. When discussing women who aided the Union cause during the war as nurses, hospital matrons, and in other capacities, for example, the only mention of Mary was in a footnote that observed she was devoted to the Union cause and that she demonstrated superior medical skills. Yet the footnote erroneously asserted that her quest to be appointed as an assistant surgeon was "without success," which the authors knew to be untrue. She was mentioned once in the body of the second volume, in a reprint of Grace Greenwood's 1870 snide remarks about her appearance, and in one brief reference to her assertion that women needed to go to the polls and demand the vote. Such misrepresentations of her military service and of her renowned standing in the movement stoked the fires of resentment within Mary. Subsequent revisions of the *Crowning Constitutional Argument* became more overt in their criticism of Anthony and Stanton.[16]

In spite of these disappointments, Mary conceived of a new way in which she might advance women's rights. She had been involved in New York State politics her entire adult life, and she now more explicitly aligned herself with the Democratic Party. But even the Democrats had moved slowly on the issue of woman's suffrage, so on June 21, 1881, Mary declared herself a candidate for the U.S. Senate from New York. First published in the *Oswego Times*, her declaration was reprinted in full in the *New York Times*:

> *To the Honorable Members of the Legislature of the State of New-York*:
> GENTLEMEN: The undersigned, believing her duty to her native State demands her services in the present exigency, most respectfully presents her name as candidate for United States Senator. She relies solely upon her fitness for the position, as hereinafter set forth.
> *Qualifications.*—Her understanding of Parliamentary rules, the methods of business in the various committees and business generally that relates to the duties of a United States Senator; her ability as a ready speaker on subjects of legislative import; her ownership of a brain that is never made abnormal by the use of anodynes or stimulants; her ignoring attire that destroys health, ruins morals, and deranges finance; her moral courage and moral worth—these combined excellences guarantee both faithfulness, and fitness, and she modestly submits that your honorable body will do yourselves credit by electing her to the position of Senator from the State that she has so long honored by efforts in noble causes. She is most respectfully yours, &c., Dr. MARY E. WALKER

Mary Walker thus became the first woman in the United States to run for the Senate. Her father would have been proud—but state Democrats were not quite sure what to do. Although she could not garner the support of the party for her candidacy, she made an important demonstration of her belief that women's rights were accessible if women insisted on enacting them.[17]

The race for the U.S. presidency in 1879 had been particularly vitriolic. During the campaign Charles Guiteau, an erratic man who had been involved in New York State politics for a number of years, became active in support of Garfield. Thrilled with Garfield's election and believing it would insure an appointment for him in the new administration, Guiteau moved to Washington, D.C. In spite of a seemingly unending campaign of letters to Secretary of State James G. Blaine and others, Guiteau's requests for an appointment went unanswered. If his behavior was erratic before, he now became zealous in his belief that Garfield must be removed from office. On July 2, 1881, Guiteau shot Garfield. Guiteau was immediately arrested and jailed. A cadre of physicians, including Mary's friend Dr. Susan Edson, attended the president, but infections developed in his wounds. He lingered for several months in agonizing pain, dying on September 19.[18]

On November 14 Guiteau's trial before Judge Walter Cox at City Hall began. Although he was sentenced on January 25, 1882, the question of his sentencing lasted until May 22 and became as much about public performances as about the law. George Scoville, Guiteau's brother-in-law, served as his counsel. Guiteau resisted the insanity defense and often countered his attorney in an attempt to speak directly to the judge. Mary's interest in criminals' insanity and the relation of the law to an insanity defense was renewed by the case and by her association with several key players. With Guiteau's conviction, the battle centered on whether or not he would be executed, based on his mental status. Mary joined a number of neurologists who believed Guiteau was mentally imbalanced, and she became one of the outspoken opponents of the execution of the criminally insane. The prosecution had as their primary medical witness Dr. John Gray, superintendent of the Utica State Hospital and editor of *American Journal of Insanity*. Gray hedged on whether or not Guiteau was insane, but he argued that because someone's mind was a "bit off" or he was a "crank," he was not relieved of responsibility, and such a criminal should be punished in the same manner as other perpetrators. Twenty-one physicians testified at the trial for both the defense and the prosecution, with widely diverse ideas about Guiteau's sanity. Gray used his journal to publicize his position, while the *Journal of Nervous and Mental Disease* published trial testimony that supported the insanity claim. Thus Mary stepped into a quagmire of medical jurisprudence; but she had come to the conclusion that the death penalty for the insane was immoral, and she immersed herself in the debate.[19]

"I think it would be a burning disgrace to the country," she declared, "if that man should be hanged. He is a monomaniac on that subject, and he has shown himself to be insane throughout the trial. His hanging would disgrace me and all other citizens." Mary acquainted herself with family members, including the poet Frances Scoville, Guiteau's sister and his attorney's spouse. Throughout the winter and spring, Mary worked tirelessly with Frances in an attempt to halt Guiteau's execution. Both women toured the region in the hope of securing supporters for the cause. Mary offered her services as counsel to Guiteau, who wanted to discharge George Scoville for incompetency, but he declined Mary's help. In the spring Guiteau published *The Truth and The Removal*, his rambling accounts of the second coming of Christ and of his justification for killing Garfield, in which he asserted, "I was God's man to do it." Frances Scoville and Mary hoped to collect enough signatures on petitions to sway President Arthur to their way of thinking. It was an ardently fought battle, but in the climate of the moment, it had no hope of success. On June 28, Mary went to the White House in an attempt to convince President Arthur to stay the execution, but she was not granted a meeting with him. Two days later, Guiteau was executed.[20]

Although the Guiteau trial was Mary's primary focus over the winter and spring, she did not abandon her other causes or her social activities. In spite of the fact that they held differing views about the Guiteau case, Mary and President Arthur liked one another, and she took time out from her activities for her annual attendance at the President's New Year's Day reception. After speaking with Arthur in the reception line, she spent the evening in the East Room, thoroughly enjoying the celebratory start of the new year. She also spent an evening at Ford's Opera House a few weeks later at which the famous medium Annie Eva Fay performed. When there was no response to the call for two gentlemen to sit on the stage to verify Fay's performance was without trickery, Mary rose from her seat in the orchestra section and asked if a lady would do. The crowd was delighted, and thus she and two others became the audience participants. She had a grand time.[21]

In the new year Mary continued to seek government support for the establishment of an asylum for impoverished women and children, petitioning the District Committee for a lot on which such a building could be erected, but the petition was tabled. Equally frustrated at her failure once again to receive an increase in her pension, she admonished the Pension Committee for recommending pensions for the widows of ex-Presidents while the petitions from herself and others who had actually served in the Civil War languished. To specifically name the recently widowed Mrs. Garfield as one of the questionable pensioners did little to advance her case. She decided to try once again for appointment to a government clerkship, and this time she was successful. On May 1, 1882, she secured the position of mailroom clerk in the Interior Department's Pension Office, which added a welcome supplement to her medical and pension incomes and increased the public's awareness of women holding government clerkships—and the appointment came with no demand that she wear a dress. By September, she had received a promotion in the mail division.[22]

In the midst of her success, George Scoville, defense attorney in the Guiteau case, filed a countersuit to his wife's petition for divorce on the grounds of cruelty. Enraged by Frances's charges and exhausted after months of a sensationalistic murder trial, George brought a cornucopia of complaints against his wife, charging her with "unchaste and unwifelike conduct," insanity, and moral depravity. He claimed that she had affairs with five men since the end of the trial, was counseled by George Frances Train to leave her husband, and that she was influenced in her actions by Mary and several men. It was an attempt to defame Frances, as George made sure his charges received national publicity. His defensiveness may have come not only from his dismay over her desire for a divorce but also because she felt that her brother's case had been lost because of George's poor performance at the trial. Fortunately, Mary did not have to further involve herself in the case. It was soon moved out of the public arena.[23]

She spent the Christmas season in Oswego where she gave a free lecture on "Prevention of Throat and Lung Troubles" at the courthouse. When she returned to her position at the Pension Office in early 1883, however, the situation quickly became untenable. Mary had addressed a Women's National Labor League meeting in September, recommending that women seek clerkships in government departments—except for the Pension Office, declaring that working as a clerk in that office "involved a great shock to the sensibilities and moral stamina of ladies." In January her supervisor, D. L. Gitt, sought her dismissal, claiming she had missed 112 days of work in her first year on the job and that she was "high tempered and abusive . . . aggressive and insolent." Mary was undoubtedly an opinionated employee, but her work record counters much of Gitt's assertions. If she had missed as many days as he claimed, it is unlikely she would have been promoted, as she had been in September. Her personnel rankings ranged from 5.5 to 7.0 out of 7.0; a notation showed that she was ranked between 5.5 and 6.5 for speed and accuracy and 7.0 for punctuality. She had no problems with her coworkers; in fact, she aided them as a physician, sometimes writing prescriptions and occasionally lending them small amounts of money. As charges emerged, the political basis of Gitt's attempt to have her fired was also revealed: he claimed that she spoke disrespectfully of President Garfield. On February 13, A. N. Fisher, Chief Clerk, followed Gitt's advice and sent a postcard to Mary at her work station, which insured that anyone in the system could read his admonitions as the card wended its way to her desk. Fisher said it was reported to him that she declined "to perform *some* of the duties assigned you, and *profess* your inability to perform *others*, and it is represented that you are of no assistance to the Mail Division." He declared that he saw no option but to request the commissioner dismiss her, though he would allow her to respond first.[24]

Mary responded in full, beginning with the observation that other individuals who remarked on Gitt's incompetence had been fired. She catalogued the significant number of errors in mail handling that she observed during her tenure in the department, asserting that under Gitt's management, over one hundred errors a day were discovered, including unsigned receipts for special deliveries and addresses with no company name included. Charges flew back and forth, including a claim by Mary that she caught Gitt and a female employee in a compromising position. By May the situation was so strained that Mary was granted a thirty-day leave of absence for illness. Gitt and Fisher were intent on her removal, and on July 13, newspapers reported that the commissioner fired her. Several newspapers hailed the decision, claiming she was fired for incompetence. However, the *New York Times* had undergone a change in editorship in April, and rather than simply publish Gitt's assertions, its reporters now investigated the charges and discovered that, in addition to her high job performance, monthly reports revealed she was not classed below excellent in deportment throughout her time in the clerkship. In an interview that appeared in the *Times* a few days later, Mary said of the firing, "Positively untrue. The newspapers have been talking about it most unfairly and most persistently." The reporter then asked if she thought women would ever be elected to office. "Indeed, Sir," she replied. "I expect to live long enough to be elected to Congress myself. My familiarity with the ins and outs of political life peculiarly qualify me for the position. . . . It is evident that the framers of the Constitution intended to make this a pure republican Government, instead of a half-jointed one as at present."[25]

The media backlash was especially vicious. One Bismarck newspaper claimed that she committed suicide by drowning herself in the Potomac because of "blighted love" and celebrated her supposed death with the headline "Gone at Last." Mary continued to insist that she had received no formal notice of termination, and she planned to return to her position at the Pension Office as usual. She had a handwritten note claiming Gitt refuted his suggestion that she be fired shortly after she accused him of the affair with a female clerk. When she returned to her job after the authorized leave, however, she discovered that she had already been replaced. Since the government could not claim incompetence after her employee records and promotion were revealed by the *Times*, Secretary Teller asserted that she was fired for being an eccentric. Mary wrote to Commissioner Dudley asking for a full investigation based on the unconscionable grounds for her firing, but Dudley forwarded her request to the secretary of the Interior with the statement that he saw no cause for an investigation.

Congress had legislated that discharged soldiers with equal qualifications as other applicants should be given preference in government hiring. Since Mary had been contracted in the service, she felt she was entitled to the same consideration. She detailed the individuals who were given positions in her department, and their salaries—men and women who had not served in the military but were salaried at $900 to $1,200. The document did not persuade her employers. After her dismissal, several clerks were fired when it was discovered they were running a side business in the office, taking money from pension collection agents who wanted to learn the status of particular claims and which ones seemed likely to be successful. Gitt remained in office. Mary would never regain her position, in spite of continuing her efforts for another sixteen months.[26]

During these months, Mary prepared a bill and a memorial to correct errors she observed in the management of the post office. The bill called for mail to be delivered even if it did not have sufficient postage attached, that small items (samples, laces, etc.) wrapped in newspapers not be "disturbed" by postal employees, and that increased care be taken in maintaining labels and addresses on letters and packages; further, the bill required that if necessary such packages would be rewrapped to insure safe delivery to the addressee. The memorial related to the dead letter office and was linked to the bill, as most items sent to that office had lost labels or had been wrapped in newspapers that had torn apart. Since it was poor Americans who most often used this method of mailing items or those who did not know that the laws regarding the use of newspaper had changed, she declared, "it is the duty of Congress to so amend our postal laws, that the sufferers from these causes shall be relieved since a great Government has its greatest duties to perform to those who are in the greatest need of its just and considerate laws." She concluded that Americans needed such protections until the government employed individuals who were not tempted to classify items as undeliverable to take advantage of the thousands of items from the dead letter office that were annually put up for sale. Such documentation, which had begun while in her clerkship, undoubtedly played a role in Mary's becoming a target for Gitt.[27]

Yet there were heartening events that fall as well. She extended her practice of exploring a variety of religious perspectives by attending the Universalists' convention in Washington, and she participated in the Woman's Centenary Association meeting that was attended by several WCTU representatives. Mary and Frederick Douglass were key participants in the meeting, and she encouraged Universalists to continue their support of woman's suffrage. That autumn an unexpected windfall came her way. An unidentified man from Massachusetts left her $2,000 in his will. Ever fascinated by visual representations of herself, one of the first things Mary did was to have a photograph taken of herself in her trousers and overcoat; the tintype was displayed in a New York City photographers' window for several weeks. Her collection of photographic self-portraits, which she often shared with newspaper reporters who interviewed her, was an important aspect of her use of the visual to defy gender norms and to keep her reform agendas before the public.[28]

Mary was now an openly declared Democrat, and it took little time for Republican-leaning newspapers to begin an extended campaign that presented her as a crazed woman. Increasingly offensive sexual innuendoes appeared in items about her as well: "It is rumored that Dr. Mary Walker rides a bicycle. The afflicted vehicle is entitled to *wide spread* sympathy." The old nudity issues were again raised in the *National Police Gazette* and *Saturday Evening Post*. While many political and cultural leaders knew and admired her, the campaign to smear her often worked for the public at large. In this period several of Mary's friends began to tell reporters that she had declined twelve offers of marriage. It is true that she received numerous proposals, including several from soldiers whom she knew since the Civil War, and she had developed close relationships with Stephen Harrington and the mysterious "Doc." But the timing of this assertion was more telling than the subject itself. It was undoubtedly meant to bolster support against the disparagement of her suffrage work and her altered appearance, with a well-intended if misguided attempt to make her appear more conventional. Mary had never desired to be classified as conventional, however, and she simply ignored the criticism and continued her usual outspokenness at lectures and in print.[29]

In the spring, Mary traveled north to serve as legal representative for eighty-year-old Sarah Briggs of Newport, Rhode Island, in an estate case. Mary and Sarah Briggs became friends during the Civil War, and although they had not seen one another for several years, it was to Mary that the elderly woman turned when she was in need of legal counsel for an inheritance claim. Mary was now fifty-three years old, and she was eager to involve herself in new avenues of fighting for women's rights. The Briggs case offered just such an opportunity. Mary was in Providence for several days speaking with members of the legislature about woman's suffrage when Briggs contacted her, and she quickly took passage by boat to come to her friend's aid—only to be arrested when she landed in Newport. As usual, the police chief confirmed Mary's right to move about the city freely in her choice of clothing, and he apologized for the arrest. It was to be a season of assaults and arrests, however. Shortly after her return to Washington in early April, she was attacked by twelve-year-old Harry Childs, who threw a brick at her while she was walking in the street. The brick struck her ankle, though her boot took the brunt of the blow. She filed a complaint against Childs, and this time the judge ruled in her favor and fined Childs. She left shortly after the hearing for Pittsburgh where another old friend, Mrs. Hale, asked for assistance. Hale's husband, Dr. Edwin M. Hale, was one of America's leading advocates of homeopathic medicine and editor of the *North American Journal of Homoeopathy* and the *American Homoeopathic Observer*. Dr. Hale had apparently run up bills while in Pittsburgh that exceeded the funds he had on hand and thus had been charged with fraud. Mary consulted with Dr. Hale in the jail at nearby Claremont and then returned to Pittsburgh where she met with the men who had brought the charges. She quickly negotiated an agreement for Hale, and the charges were dropped.[30]

While in Pittsburgh, Mary granted a reporter for the *Dispatch* an interview. He questioned her on a variety of subjects, especially in relation to labor issues. As the reporter noted, "She has been intimately identified with the interests of working people for years, and has always advocated arbitration and peaceful adjustment of difficulties between employer and employe." She explained that her preference for arbitration was based on the belief that no one, especially workers, benefited from strikes and riots. She had seen first-hand the consequences for laborers in the Great Strike of July 1877, but her commentary was surprising in some ways, as she attempted to balance the needs of capitalists and laborers. "Capital and labor do not understand each other," she asserted. There are employers who keep laborers on even when their finances are strained, but "a few hot-headed leaders" encourage laborers to strike, even though "[t]here never was a strike which did not in some way injure labor." She went on to argue that "laboring men and women do undoubtedly have to work for wages much too small, but . . . reform must be brought about through the co-operation of employer and employe. Their interests are identical, and there is no reason in the world why they should be forever pulling in opposite directions." She added that arbitration avoided the inevitable destruction of property and bloodshed that befell workers during strikes, as well as the economic and bodily harm which could take years to overcome. Mary's attitudes toward the labor-capitalist tensions were rooted in her longstanding commitment to the peace movement, and her argument was in line with the Universal Peace Society's preference for arbitration over strikes. The reporter concluded by noting that the doctor intended to return to Pittsburgh soon to deliver a course of lectures on scientific topics and the labor situation.[31]

Mary had no sooner returned to Washington than she received the devastating news that her mother had died on April 25. At eighty-five, Vesta Walker had endured a long illness. Vesta had been an honored member of the Oswego community and was recognized as a pioneer settler of the region. At the funeral, Alvah

Jr. again inserted tension into the situation. A local newspaper published a long text they claimed he read at the funeral; he quickly asked for a correction, noting that the ministers, "for reasons that reflect no credit upon them," had not allowed him to speak. He was angry, too, that the article connected Mary to his remarks with a headline that identified Vesta as "mother of Dr. Mary Walker" rather than the mother of several children. The situation did little to comfort the family in its sadness and loss.[32]

Good news awaited Mary when she returned to Washington; she was granted a patent for a system to teach orthography. Her method focused particularly on words that sounded the same but were spelled differently (such as "slay" and "sleigh") and used visuals to help students memorize the difference. Both her father and brother had been inventors, and Mary continued the family tradition in several instances throughout her life. She was inventive as well when it came to helping others. President Cleveland's daughter suffered from cerebral palsy, and through Mary's negotiations, Dr. Anna Easton Lake of Baltimore received the presidential appointment as their daughter's physician. Mary had been friends with Lake for years, and she believed Lake, who specialized in treating physically disabled children, would be effective in treating the Clevelands' daughter.[33]

During the summer Mary helped organize a dress reform convention in Syracuse. Mary, Dr. Lydia Hasbrouck, and Dr. Mary York of Dansville were among the speakers. The convention offered free admission during the day and charged only a fifteen-cent fee for the evening lectures on health and dress. By mid-August, Mary determined to embark on another lecture tour that would again take her across the country to San Francisco. Passing through Cincinnati on her way, she was asked by a reporter about her attitudes toward marriage. "I have had men, intelligent and wealthy men, come to me and say, 'Dr. Walker, I respect you, I respect your intelligence and good sense, and I believe if you only dressed like other women I would love you and ask you to be my wife,'" she replied. "Well, do you know what I told them? I said, 'There are plenty of women in the world who dress just as you want them to; go and marry them.' I don't want any one to marry me for my clothes, or because when I am dressed up I look well. If I marry it must be from the highest motives." For all that Mary remarked on her belief in marriage, her individualistic lifestyle cast her in the public mind as an aberrant woman. She resisted such attitudes whenever possible, but the personal cost of increasingly virulent public outrage was immense. Critics attacked her for being too "masculine." Some also began to spread rumors about her acquaintance with President Cleveland. "If the discourteous paragraphers speak truly," *Life* magazine whispered, reprinting a rumor spread by *Puck*, "Dr. Mary Walker has the best claim to the title of First Lady in the Land." She was either the sexually aberrant she-man or the wicked seductress. These rumors made for a better story than Mary's own comments about the sacredness of marriage or a woman's right to independence. Her critics' fears were rooted in the fact that many young women were increasingly attracted to Mary's ideas. The *American Catholic Quarterly Review* revealed as much when they intoned "[o]nly a few years ago it provoked laughter to hear . . . that Dr. Mary Walker had appeared on Broadway in male habiliments *cap-à-pie*. But now it is quite ordinary to hear of ladies, gentlewomen, daughters of some of our country's best men, not, indeed, imitating Dr. Mary Walker's exceptionable attire, but mounting the rostrum" to lecture on women's rights, spiritualism, and other subjects on which Mary often spoke. The recognition that she was making inroads for reconfiguring women's roles in society sustained her against the onslaught of criticism.[34]

That fall Mary met for the first time another women's rights activist who had also survived outrageous public condemnation over the years—Charlotte Perkins Gilman. On the cusp of some of her major work, Gilman wanted to meet the famous Dr. Mary, and so arranged a visit to Mary's home when she came to Washington in November. Through the afternoon the two women discussed a variety of political issues. Gilman reflected on the meeting that evening in her diary. "Like her," she remarked about Mary, "but am not converted." The conversion reference was undoubtedly to Mary's brand of dress reform; Gilman preferred "beauty in costume," and a few days after meeting Mary she wrote an article on the subject, "The Dress of Women." Gilman's remarks about meeting the pioneer suffragist perfectly captured the nature of both women—admiring of other activists but absolutely unwilling to compromise their own beliefs.[35]

The year 1887 demonstrated just how little attention Mary would give to critics who wanted to curtail what she would say and the venues in which she chose to express her ideas: she booked a major lecture tour at entertainment museums in the Northeast and mid-Atlantic states. She began such lectures on a small scale two years earlier. Certainly the economic factor was part of the attraction, but she was equally excited about the possibility of offering scientific lectures to mass audiences. Not since her time in Great Britain had she been able to reach such large middle- and working-class audiences. Suffrage lecture tours were important to her, but they tended to draw a limited range of attendees. She saw lecturing at the dime museums and popular lecture halls as an opportunity to spread her ideas to thousands of American citizens. While the newspapers went wild with proclamations of Mary's "decline" for lecturing in such low-brow institutions, her own reasons for doing so were clear:

> I am of the opinion that the crying need of the masses is a better and more thorough scientific education than they at present receive. Now, you may think it strange that the first woman in the country to assert her right to vote, the first woman in the country to vote in a political caucus, the first female surgeon to serve in an army, and the woman who was complimented by Charles Sumner

should lecture in a dime museum, but I tell you the time is not far distant when the greatest scientists in the country will adopt the stage of a dime museum as the best place from which to disseminate knowledge. I want to instruct a class of people who cannot afford to patronize high-priced lectures.

She appeared at a dime museum in Philadelphia in April, and she soon expanded to amusement halls owned by M. S. Robinson, whose best-known museum was the Wonderland in Buffalo. The negotiations for how these lectures would be advertised were time consuming because she wanted to control the content of all advertisements in which her name appeared. She also preferred the stage to be set as a parlor so it would appear she was having an intimate conversation with her audience.[36]

Dime museums varied widely in their entertainment and propriety, but Robinson's museums were particularly well-managed sites that blended popular figures, educational events, and the sensational. Mary was drawn to Robinson's museums because of his attention to female attendees. In advertising the Wonderland, Robinson presented a "Visitors' Guide" that led the reader on a virtual tour through the variety of entertainments available. Before detailing the attractions, the flyer headlined its assurance that "Ladies can visit Wonderland without an escort. Tickets will not be sold or admission given to any improper characters." There was an art gallery and four elegantly furnished "Ladies Parlours." On the second floor were the lecture parlors. Comedies, dramas (especially those with murder scenes), wax figures, illusionists, trained bird acts and musicians competed with serious lecturers for the audience's attention in the various auditoriums. Robinson also emphasized his interest in attracting working-class attendees; on Saturday evenings, Robinson maintained the daytime ten-cent price "in order to allow people who are employed during all the afternoons of the week an opportunity to see Wonderland." Mary's participation was prominently noted in the ads, and her lectures included "Curiosities of the Brain," "Human Electricity," "Causes of Unusual People," "Beauties, Uses and Injuries of Tobacco," "Science of Dress," "Woman's Franchise," and "The Great Labor Question." By offering these lectures every four to six months, she reached a wide audience over the next few years.[37]

In the early fall NWSA leaders presented a document to the president of the United States that proclaimed women had the right as citizens under the Constitution to enfranchisement, as Mary had argued in *Crowning* for the past fifteen years. Rather than the usual argument of a need for a constitutional amendment, they protested the injustice of ignoring their rights under the law and demanded that "hereafter the Constitution of the United States shall be interpreted in accordance with the simple words in which it is framed." The document was signed by Anthony, Gage, Lillie Devereux Blake, and other officers of the NWSA. Although publicly they primarily argued the necessity of a constitutional amendment, the "Protest" signers never actually abandoned the belief in their constitutional rights. In reality, their dissatisfaction with Mary was the matter of her attire and outspokenness. For all of her differences with the NWSA leadership, Mary maintained a strong following within the suffrage community. In a poll taken the year before in which respondents were asked to name America's greatest social reformers, Frances Willard and Stanton tied for first place among the women reformers, followed by Mary, and then Lillie Blake, Ella Church, and Anthony. At the same time Mary was involved in her own endeavors for women's rights on national and personal levels. After securing all rights for herself, she brought out a second edition of *Unmasked*.[38]

She also attended President Cleveland's White House New Year's celebration, wearing a red rose in the lapel of her Prince Albert coat. She and Cleveland heartily greeted one another. As the newspapers acknowledged, "it was the meeting of two reformers." One of her first activities in the new year was to attend the lengthy Senate hearings on a bill to prohibit the production and sale of alcohol in the District. The bill split politicians and women activists alike. Nebraska attorney Ada Bittenbander and WCTU founder Frances Willard spoke on behalf of the bill, but Mary joined its opponents. Although she supported temperance, she believed it would be impossible to enforce a complete ban on alcohol and favored a substitute measure that would prohibit alcohol consumption by minors. At this time Mary also met with legislators about woman suffrage. Thus when a Women's International Council, which included suffragists and their opponents, was held in Washington in March, she was eager to express her opinions. Attendees included Stanton, Anthony, Gage, Dr. Caroline Winslow, Phoebe Couzens, Clara Barton, Caroline Dall, Isabella Bageiot of Paris, Lady Ashton Dilke of Newcastle, Alice Moore of Ireland, Mrs. Ormiston Chart of Edinburgh, and Pundita Ramabai Sarasvati of India. In conjunction with the gathering, Stanton was granted permission by the House Judiciary Committee to read a statement on behalf of woman's suffrage, which returned to the call for a constitutional amendment. After Stanton's declaration was read, Mary attempted to express her own opinions, asserting she represented more women than Stanton did, but the committee refused to hear her. The leaders of the council then banned Mary from their meetings. Not all participants agreed with the action. The politically moderate Ethel Ingalls published a generally favorable eight-page report on the women's congress in the *Cosmopolitan*, but she noted a new "conservative conciliatory spirit never before manifested" by the NWSA suffragists. Ingalls cited two cases for her assertion: the inclusion of anti-suffragists at the convention, and the exclusion of Dr. Mary Walker. Although Ingalls preferred the soft, feminine style of Clara Barton's activism, she observed that while most of the early suffragists had once worn Bloomers, "in this convention, the 'bloomers' have all been nipped in the bud; not only were all such costumers forbidden to appear, but Dr. Mary Walker, who was formerly one of its chosen members, was denied entrance to this select Congress, and was not admitted to the hotel where the suffragists made their headquarters." Ingalls slyly concluded that this selectiveness was surprising since "on the platform, and in the boxes and seats of the Opera House, were numerous costumes from Worth, Redfern, ladies' tailors, and the artists of the world."[39]

In response to her rejection, Mary published a new edition of the *Crowning Constitutional Argument* in the radical *National Free Press*, whose motto was "Fearless in Exposing Official Corruption; and Devoted to the Welfare of the People." She was especially upset at being excluded from the Women's International Council's "Conference of the Pioneers" of the suffrage movement. This latest version of *Crowning* reiterated the historical overview of republicanism, the constitutional reference to "We the People" and not just to men, and Charles Sumner's praise of the document when he first read it. But now it also included challenges to those who for several years attempted to silence her:

> And now, in justice to my friends who are told as a reason why I am not attending the Council here, that I am a *"woman's franchise backslider"*—After all these years I deem it my duty to speak what hundreds in Washington knew at the time.
>
> The first time my C.C. Argument went to Congress was through Hon. Mr. Teese of N.J.
>
> This was the day before a Woman's Franchise Convention in Lincoln Hall in Washington.
>
> In my speech I stated my Argument, and the whole audience was with me.
>
> Years of jealousies on various grounds culminated by concert action of Susan B. Anthony and Elizabeth Cady Stanton in a most shameful scene on the platform as I at a proper time in the proceedings, when volunteer resolutions were called for, began to offer a Resolution of thanks to Hon. Mr. Teese for introducing my Bill to protect woman in her suffrage, her constitutionally guaranteed right. I learned afterwards that there had been the greatest consternation regarding the honors that would come to Dr. Mary Walker if she was not disgraced, and suppressed, and that the only way they could do this effectively, was to stick to an Amendment to the constitution, and impress the women all over the country that there was no other way to get their right.
>
> As I have presented my Argument to many thousands through my speeches on Woman's Suffrage, I have to-day a far greater following, simply because truth is bound to triumph. Wounded error is now writhing among its blind worshipers.
>
> The Supreme Bench will ere long declare the supremacy of the Crowning Constitutional Argument, and the work is done.
>
> Let monuments be erected to the women in New Jersey and to Margaret Brent of Maryland.
>
> My tears of gratitude are for those grand women, whose bravery and womanly grandeur made this an *Unlimited Republic*.[40]

While Mary certainly exaggerated her standing as having more followers than Anthony and Stanton, her opponents were equally guilty of diminishing the significant role she continued to play in advancing the cause. On the one hand, Anthony and Stanton felt their control of the suffrage movement waning. So many woman's suffrage and reform organizations had emerged by the late 1880s that no single group could legitimately claim to represent the majority of women. Stanton, Gage, and others were particularly concerned about the evangelical contingency that seemed to have gained control of the NWSA. On the other hand, Mary was also guilty of exposing an internal fight that had raged at the council. British politics had split feminists over whether or not to attend the women's congress in Washington. A conservative social purity movement in England had evolved after a journalist exposed rampant child prostitution in the country; Radical suffragists opposed the repressive policies of the National Vigilance Association that emerged in response to the exposé. Stanton had been in England at the time it was being organized, and she sympathized with the Radical feminists. Both Radical Sir Charles Dilke and Irish Nationalist Charles Parnell opposed the repressive policies, but the fact that both men had been named as correspondents in very public divorce cases only fueled the debates over social purity. Thus the results were explosive when the British delegation to the women's congress included both Radicals and social purists, as well as Lady Ashton (May) Dilke, Charles Dilke's sister-in-law. Stanton supported Dilke's inclusion, although it led Radical Helen Taylor to withdraw from participation. This incident became known as the Taylor-Dilke dispute and foreshadowed the split in the British suffrage movement that would come by the end of the year. By exposing these issues in the American press, Mary presented what she viewed as the two-facedness of the NWSA itself. The exposure did nothing to advance the suffrage cause.[41]

It was especially painful for Mary when, a few months later, Belva Lockwood spoke out against her, asserting she had no sympathy for Mary's ideas on suffrage or in her choice of dress. But Mary continued to voice her opinions, and in April she joined a group of African American friends in celebrating the twenty-sixth anniversary of emancipation. Here, too, political differences led to splits among activists who supported different political candidates; thus rival meetings were held. Frederick Douglass spoke eloquently at the Republican gathering, insisting that emancipation had not been fully gained, and he nominated Justice Harlan as the African Americans' candidate for the presidency. Lockwood and a large crowd attended the meeting. The message of unfulfilled emancipation was similar at the rival meeting, at which Mary had been invited to sit on the stage with James Langston, ex-minister to Haiti, Rev. W. H. Phillips, Bishop Johnson, A. J. Jones of Petersburg, Mrs. E.V.C. Miller of South Carolina, and S. B. Wall, who presided. Here Senator John Sherman was nominated as president and John Langston, an African American candidate, for the House of Representatives. After participating in the emancipation celebrations, Mary scheduled lectures on suffrage in Washington. At the end of October, in preparation for the upcoming presidential election, she sent an impassioned appeal to "the great sisterhood all over the land" to go to the polls and register to vote. The appeal was published throughout the United

States: "Sisters, step into your own ballot sphere, and the day is near when all men will arise and call you blessed." The concluding remark effectively shifted woman's "sphere" from the household to the polling station. Mary was feeling invigorated, and she shocked politicians and the public on March 6, 1889, when she walked onto the floor of the House of Representatives and ascended to the Speaker's desk, where she pronounced that it would not be long before the Speaker of the House would be a woman and that she would recognize not the "gentleman from Indiana" but the "*lady* from Indiana." She was in full voice, espousing women's rights, when the doorkeeper arrived to escort her out of the hall. Thus Dr. Mary Walker became the first woman to *speak* from the desk of the Speaker of the House.[42]

A few days later she headed to Boston for a series of lectures at William Austin's Nickelodeon museum in what was clearly a well-staged publicity stunt but one that Mary seems to have taken seriously. Her role was to make a medical study of Josephine Marie Bedard, dubbed the "Tingwick Girl" for her performances at the Nickelodeon, who claimed not to have eaten for seven years. Within ten days, all of Boston was abuzz with discussions of the Tingwick Girl, and it was announced in the *Globe* that anything Dr. Walker could report "from her own observations of the case will be of great interest from a scientific and popular standpoint." Mary and the nineteen-year-old Bedard were seen everywhere together in Boston, and after several days Mary declared she had seen Bedard intake only water. By the time Mary and Josephine appeared together on stage, they drew over five thousand people. Finally, however, Mary announced to an audience that she had discovered that Bedard had been sneaking food. It was a ridiculous event all around, and Mary became part of the ruse. From there she moved to Austin and Stone's Museum in Boston where she returned to her usual lectures on health and dress reform. These later performances were a welcome interlude from her exhausting work in Washington, and she was reaching a large number of Americans with her appeals for reform.[43]

The 1880s included many challenges, but by its end Mary had run for the U.S. Senate, published her opinions on women's rights and the need for men's moral reform, and resisted every attempt to silence her. She was now moving into an era in which she would develop provocative new means for aiding women in gaining the kind of independent life she so thoroughly enjoyed herself.

CHAPTER 11

A Pragmatic Utopia

At the beginning of the 1890s, Mary's commitment to political causes spiderwebbed into a grid of interrelated work for women's rights. Although the usual criticisms continued, newspapers now published as much about her ideas as about her appearance. In part, attitudes about unconventionality were changing, and in part her bouts of ill health drew forth sympathy even from those who disagreed with her activism. In the fall of 1889, Mary fell, injuring her leg so badly that it would take more than a year to heal sufficiently, although never fully. As late as April 1890 bed rest was still required for her recovery, and national sympathy evoked rare comments from Mary about the personal costs of activism. "The world has thought me hardened and brazen," she acknowledged to one reporter, but it was mistaken: "I have never seen the day when it was not a trial to me to appear in public in a reform dress. Every jeer has cut me to the quick. Many times have I gone to my room and wept after being publicly derided. No one knows, or will ever know, what it has cost me to live up to my principles, to be consistent with my convictions and declarations; but I have done it, and am not sorry for it."[1]

The statement was surely heartfelt, considering the decades of ridicule she had faced; but she was also adept at recognizing opportune moments. The Harrison administration enacted the Dependent Pension Act in June 1890 allowing veterans who could not perform manual labor to receive pensions. Mary and her congressional supporters viewed it as an avenue for increasing her pension, since she was now disabled from the fall. One of the most extensive interviews of these months appeared in New York's *Hornellsville Weekly Tribune*, accompanied by illustrations of her medical work during the war, lying abed in her current illness, striking out belligerently, and standing with President Chester Arthur. She was interviewed sitting up in bed, dressed in her usual shirt, using the effect to argue against the government's ill use of one who had served its cause so well. The reporter, Robert Graves, asked her to speak about her life, and she immediately turned to incidences of her selfless service to wounded soldiers at Warrenton in the early years of the war. Newspapers across the country pronounced assurances that the Senate would confirm the House's appropriation to her of a $2,000 pension payment, but as usual, such expectations were wrong. Graves was more interested in Mary's personal life. A rumor had emerged that the unmarried President Arthur had proposed to her. Although Graves believed it was a prank because it was reported the proposal came in a letter, Mary asserted that Arthur had proposed to her several times. Most of President Arthur's papers were destroyed at his request the day before he died, so few of his private papers survive; but Mary believed the proposals were sincere.[2]

In the midst of her own health problems, Mary's brother Alvah Jr. died on May 17 at the age of fifty-six. Their relationship had been strained for many years, and Mary did not return home for his funeral. When his death was announced, the local newspaper said no information about services was available, and no record of a funeral remains. His death added to Mary's sense of advancing age, and she became adamant that she receive compensation from the government for her war services before she died. Over the years it became less an issue of money than of recognition and acknowledgment. By the summer, when the $2,000 pension was not approved—for the fourth time, the House approved payment only to have it tabled in the Senate—Mary and her supporters returned to their original request for $10,000, this time with an important ally, Senator William M. Evarts, who introduced the bill. Evarts was well-respected, and he had just successfully introduced a bill to incorporate the American National Association of the Red Cross, with Clara Barton among its incorporators. Mary worked untiringly to gain support for her claim. In August she wrote a nineteen-page account of her wartime activities as a basis for the petition. She and her congressional supporters had by then decided against filing a typical pension claim; instead, they prepared a petition seeking "pay for services rendered and money expended as a surgeon in the army." Rather than an increase in her pension of $8.50 per month, she asked for a flat $10,000 payment that would compensate her and end the time-consuming process necessary each year to seek an increase in the pension. Although rumors abounded throughout her life that she was writing an autobiography, this pension-related petition constitutes the only autobiographical narrative Mary ever published. It was a collage of narratives. One framed the collected versions of her volunteer and military service; a second, entitled "Statement," was largely anecdotal and episodic rather than chronological, yet informative of her activities in those years; and a third, "Affirmed Statement," presented the more subdued, date-and-place narrative expected in a petition of this sort but also included anecdotal segments and critiques of government actions. Also embedded in the latter was another version of the *Crowning Constitutional Argument*.[3]

Shortly after the bill was sent to Congress, Mary returned to Oswego in the hope of more fully recovering her health. Absence from Washington did not keep her from responding, however, when she learned in September that her petition had been denied because she did not "dress like other women" and that one Senator had proclaimed he was offended by the "vulgarity of a woman dressing like a man."

She quickly penned a mock petition that satirized Congress and conventional attitudes toward women's clothing. It was a scathing attack on the gender inscriptions she had been fighting all of her life. It surprised her to learn her choice of clothing was the reason her bill had not passed, she mockingly wrote, since "there is no national costumer elected or appointed under existing laws"; thus her petition proposed the establishment of such a position through an amendment to the Constitution, satirically challenging both the clothing issue and the idea that women's rights needed a constitutional amendment. How odd, she noted, that "American squaws" dressed very much like their male counterparts and yet were granted an annual payment from the U.S. government. Further, fashions for women at present could not be accepted in America unless they were designed in Paris and met tariff considerations, so it was incumbent upon her to propose to the Fifty-first Congress a bill to "be passed as one of the 'graceful acts'" of their session:

> Be it enacted, That the Constitution of the United States be amended so as to read: That a National costumer for the women of the United States be selected from some foreign court whose special duties shall be to devise costumes for every woman in the United States and Territories that shall seem appropriate to him, and that this act includes squaws as well as all other women; and
>
> Be it further enacted, That whoever disregards the fashion plates in a National magazine published by said costumer shall have no appropriation from the Government of the United States, and their men relatives shall be debarred from appropriations, pensions, etc., during the life time of such women, and,
>
> Be it still further enacted, That the salary of costumer shall be $10,000 per year, and the magazine published at the Government office once in three months and sent to every woman in the United States free of expense.

The petition was published in all major newspapers. At its core was a wonderful satire of normative thinking, but it was marred by its conventional use of "squaws." As much as Mary argued for equality for Euro- and African American women, she did not recognize her own biases in such language.[4]

When seeking support from Congress failed, Mary determined to try another tactic: she called a convention in October in Weedsport, New York. Ella Sturge, B. Barnes, and Mrs. E. Chaffee constituted the committee that nominated her as an independent candidate for Congress in the 27th District. Certified copies of the nomination were sent to the secretary of state and the county clerk, but new election laws prohibited her name from appearing on state ballots. The situation raised consternation among Democrats, with whom Mary's alliance was well known, and ridicule from Republicans. How far she could have taken this second campaign for the Senate is questionable, but she had no chance to pursue her goal. By December she was again bedridden from complications to the healing of her leg, and word spread throughout the country of her impending death. Biographical essays appeared, citing her many accomplishments and the debt the country owed her.

As Mary began to recover, she made it known that she was determined to survive until she could obtain justice from the government. By mid-December a new bill was prepared, and she again wrote letters to influential friends seeking support for $10,000 in lump-sum compensation. Although to no avail, Mary continued her actions both behind the scenes and in the public eye, with constant pressure on Congress through increasingly supportive commentaries in national newspapers to which she granted interviews over the next years.[5]

She spent the winter of 1890–91 in Oswego, rarely venturing out of the house. Through the frigid winter months she turned to her pen. One of the results was a long letter to the editor of the *Philadelphia Inquirer*. During her recent illness, the paper had published an appreciative piece about her, and she responded, thanking the paper.

"That the most intelligent all over our land have an appreciation of a liver of principles, written and spoken, all the days of more than ordinary life time," she added, "is attested in by personal letters of regret that the life of her who writes you can not last many years at most."[6]

By late February Mary was well enough to return to Washington, where she became immersed in the infamous, decades-long Myra Clark Gaines lawsuit, which rivaled Dickens's *Bleak House* for its interminable meandering through the courts and the decimation of the estate by legal fees. The case had been in the courts through generations, beginning in 1834. Gaines, the daughter of a wealthy New Orleans businessman, sought legal recognition as heir to her father's estate. There were claims of two wills, fraud, and other allegations. By the time Belva Lockwood entered the case as an associate of attorney Walter K. Griffin, Gaines had died and the battle was between Maria P. Evans, a friend of Gaines's represented by Griffin and Lockwood, and Gaines's grandchildren. When court was called to order on March 23, 1891, Griffin surprised everyone by calling Mary as a witness. Mary met Gaines in 1869 during an earlier stage of the dispute, and they became good friends when Mary visited her in 1870. During that time, Gaines asked Mary to look at her will; Mary testified it named Evans and another woman as beneficiaries. Mary cautioned Gaines that the will would be contested if her grandchildren were not named as heirs and, as it was not dated, encouraged Gaines to have it properly executed. She also confirmed that the will naming Evans as heir was in Gaines's distinctive handwriting. When the court finally ruled in favor of the grandchildren, the once magnificent estate purported to be worth $35 million had dwindled to $100,000.[7]

In September Mary returned to Austin and Stone's Museum for another week of lectures. Through her work with the museum she had come to enjoy Boston, and in the 1890s spent an increasing amount of time there, returning only periodically to Washington. But by the end of the month she was involved in a murder trial that would endanger her life, lead her to develop an extraordinary conspiracy theory of murder and greed, and embroil her in legal matters for the next three years. For decades she had been persecuted for her choice of clothing and her outspoken demands for radical reforms in American culture. She could not walk on the street without being followed; she had been arrested numerous times for her appearance; and she had been chased and had objects thrown at her by men who felt her clothing threatened their status quo. After a lifetime of such treatment, she began to believe that numerous conspiracies were being enacted against her. In each instance where she charged conspiracy over the next decade, there would be both substantial evidence to suggest wrongdoing and a sense that Mary exaggerated many points because of a growing sense of persecution.

On the evening of July 17, 1891, twenty-five-year-old Christie Warden was walking near her home, about a mile outside of Hanover, New Hampshire. As her family told the story, Christie was with her mother Louisa Warden, sister Fannie, and a female friend when a man jumped in front of them, grabbed Christie's arm, and declared, "I want you." When Mrs. Warden and Fannie attempted to intervene, the man shot at them, missing both although in close range. He dragged Christie into nearby bushes where he shot her twice in the head and then fled. When help arrived, Christie's nearly nude body was discovered. The family identified the murderer as Frank C. Almy, a hired man who had been employed by them for nearly a year. The case became nationally sensationalized, with the family, police, neighbors, and others adding so many versions of events that the accuracy of anyone's statement remains suspect. The official story was that while authorities spent a month looking for Almy, he was hiding the entire time in the Warden's barn where he was finally captured. A convoluted process of determining aliases and true identities began, and the man arrested for the crime was discovered to be George Abbott, an escapee from the state prison where he had been serving fifteen years for burglary. Abbott was quickly found guilty and sentenced to die, based on the Wardens' identification of him as the man they knew as Frank Almy.[8]

Mary followed the unusual case closely from its beginnings, and she began to suspect that there were flaws in the story the family was telling about Abbott. Descriptions of the murderer had been widely spread through the newspapers before Abbott's capture, and there were several features about the arrested man that did not coincide with those original descriptions. At the same time, Mary became reacquainted with Arthur D. Snoad. In mid-May she had hired Snoad to work on her farm for a few days. On July 18—the day after Christie's Warden's murder—Snoad returned. He appeared to have come a long distance, was exhausted, and his clothing was in disarray. Snoad remained at her home for a month, and Mary began to suspect that he was actually the man who called himself Frank C. Almy and who killed Warden. A series of discussions with Snoad initially raised her suspicions. She claimed that before the murder occurred, Snoad told her that he was returning to his previous place of employment and declared he had an argument that would convince Christie, a young woman with whom he had fallen in love, to return with him. Mary also knew he had purchased a gun in preparation for his trip. Based on this discussion, Snoad's physical appearance, and other comments he made, Mary suspected he was actually Frank Almy.[9]

Was Mary's imagination leading her into a quagmire of misidentification, or had she actually stumbled onto Christie's real murderer? Most newspapers proclaimed her a crank, but their sources were members of the Warden family and associates such as Sheriff Brown—people Mary eventually accused of a conspiracy to murder several people, herself included, in order to receive the $4,000 reward money for locating Almy.

Beginning two weeks after the murder, Mary wrote four letters to Christie's father, Andrew Warden, informing him of her concerns that the wrong man had been arrested for the crime. She also requested that a detective be sent to Oswego to determine if Snoad could be identified as the real Almy. This was not an unusual request; during the search for Almy, detectives had been sent as far as Connecticut and Indiana to determine the truth of citizens' claims that he was in their vicinity. Two years earlier, Mary had become friends with a detective employed by Austin and Stone's Museum, and in late September she asked for his assistance to check Snoad's identity and to negotiate with the Boston police for her. She wanted the police to arrest Snoad immediately, fearing her life was in danger. After meeting with the detective, Police Inspector Robinson met with Mary at the museum. She explained that she had information about a crime; if he would sign a contract, she would split the reward money with him as an inducement for an immediate arrest. Robinson later admitted that he "made a scrawl, giving her the impression that I had signed my name." Believing he had agreed, Mary revealed her suspicions. After the fact, Robinson insisted he never believed her, but at the time he simply told her that he could not become involved, and "if she really believed her story to be true the authorities at Hanover, or of the county in which that town is located, were the ones for her to see." Thus, having finished her lecture series in Boston, Mary headed for New Hampshire. After an unsatisfying meeting with local police, she hired a carriage and went directly to the Warden home, arriving on the evening of September 30. Newspaper accounts, based on information from the Wardens, declared that she refused to identify herself and was a "mystery woman" who wanted to sleep in Christie's bed for the night. Mary's harrowing account of what happened that night was never reported in the newspapers, but it was filed as part of the legal documents in the case. It is very likely that Mary, drawing on her Spiritualist beliefs, wanted to sleep in Christie's room to see if she could draw forth information about the murderer's identity.[10]

When she arrived, the house was full of people—Christie's parents, Andrew and Louisa Warden; her uncle, Oscar Warden; her grandparents, Mr. and Mrs. Flint; and several neighbors—but most were sent outside shortly after Mary's arrival, and only the family and their friend Charles Hewitt remained. Although Mary did not immediately recognize Oscar Warden, he knew she was the famous Dr. Walker. They had met in California several years earlier, he reminded her, when he had attended her lectures; when she was called in to treat a patient at the Whitcomb Ranch on the Sacramento River (probably Katy Barrett), Oscar was there as well, and they had seen each other on a daily basis for six weeks. She spent the evening and most of the following day with the Wardens, but not of her own free will. That evening, the Wardens grilled her with questions; occasionally, two or three of them would leave the room to talk quietly among themselves. They may have been trying to assure themselves of her identity, Mary recognized, but she presented ample proof: she could recount the content of the letters she had sent to Andrew Warden, and she produced several documents with her name and address on them. More importantly, Oscar had already recognized her. He questioned her specifically about who knew she had come to the Wardens' home; she unwittingly explained that only the hack driver who brought her knew of her whereabouts. When Mr. and Mrs. Flint left the room shortly thereafter, Mary was brutally attacked. Oscar later claimed it was because she was an unknown intruder, but Mary felt his real intent was to murder her because she discovered the family's plan to substitute Abbott for Almy and collect the reward. As she recounted, Oscar's

> first move was to grab my left hand and thrust against my throat. My resistance was such that I could speak, and not having the remotest idea of a reason to kill me, I declared twice, that I was Dr. Mary Walker, with the effect of having more force and fierceness if possible, in the blows in my face to hasten death. . . .
>
> There was such a strain all over me in my efforts to resist the choking with one hand, and the effort to pull his hand down and out with the other while he struck holding my right hand as the shillalah, that I could not make an outcry, but when Charles Hewitt held my right hand by Oscar Warden's order, and Oscar struck my lungs such a fierce blow, that I felt the deafness of death, and the dying-away sensation, my thought, not that I might be dead but that they three would outrage my dead body, caused me to make the desperate effort to yell, "Grandma, they are killing me."

In spite of her diminutive size, Mary's years as a surgeon and a woman who often worked her own farm had made her arms and hands far stronger than Oscar anticipated. When she yelled out, Mrs. Flint came quickly into the room and saw that their guest's clothing was spattered with blood. Mary's nose was possibly broken, her mouth was "jambed to one side," and she had a hemorrhage of the lungs. Mrs. Flint helped her to the couch, but Mary was not allowed to leave the house.[11]

The following day, Sheriff Brown was called to the Warden home—and Mary was arrested as an unknown trespasser. Even when her identity was clarified, she was held for an additional two days. Newspaper reporters were told that she was not released because she had gone beyond the endurance of the law by disturbing the grieving family. Disdaining her treatment in New Hampshire, Mary damned the entire state and returned to Boston, where she stayed with friends, Drs. Lillian E. Landis and Simon Mohler Landis. The *Boston Globe* alone reported that she had been attacked by Oscar Warden and that she still had "an ugly cut on her upper lip" four days after the beating. In an interview with a *Globe* reporter, Mary asserted that Oscar attacked her because she was wearing pants, and that she did not identify herself immediately upon arrival because she was too tired.

It is likely that Mary told an edited version of events because she feared for her life, both from Snoad and now from the Wardens. Yet she continued because she noticed several things while in the Wardens' home that made her question even further their claim that George Abbott was Almy. She believed Abbott had been duped with the promise that he would receive part of the reward if he agreed to impersonate Almy after the murder. Additionally, according to Mary, Grandpa Flint stated that he did not believe the right man had been arrested. Details of Abbott's own statements also seemed suspicious. When arrested, for instance, Abbott repeatedly declared he was "Frank C. Almy." It made no sense to Mary that under such circumstances a perpetrator would include his middle initial—unless he had been instructed to say the name precisely in that manner. She also questioned why Andrew Warden was allowed private jailhouse interviews with Abbott. "A father of a murdered daughter, must have unusual reasons for desiring private interviews, with his daughter's murderer," she declared, "and a warden of a prison must not only know why such unusual interviews were desired, but would not be likely to allow them without promises for the future by Mr. Warden, as were satisfactory to the warden of the prison."[12]

Mary's evidence was as much innuendo as fact, yet the trial of Almy was itself precedent-setting in its manipulations of the law. When the Almy case began in November 1891, Chief Justice Charles Doe presided over the trial himself rather than have a jury; with Almy-Abbott's guilty plea, the trial centered only on the degree of the crime. After hearing the cases presented by both sides, Doe made a unique decision. While deliberating, he had Abbott sent to the state prison in Concord. Thus when he rendered his first-degree murder verdict in court, Abbott was not present to hear the sentence pronounced—nor to have the required opportunity to declare why he should not be sentenced, in spite of the fact that the U.S. Supreme Court had ruled seven months earlier that "it should appear of record that the defendant was asked before sentencing if he had anything to say why it should not be pronounced." Thus if Abbott wanted to finally express his innocence and reveal the conspiracy, as Mary contended, the court assured that he had no opportunity to do so.[13]

Although she had not abandoned her zeal to have Snoad recognized as the real perpetrator, Mary returned to New York after the first of the year and began her usual schedule of lectures and writing. In February she attended the New York State Grange's meeting in Oswego. Mayor J. D. Kehoe spoke and musical numbers were presented, after which an audience member noted that Dr. Mary Walker was present and asked that she be given an opportunity to speak. Delighted, she spoke on women's rights and several other topics of the day. She also entered into another legal controversy. The previous December 4, Henry Norcross attempted to assassinate the multimillionaire Russell Sage. Norcross had demanded money from Sage, and when his demands were refused, he devised a plot to kill Sage with a dynamite bomb. Sage escaped, but Norcross was killed in the bombing. Sage appeared at the New York coroner's office on the morning of March 12, 1892, because he read in the papers testimony given by clerk W. R. Laidlaw at the Norcross inquest that he felt dramatically differed from his own account of the explosion. He came seeking the stenographer's record of Laidlaw's remarks in the hope they would prove useful in countering the lawsuit Laidlaw had brought against Sage, in which he claimed that Sage used him as a shield during the bombing. Sage denied the charge, noting that he received more than forty wounds himself from the explosion. To everyone's surprise, Sage also revealed a letter he received from Mary in which she declared that she had known Norcross and considered him a dangerous Nihilist. She explained that she had written both to Mrs. Astor and Sage's wife seeking support for her pension claim, but her letters went unanswered. According to Sage, Mary declared that if he and Mrs. Astor had had the courtesy of answering her letters, "this bomb throwing business might have been averted. I knew Norcross to be a desperate character and that he contemplated making an attack upon yourself (Sage), Gould, Huntington, and Vanderbilt. But I concluded not to interfere. I might have warned you in time, but you would not notice my letters." It was an extraordinary lapse of judgment on Mary's part, and it revealed the increasing anger she felt over her failure to receive the recognition she felt was her due. Although Sage gave Mary's letter to the police, no further action was taken.[14]

Mary had long been immersed in Democratic state politics, and in June when the Democratic convention was held in Syracuse, she was seated among the Oswego delegates. But her goal was larger: she wanted to be a delegate to the national convention, which would be one way to vote in the next presidential election. The Republicans had a woman delegate from the Territories, and Mary reminded Democratic Rep. Henry R. Beekman, "Every one knows me, and I have influence. It will be worse for your party if you don't give me this honor, for there are thousands of women's rights women who are friendly to me who will work against you." One Oswego newspaper deemed her the "Greatest Female Democrat in America." When she was not selected as a delegate to the national convention, she called a nonpartisan meeting for the evening of June 14 at the Oswego City Hall with the purpose of electing one Democrat and one Republican woman as delegates to the Chicago convention. She, of course, was to be the Democratic delegate.[15]

As delegates gathered at the train station for the trip to Chicago, Mary joined them, spoke on behalf of party unity, and boarded the train. The evening before the convention opened in Chicago, she was among the many Democrats holding forth in the lobby of the Wellington Hotel. Although she had been a longtime supporter of Cleveland, her motto was now "Any one to beat Cleveland." It is likely that Cleveland's veto of a veteran pension bill in 1887 was the key factor in her split with the candidate. She soon allied herself with Cleveland's chief opponent for the nomination, Senator David H. Hill of New York. Hill was a likely choice for Mary, as he had been governor of the state, an associate of Samuel Tilden's from his earliest days in the Senate, and had always faced vituperative opposition from Republicans, but, as the *New York Times* proclaimed, he had "the increasing commendation of the people." When his name was mentioned from the podium, the entire New York delegation burst into applause. As the convention continued, Mary met with several groups of delegates from other states, to whom she declared, "I live in Washington, and I have opportunities to inform myself upon subjects pertaining to the administration of government affairs. Mr. [Adlai E.] Stevenson I don't know much about. He may be a good man, but I don't think Cleveland is. Harrison will, I think, be elected." When questioned how a Democrat could say such a thing, she explained that she felt the Democratic platform was not as good as it should be and, if she had been allowed to speak at the convention, many would have been persuaded not to support Cleveland. She was not allowed to vote as a delegate, but her opinions were heard by many Democrats and reported widely in the newspapers.[16]

Before leaving Chicago, she laid the groundwork for another of her goals—to have a costume department under her direction at the World's Fair planned for 1893. She wrote to the director general of the fair about the possibility, and Mrs. Potter Palmer, president of the Board of Lady Managers, said, "the dress reform movement has attracted so much attention of late that it might be productive of much good." Palmer added that Mary "has given much thought and attention to the subject, and I have no doubt she would make it a success." By July 1892, thousands of invitations to attend the exposition had been sent out, and members of Congress were asked to provide a list of twenty to fifty prominent citizens who should receive invitations. Very few women were on the list, but Mary, Susan B. Anthony, and Belva Lockwood were included. That summer was a busy one in terms of Central New York Democratic activities as well. In August she returned to the area to find the cities of Mexico and Pulaski vying for her appearance at their Democratic conventions. Longtime acquaintance Judge C. N. Bulger sought an interview with her and requested she attend neither so as not to create undue competition between the Cleveland and Hill factions, but when other leaders discovered Bulger's interference, they quickly sought her out. H. C. Benedict was especially ardent in his desire that she take the 12:30 P.M. train to Mexico, but it was a ruse—Benedict was a Cleveland man, and he knew that the train which Mary and other Hill supporters boarded did not stop at Mexico, and thus she was thwarted from speaking at the convention.[17]

Later that year, Mary became embroiled in a lawsuit brought against her by a laborer, Charles Peck, whom she hired to do some work on her house. They had a disagreement about the quality of his work, and he brought charges against her for slander, claiming she said he was dishonest and that he had taken boards and hay from her barn. He sought $1,000 compensation. Mary had an agreement with her attorneys at Whitney and Bulger that she would defend herself in any cases in which she sought their advice, but the judge informed her that a New York law denied the possibility of self-representation if a lawyer had been used at any time during a trial. Bulger spoke eloquently on her behalf. She lost the case, but the jury awarded Peck only $50 and court costs and the judge denied his motion for a new trial. Never one to be foiled when she felt wronged, in January Mary went to the Albany legislature on what she termed "a mission of justice" to have two bills presented. The first decreed that no charge of slander could be made if accusations of theft were based on reasonable grounds. The second declared that sex would not disqualify women for jury duty if they met the same qualifications as their husbands. She spoke on behalf of the bills before the state senate judiciary committee on January 31. Neither bill was advanced by the committee, but there was a moment of comeuppance when, six weeks later, Peck was again arrested on theft charges.[18]

Mary was so immersed in these activities over the winter that she barely had time to celebrate the fact that on November 26 she turned sixty years old.

Mary left Oswego immediately after speaking before the judiciary committee, spending a few weeks in New York City where she attended a performance at the Imperial Music Hall. She had a box to herself, until a reporter for the New York *World* joined her. She explained to the reporter her disdain for people who denigrated actresses: "Now these poor girls who have to work so hard for a living have relatives . . . There is that young lady who sings naughty songs. She does it for a livelihood. She's got a sweet face, and she looks like a dear little woman. Bah! for the opinions of society." She added, "I like the theatre. Its mimicries bring newer and brighter thoughts into the gloomy actualities of life." While in the city she also gave a series of lectures about the renewed fashion interest in crinolines. *Godey's* illustrations of the latest Paris fashions showed women whose waists tapered to a pinpoint, thus creating an extreme exaggeration of the hour-glass figure. In her lectures, Mary noted that she had tried on both hoopskirts and corsets in order to understand how it felt to wear them, but she concluded that, in spite of the lighter weight of the new styles, crinolines still affected the body in unhealthy ways, and their habit of swaying up as a woman climbed onto streetcars or ascended steps made them immodest to wear. She satirized their size as well, "Why, rapid transit will be impossible; ten women will fill up a car, men will get tripped up, and all sorts of trouble will follow if hoopskirts become the fashion." Her own clothing, she noted in contrast, was modest, convenient, and utilitarian, and she recommended her style for the general use of women everywhere.[19]

In this era Mary published one of her most self-revealing essays, "Why Women Should Wear Trousers." Humorous and self-aggrandizing, it is a notable record of her own life choices. If women had embraced "justice physically" from the beginning of the suffrage movement, she asserted, they would have been far less impeded physically and mentally in enacting the vote for women. Women who do not respect their own opinions, lack self-reliance, and travel only well-worn paths will never understand pioneers like her:

> Such cannot comprehend motives for sacred and holy endeavor by those who could not respect themselves while living a life that is an age back of their birth

any more than the elocutionist could be connected with the boy in the apple-tree. Onward the thinker, the reasoner, the philosopher must go, not liking brambles, sharp rocks, wild beasts, or whatsoever impedes; not liking martyrdom any more than the most timid, but respecting self too much to relinquish what is right, what is duty, what abilities have been given to establish!

There is nothing as enslaving as the petticoat, she insisted, and "no woman is out of her doll-babyhood who is in petticoat trammels instead of trousers."[20]

In the spring of 1893, Mary's interest in the Christie Warden murder case was reignited when she located a man she believed to have been with Snoad in Hanover. She wrote to the secretary of state and governor of New Hampshire about her discovery and outlined it in a long narrative she titled "Mistaken Identity" to explain the fraud that had taken place and to stop the execution of the wrong man. When she learned a few weeks later that Abbott's execution was scheduled, she boarded a train for New Hampshire. She telegrammed the governor, asking for a stay until she could present her argument, and for protection from Oscar Warden and others who she said had threatened her life if she came, but the governor did not respond. The train was delayed by engine trouble, and when Mary arrived on the afternoon of May 16 she was devastated to learn that Abbott had been hanged that morning. It was an ineptly conducted execution at the state prison, with a rope too long to instantly break Abbott's neck; several men had to step in and pull the body up, as the length of the rope allowed his feet to touch the floor when the hatch dropped. It took *fourteen minutes* for death to occur. Abbott asked twice to speak before he was hung, but the sheriff refused. Accounts of the hanging indicated that even as the rope was being placed around his neck Abbott tried to speak, but the sheriff quickly pulled the hood over his head. Nor did the sheriff take time to make the usual proclamation about the reason for execution. Instead, he proclaimed, "I now move to execute the sentence of the law, and may God have mercy on your soul," and hit the bar to open the hatch.[21]

Mary sent a request to the governor to claim Abbott's body. When the governor refused her request and would not meet with her, she held forth in the statehouse lobby for more than hour, relating her theories about the case and her opposition to capital punishment to reporters and a crowd that had gathered. Some newspapers found her story about a conspiracy "interesting and plausible." She explained that Abbott was not Frank Almy; the real murderer had escaped by swimming the Connecticut River and then traveling across land on a series of stolen horses. His arrival at Oswego, New York, coincided with her need for a man do some work on her house, and she rehired him, with no idea of his real identity, she explained. She identified her evidence as letters, a series of circumstances he revealed that coincided with his being in Hanover at the time of the murder, and the fact that he was suffering from varicose veins, which the Warden family said Frank Almy had but which George Abbott did not. A few days later she offered more details to the public about her belief in a conspiracy, explicitly charging the Warden family and several prominent officers, including the sheriff, with plotting to substitute Abbott for Almy in order to claim the reward money.[22]

The *Daily People and Patriot* ran a lengthy front-page story in which they detailed how Mary came to discern that her laborer was the real murderer. For the first time in public, she identified the man by both his assumed name, Arthur D. Snoad, and what she asserted was his real name, Henry L. Norcross. It was, she claimed, actually a companion of Norcross's who had been killed in the Sage bombing. Snoad passed himself off as an Englishman and was polite and agreeable while in her employ. While staying with her, however, he said that Sage and other millionaires should be blown apart with dynamite and that he had worked for a man named Almy in New England as well as having a lover named Christie. She sought his immediate arrest but was unsuccessful in securing the cooperation of the police. He left her employ shortly thereafter but returned on the evening of July 18, 1891, entering her back door, saying he was fatigued from a long journey. He also asked her to examine his legs, as he was suffering from what Mary termed "the worst kind of varicose veins from his knees to his ankles." She prescribed black silk stockings for his legs. "You will remember," Mary told the paper's reporter, "that when he dynamited Russell Sage he wore black stockings" and reminded him that George Abbott had no varicose veins. Snoad also had a rash on his back; when she examined it, she told him it looked like water rash. His explanation was that his clothes were soaked during a storm while he was on a lake cruise. She later discovered that no excursion boat had been on the lake the day he claimed to have been aboard. But it was learning details of the clothes worn by the murderer, which precisely fit those of Snoad himself, that convinced Mary. It was then that she determined to contact Andrew Warden and the long process of attempting to have Snoad-Norcross arrested as the true perpetrator began. She also indicated she still had in her possession a knife that belonged to Snoad. When the *People and Patriot* reporter questioned Mary about the fact that Abbott had confessed, she countered that many conspirators confessed to crimes they did not commit in order to profit from a confession and cited a recent New Hampshire case of a false confession. She was sure the Wardens hired Abbott to pass as Almy and that Sheriff Brown was part of the conspiracy. Abbott believed he would be acquitted, and she noted that he tried to make a statement from the scaffold but was thwarted from doing so by the sheriff.[23]

On June 7, after weeks of going to the statehouse to request a meeting with the governor, Mary was finally admitted to his office. For two hours she explained her theories, after which the governor said he would take the matter under advisement, and she returned to her hotel to await his response. The next morning, the governor simply sent word that it was too late to take any action in the case. Angry and disgusted, Mary left for the northeast.[24]

After spending a few weeks in Boston, Mary returned to Oswego. In the fall, Syracuse papers picked up the details of the interview in the *People and Patriot*; she immediately went to police headquarters in Syracuse to have Snoad arrested. He gave the police a rambling story of his movements, claiming he had come to the States from England about ten years earlier and that he had never been in New Hampshire. He could not offer an alibi for his whereabouts when Christie Warden was murdered, however. The authorities believed Mary's evidence was strong enough to arrest Snoad, and he was held in a Syracuse jail while they investigated the charges. More details came out at this time: in addition to telling Mary he worked for a family named Almy in New Hampshire, Snoad revealed he was born in Wilton, New York, and had a grandfather who died in an insane asylum, a history that paralleled that of Norcross. On October 10, Snoad retaliated by filing a $10,000 slander suit against Mary. At the same time she filed for rights to the reward money, since she was the one who identified Snoad as the true culprit. Over the next few months, Mary moved back and forth between Syracuse and Hanover, fighting against Snoad's lawsuit and for her reward claim. She filed a petition with the chief justice of the New Hampshire Supreme Court requesting a grand jury be called "that she, according to common law, may have her right to go before that body to state grievances that have been denied her in consequence of threats, and to such extent that she was not safe in the State of New Hampshire." She knew that legally a Grand Jury could be called during the entire session of the court. The judge allowed the motion to be filed but told her that it would be denied because only extraordinary circumstances would warrant such action. A total of twenty-six people, including Mary and the group at the Warden house the night she was beaten, would eventually file a right to the reward. Consequently, the supreme court decided that hearings would be held in January to determine who had a legitimate claim to the money.[25]

When a *Nashua Telegraph* reporter interviewed Mary in mid-November, he observed that she was "one of the most pleasant and courteous persons to interview that can be imagined." He found notable her commitment to the "ennobling or elevating of her fellow creatures" and asserted that her ideas about how to advance the betterment of society were "far ahead of the majority of people." She discussed the breadth of subjects on which she lectured and noted that her love of justice and equality had developed initially through her involvement in the abolition movement. On the subject of religion, she explained that she was a member of the Methodist Episcopal Church early in life, but "[n]ow I am a member of every Church in a sense. I have lived to see good in every church, to see good in every kind of association and to affiliate with every thing that is for the good and elevation of humanity. I am not cramped in any station and willing to stagnate there." She concluded with an expression of her strong opposition to executions and hoped that her legal challenges in the Almy case would induce New Hampshire to revoke capital punishment. Within weeks, she was headed north once again.[26]

On the morning of January 8, 1894, Mary arrived early at the Syracuse courthouse, ready to defend herself in *Snoad v. Walker*. More than one hundred lawyers and spectators crowded the courtroom. Mary knew well how to work the press. Before her case was called, she took a seat near the reporters' table and was soon engaged in friendly conversation with them. She made it clear that since she was just returning from New Hampshire she was not ready for trial, and everyone expected her to move to have the case delayed. When the time came for her to speak, however, she declared:

> If your honor please, I would like to make a motion in a very unusual case. I am the attorney for one Mary E. Walker, who has been sued in this court. She is unable to procure counsel for herself and I therefore appear for her. She is charged in this court with having said that Arthur D. Snoad had insane spells, during which he committed murders and that he was the person who made the dynamite with which Russell Sage was blown up. Now, as Mary E. Walker's attorney, I think that this is not the proper place to try those charges, and I ask that this court order that both Arthur D. Snoad and Mary E. Walker be taken into custody and that a commission in lunacy be appointed to examine both and determine which, whether Arthur D. Snoad or Mary E. Walker, is the lunatic.

Judge Williams was no less stunned than the spectators. His initial reply was that he was not sure he had the authority to do so, but as Mary pushed her motion, he admitted that in such instances he usually sided with the defendant. "I am the defendant, your honor," she quickly replied, and a burst of laughter filled the courtroom; the judge blushed at having thus been cornered by his own questioning. After thinking for a moment, he declared that a written request in the format required by state statutes would be necessary to consider such a motion. "I am afraid you could not do that," he concluded. "No, perhaps not," Mary agreed but quickly added, "I think under the circumstances some attorney here ought to volunteer to help me." As she sat down, several attorneys rose and seated themselves next to her. In a short while, she requested that her case be reserved until the fourth week of the term, and the court agreed. Afterwards she conferred with attorney M. F. Dillon and told reporters she would have the papers ready by the time the trial resumed. To have a commission in lunacy established would have, by its very creation, offered concurrence with Mary's assertions that capital crimes should come under the venue of physicians, which was integral to her anti-capital punishment arguments.[27]

No commission was called. Mary therefore presented her answer to the charges nearly two weeks later, simply stating she had not used false or malicious defaming words in relation to Snoad's character, but rather the charges she had made against him were

> true and that plaintiff is Henry L. Norcross, and was the murderer of Christie Warden, on the 17th day of July, 1891, under the alias of Frank C. Almy, and that

he did have dangerous materials in his brokerage office, at No. 12 Pearl street, Boston, Mass., between the time he left Oswego, N.Y., on the first day of November and the third day of December, 1891, when the bomb was dropped in Russell Sage's office, probably accidentally. That plaintiff did leave a letter locked in his safe, in his office at No. 12 Pear street, Boston, Mass., stating that he was going to New York city and that he would not be seen again, if he did not return with a million of dollars—not even his remains would be seen. That plaintiff told defendant that he had a patent for elevated railroads, and that he had a partner in Boston, and wanted money to pay half of his office rent. His partner, plaintiff believes to have been Arthur D. Snoad, an Englishman, who closely resembled himself, and who for some reason wore his clothes on the bombing occasion in Sage's office, as those clothes were the same worn at her house, in Oswego, N.Y., except hat and trousers.

The document concluded with a demand that all charges against her be dismissed and the plaintiff be responsible for court costs.[28]

On February 3, the case returned to court. Mary drew on her Spiritualist beliefs as part of her testimony. She told the court that on the evening of Snoad's return, he retired to the upstairs room where she had laborers sleep, but he was clearly agitated and talked in his sleep. On the second night, she testified, the spirits of two girls in white appeared above Snoad as he slept. When the judge interrupted to ask if she believed in ghosts, Mary countered, "Do you believe that Christ came back?" After a long argument about Spiritualism and Christianity between Mary and the judge, she was allowed to continue. In spite of the judge's occasional urging to hurry her testimony, it lasted through the evening. Mary's closing arguments took half an hour to present, and then Snoad's attorney, Harrison Hoyt, rose. He demanded that the jury find for the plaintiff and with a verdict large enough to "close her mouth effectually." When Mary called out, "You can't do that," the spectators broke into laughter. Hoyt asserted that either greed or passion had made her obsessed with Snoad: "Did there awaken in that little heart of hers during the month and half that Snoad was with her an affection which was not returned?" "That's too silly," Mary replied. They continued to volley comments back and forth in spite of the judge's warnings. Finally, Hoyt concluded his arguments, and the jury retired to consider the evidence. It took only thirty minutes for them to come to a verdict. They found in favor of Snoad—but awarded him only *six cents* in damages.[29]

Although Mary was not attending NAWSA meetings in these years, other women were speaking out in opposition to a constitutional amendment. At the February 1894 convention, Sallie Clay Bennett, a journalist from Richmond, argued against the tactic. Instead, she argued, "We should demand protection in the right already guaranteed by the United States Constitution. Even when asking for municipal suffrage, we should never fail to assert that it is already ours under the Constitution and that there is strength enough in our National Government to protect every woman in the Union, provided the men had interpreted the laws right." Had she been present, Mary would have cheered Bennett's assertion; but with the Snoad trial finally completed, Mary's attention was elsewhere. She was relishing the renewed interest in dress reform. A man from Texas wrote to Eugene V. Debs's *Locomotive Firemen's Magazine*, recalling Mary's determination to withstand ridicule and live her principles when she was in Texas in the 1870s. "It took some years," he remarked, "for San Antonio freethinkers to comprehend her policy," but the change was now evident throughout the country.[30]

By mid-June the final settlement of the Almy reward monies were due, and Mary headed to New Hampshire once again to argue the merits of her claim. As she was passing through Springfield, Massachusetts, she began to feel that she was being followed, so she stopped at police headquarters to ask for protection. The Matron on duty allowed her to sleep there for the night, and the next day she asked the sheriff if a deputy could escort Mary the rest of the way, but he refused. In spite of her fears, Mary boarded the train the next night and continued on her way. She arrived in Lebanon in time for the special supreme court session that was being held by Justice Smith to hear the claimants for the reward. There were now only five claimants. When her time to speak came, the judge insisted that nothing she could claim would influence him, but she presented her argument that the wrong man had been executed and the Wardens and the sheriff had conspired in the deception. The attorney general then moved that all of the claims be dismissed, saying all five of the petitioners had simply furnished information or, in the case of county officials, performed duties that were required of them. To no one's satisfaction, the judge instead announced that the case would be deferred until the supreme court met again in December.[31]

On her return north, Mary stopped in Worcester to offer lectures on women's rights. Their success increased her desire to do more lecturing than she had in recent months. One of her lectures focused on the connection between love and murder, drawing on the Christie Warden case and others. When she left Worcester, she stopped in Fitchburg to tend to some legal matters, and a local reporter sought her out. The reporter lamented the "morbid sentiment" attached to some criminals, the slowness of trials, and the long time between conviction and execution. Immediately, Mary countered his assertions. Capital punishment was no punishment at all, she proclaimed. Life imprisonment was a much harsher sentence, and she hoped soon to begin a campaign against capital punishment. She knew the isolation of imprisonment; she could think of nothing more devastating to the human will and believed it was a stronger deterrent of crime than execution. Her comments created such interest that she was invited to return to Fitchburg in early October to lecture, and the ticket sales were brisk.[32]

After lecturing in Massachusetts and Connecticut, she headed for the World's Food Fair in Boston where she lectured twice a day, drawing large crowds and good reviews. Mary began her campaign against capital punishment with a lecture on the subject at Faneuil Hall on November 4. Although she drew only a small crowd, the lecture was covered at length in the newspapers. Dr. P. P. Field, a leader in the People's Party of Massachusetts, introduced Mary. She forthrightly declared her position: "It is terrible that the people of this state should sanction hanging entertainments. That's what they are—stag party wine entertainments wherever there are executions." Capital punishment will never prevent crime, she declared, arguing that the act of execution itself created state-sanctioned murders. Nor was electrocution, as New York State used, any better than hanging—"It is simply a compromise on hanging, with which the people had become disgusted." Criticism was not enough, she declared; action must be taken. "What I want to see enacted is a law to place murderers in state prisons for life. The power of the pardon should be taken away from governors and vested with the judges of the supreme bench." Further, the abolition of capital punishment would eliminate the execution of the innocent: "If a prisoner's innocence is ever established, restitution ought to be made. He should be paid a sum equal to what he would have earned in whatever occupation he was employed when imprisoned." As a Spiritualist, Mary also felt that murderers could have influence after death and thus execution empowered them in unnatural ways: "The spirit of an executed man will do all the harm it can for sake of glorying over its revenge." She also challenged the state's role in executions: "The state of Massachusetts works on the same principle. It hangs for revenge—for punishment. A person should be confined only for the sake of safety to his fellows. He should work for his own support and that of his family. He should be surrounded with flowers and pictures, and above all good books, so that when he gets freedom, either by pardon or death, he will not leave with feelings of hostility to humanity."[33]

Shortly after her lecture, Mary returned to New Hampshire for the fifth time on business related to her claim for the Almy reward money. Expecting to hear a decision, she attended the supreme court session in Concord on December 11, but the justices reported that the case had not yet been prepared for presentation to the higher court and assured claimants it would be ready by the March term. In July the court rendered its verdict: Louisa Warden was granted $500, and the remaining $3,500 was split between Sheriff Brown and a Professor Whitcher. Mary's claim for a portion of the reward was denied. Before she left the state, however, she visited Louisa Warden, inviting her to go with Mary before the state legislature to plead for the abolition of capital punishment. Although Warden was unwilling to do so, she raised another issue with Mary. She was preparing to leave Hanover to attend medical college and asked for advice, which Mary readily offered. It was her final contact with a member of the Warden family.[34]

Mary went to the New Hampshire House of Representatives on January 18, 1895, and filed a request with the Speaker that she be allowed to use the House for one evening the following week in order to be heard on a current bill relating to capital punishment. The request was "by unanimous consent laid upon the table." However, Mary had the consolation that, because of the bungled hanging of Abbott, the New Hampshire legislature soon thereafter abolished the death penalty except when the jury itself called for execution. No jury made such a recommendation until 1916, effectively eliminating execution in New Hampshire for more than twenty years.[35]

As the new year began, Mary's emotions surged and plunged. She was pleased that an increasing number of magazines and newspapers sought her opinions on subjects of the day, and yet once again she felt she must enter into a legal dispute.

This dispute was on a more personal level than the nationally publicized cases in which she usually engaged. Upon the death of her paternal aunt and namesake, Mary Walker of Greenwich, Massachusetts, Mary was stunned to learn that everything had been left to Greenwich relatives. She immediately traveled to Massachusetts to investigate and soon came to believe that the revised will allotting the estate to these relatives was a forgery. She had seen the original will written by Aunt Mary; it left everything to Vesta Walker, with only selected household items to other relatives. Once again a conflict led her to envision a conspiracy. She asserted that the signature on the revised will did not appear to be her aunt's and there was no intact seal on the original will. When no satisfactory explanation came from her relatives, she filed a lawsuit contesting the will as a forged document. She pleaded her own case, but the court found against her. Her loss was greater than a legal decision, however. Her Greenwich relatives had been her supporters for decades; she always traveled to Greenwich when she needed a reprieve from public outcries against her reform arguments. While she remained close to her Aunt Vashti, the lawsuit created a rift and such stringent animosity from her remaining Massachusetts relatives that she became fearful of confrontations with them. It was the end of one of her most important family connections.[36]

The contentions of the past few months abated, and Mary spent a comfortable summer in Oswego, participating in local events and giving occasional lectures. The rest of the year was a time of planning for Mary. She had been mulling over ideas for several years about how best to advance women's independence and abilities to govern. Through these endeavors she was able to draw herself out of the psychological miasma of conspiracy theories and legal entanglements. Her plan was announced in October 1895. In a carefully crafted broadside that was reprinted in newspapers throughout the nation, Mary announced the founding of *A Colony for New Women*. This document was one of her most important writings in the 1890s. She consulted several of Oswego's progressive women about the project before it was announced, and their approval encouraged her to proceed. She had legal documents drawn for the colony that would utilize all thirty-five acres of her Oswego property. The community's goal was to train women in agricultural skills so they could be financially independent. The financial panic of 1893 and the departure of many young men from the rural northeast left their female counterparts vulnerable to lives of poverty and isolation. The Colony sought to offer new advantages to working-class women: "We will live in a large, commodious farm house.... Every member will have her own room. Portieres will take the place of doors. Steam will be employed for heating purposes, and there will be bathrooms and every convenience to be found in a well-regulated and modern house." Each member would be given a share in the profits of the Colony, and a portion would be held in a general fund for improvements and the purchase of adjoining lands as the Colony grew. Any women of good character between the ages of fifteen and thirty-five were eligible for membership, and they were expected to make a three-year commitment to the community. After three years, if a member chose to "retire" from the Colony, she would be given seven-eighths of her earnings, with one-eighth deposited into the general fund.[37]

Perhaps most important in the planning of the Colony was its goal of educating women to govern themselves. "I expect lots of politics in the community," Mary wrote, "and the members will soon be able to hold their own, I warrant, with some of the so-called statesmen of the day." Mary would serve as the general supervisor of the establishment, but members would elect officers twice a year to manage all aspects of the Colony. There would be an auditing board to handle financial matters, an improvement board dedicated to insuring maintenance and progress in the Colony's development, and a governing board. A chairman would be elected for the governing board, with the responsibility to report any infractions of the rules by members. As in any community, discipline would be necessary. Two judges would be selected; one would have authority similar to a police magistrate, while the other would serve in the more traditional capacity. Anyone accused of infractions would be tried by a jury of five; if they were not satisfied with the judgments of the "lower courts," they would have an opportunity to appeal directly to Mary herself. "I will sit as a court of last resort," she explained, thus granting herself not simply general directorship of the Colony but a position as supreme court justice. The rules of evidence for the Colony's courts were patterned on those that governed New York's state judiciary. However, there was a very distinct difference to the Colony's sentencing for those who committed infractions: "There will be no imprisonments; all punishments will consist of withdrawal of privileges for a certain length of time. If we should get into our fold undesirable women, who flirt or gad about with men when they go to market or on other occasions, they will, after suitable warning, be expelled." Having endured imprisonment during the war and more recently being held for several days in a New Hampshire jail, Mary would not countenance such harsh treatment in her utopia.[38]

The educational benefits of the Colony were to be many. The property already boasted of several acres of strawberries, an apple orchard, several hundred pear trees, and four acres devoted to a vineyard. The members would learn to tend all of these sections, but "it will not all be farm work," she promised. "There will be many hours each day for study, and the curriculum will be as broad and extended as that in any of our universities. There will be frequent lectures in a large assembly room that I propose to have, and current literature, politics and questions of the day will be discussed." There would be bicycles for the members to ride as well as horses—and the women would be expected to forego side saddles: "My girls will ride astride, as do the men, and I predict that three years of life in our institution will make the members the peers of any man physically or mentally." She had no intention of making rules "that defy all the laws of nature [or] exact pledges binding for life," although members would be expected to wear a reform dress. "I expect that many of those that come to us will go forth from our tutelage to enter the homes of men to become wives and mothers. When such times come they will know how to be both, and how to raise and educate families that will reflect credit upon the nation of new women." The beautiful site would become, Mary predicted, "a perfect garden of Eden, but without an Adam."[39]

National newspapers and magazines exploded with responses to Mary's project, and word spread through the United Kingdom, Europe, and Australia of this unusual plan for women's advancement. The majority ignored the complexities of the proposal and satirized the concept of developing "an Adamless Eden," but a few periodicals took the project seriously. The *Daily Northwestern* called it a "scheme for bloomer girls" and emphasized the requirement of celibacy, but they detailed the plans for a common house, boards and judges, and profit sharing. Even more balanced was W. D. Inslee's interview with Mary for *Metropolitan Magazine*. As she told Inslee, the idea for a Colony had been percolating in her mind for many years. "Every woman must do something to be somebody," she explained, and she envisioned the project as primarily for women who would be living in rural areas, marrying farmers, and struggling to make a living unless they had an opportunity such as her "training school" would offer. She quickly reneged on the requirement of wearing reform clothing, and Inslee reported that she was presenting a new wife's school, although that was not a term Mary ever used. Inslee remarked on her amazing level of activity. She worked the farm, cared for an elderly woman who had been in her family for many years, served the community as a surgeon, physician, and dentist, and was a prolific reader who had a "small but excellent library." He concluded that there were many places more pretentious than Mary's home, "but there is no place where content and peace are more in evidence."[40]

Most damaging to the possibilities of her plan was a satire of the Colony that the extremely popular humorist Bill Nye published in the *Boston Globe* and which was reprinted widely. Illustrating the article with images of aging women plowing and young women in ridiculous costumes with "harem pants," Nye declared, "Plowing will be done by middle aged ladies in peasant costume and Tyrolean red morocco slippers. . . . Turkeys with pale blue watered ribbons will eat bird seed and cuttle bone. . . . The milkmaids will dress picturesquely in beautiful white tarlatan chemisettes and duck trousers," and on and on. Although as Inslee noted at present Mary lived in a "colony of one," she was able to enact a small version of her ideal over the next several years. No lodge was built and the goal of seventy-five members was never achieved, but there were several women who stayed at Mary's home, learned new skills, and certainly had the opportunity to engage in political and literary discussions. If it was ultimately an unachievable goal, it was a remarkable gesture of envisioning how to bring the New Woman philosophy to the working classes.[41]

On November 15 Mary learned that her Aunt Vashti had died, and she traveled to Greenwich to settle the estate, which she managed to do without any major confrontations with surviving relatives. In early January 1896 she began her return trip to Oswego, stopping one night in Rome to see old friends, where a *Rome Sentinel* reporter arranged to interview her. "I have great love for the Romans. . . . Next to my native place, Oswego, there is no place for whose people I entertain such a feeling of regard as I do for the people of Rome," she remarked. She also discussed her medical practice as a registered physician in Washington and New York. She advocated dress reform, and then the subject of her age arose. "If people want to know how old I am," she replied, "I say I am nearly as old as Methuselah, because we live in deeds and not in years." It was a phrase she liked and would often repeat about herself in coming years. She attributed her healthy appearance to never using tobacco, intoxicants, tea, or coffee. As she looked ahead to the fall's presidential election, she declared her preference for Governor William E. Russell of Massachusetts. Young and progressive, Russell had supported several pro-labor laws during his tenure. If the Democrats would nominate him and select a vice president from the west, Mary predicted, they would sweep the elections. She intended to be at the Democratic convention again and felt that, because she had so many veterans from around the country as friends, her advocacy of a candidate would draw the veteran vote. The comment was true, but also a nice touch of self-promotion. Shortly thereafter, Captain Jack Adams gave a talk about his war experiences at the Kernwood Club in Malden, Massachusetts. Adams had been a member of the 19th Massachusetts Regiment, and he, too, had been a prisoner of war in a Confederate camp. "One day," he recalled," as we were being marched by Castle Thunder I saw a woman sitting at the window fanning herself. On one side of the fan was an American flag. Afterward I discovered that the woman was Dr. Mary Walker. I don't care whether she wears pants or not, she's all right. She wears a medal of honor on her breast that stamps that upon the mind of all loyal men."[42]

Mary stayed in Oswego only a short time, traveling in early February to Boston where she was the guest of Anna Christy Fall and her husband, Councilman George H. Fall. Both Falls were attorneys, Anna having graduated magna cum laude from Boston University Law School in 1891. In addition to the Falls' joint practice, Anna lectured throughout the state on issues relating to women and the law. George Fall was also a graduate of Boston University Law School and had been a member of the faculty since 1886. Over the next two months, Mary gave a number of lectures in the area, attended the theater to hear the Edelweiss Swiss Choir, and toured Amherst College. She also gave an impromptu speech on the evening of February 9 at the Enterprise Club of Working Girls' headquarters in Malden. The early part of her talk was autobiographical in nature. Touching on a point of importance to her audience, she explained that part of her early work with Congress to abolish unjust laws was to change the tax laws; after the war, workers were required to pay taxes on all annual incomes over $500, and she had argued successfully to have the minimum raised to $1,000. In early March she also gave a benefit lecture at the People's Temple, speaking again on her war experiences.[43]

Although thwarted in her plans for a New Woman Colony, Mary began a new quest to found a sanitarium for women. It would be four years before she published a broadside calling for financial support of the institution, but while in Boston she attended a hearing of the Aldermanic Committee on Health that related to homes for consumptives, following such arguments carefully as part of her preparations. She also revealed her opposition to the new germ theories—what she termed "that humbug theory of microbes in consumption"—that were reshaping medical research. Many allopaths, homeopaths, and eclectics alike questioned the theories in these years. Although cutting-edge work was being done at Johns Hopkins Medical School, it would not be until the 1910 Flexner Report exposed gaps in medical education that training in germ theory and other advances would enter medical education on a nationwide basis. The move to clinical research and a compendium of new discoveries in medicine beginning in the late nineteenth century were leaving physicians from Mary's generation far behind the curve of cutting-edge medical treatment. Many if not most continued to practice, but there was a notable breach between medical generations that had given rise to the required licensing of physicians in most states. Mary was licensed and continued to practice on a small scale for the next twenty years, maintaining a viable interest in "the school of prevention." Thus she planned a sanitarium that would teach prevention as well as treat patients.[44]

That summer Mary gave an address at the Cayuga County veterans' reunion in Westbury, New York. In addition to her busy lecture schedules, she attended G.A.R. reunions whenever possible. The fall presidential campaign once again drew her attention. She was interested in William Jennings Bryan's candidacy because he was a peace and temperance advocate (his spouse, Mary Baird Bryan, was a member of the WCTU), and after studying his ideas on free silver and other issues, she began to speak in his favor wherever she lectured that fall. After McKinley won, Mary maintained a cordial relationship with the Bryans, and occasionally corresponded with Mary Baird Bryan. Becoming active again in presidential politics whetted Mary's appetite for a return to Washington. By February 1897 she was in the capital, weathering a snow storm to make calls on cabinet members, and she remained in the city for several months, becoming as active as she had been decades earlier. She was an attendee at three drawing-room receptions among "the Cabinet circle," wearing her new chinchilla cape and conversing on a wide range of political issues of the day.[45]

Mary also attended the first National Congress of Mothers, which ran for three days in mid-February. It was largely an organization of conservatives; religion and the romanticization of motherhood reigned, but there were also important discussions on mothers' roles in the elimination of crime and poverty. Anthony Comstock was one of the invited speakers. He proposed a resolution to enact more stringent laws in relation to obscene literature and art, but the committee on resolutions refused to act on it. Mary attempted to speak on dress reform but was rebuffed with laughter and hisses and only a smattering of applause. Yet she enjoyed lectures at the congress, such as Julia King's on "Physical Culture" that advocated physical activity for health and character development, and Belva Lockwood's presentation of a resolution on behalf of the Peace Union. At the same time there was increased attention to the fact that Mary's clothing style, while still unique, was not as shocking as it once had been. The *Chicago Tribune* ran an illustration of her changing clothing styles from the 1850s to the present, and the *Minneapolis Sunday Tribune* published a lengthy interview with illustrations of her transformation from the 1850s reform dress to the Prince Albert coat and pants of the 1890s. The Minneapolis interview, conducted by S. R. Charles, was one of the most extensive Mary gave in these years. She traced her life from medical school to the present. "I am the original new woman," she declared, and was pleased to observe that "public opinion on the matter of dress reform is changing considerably. I do not meet with the ridicule and persecution which were so common years ago. Why! up to four years ago any woman who was before the public was called crazy. That's different now." Charles was not a sympathetic interviewer. The title of his article, "The Only Self Made Man in America," used the satirical phrase that Bill Nye had coined about Mary years earlier and which was repeated often by her critics. Charles also concluded the article with the false claim that Mary had married a man named Brown after the war. But the interview was rich in lengthy commentaries by Mary and reflected the way in which she was thinking about her life's history.[46]

She also had the pleasure of seeing two major books on famous Americans appear at the end of the decade that acclaimed her contributions to American culture and politics. A. T. Camden Pratt's two-volume *People of the Period* was published in London in 1897 and listed Mary as a pioneer of dress reform and women's rights in England. Although somewhat skeptical of her plans for the New Woman Colony, Pratt offered details about its philosophical basis. Far more laudatory was Frances E. Willard and Mary A. Livermore's *American Women*. Published with a portrait of Mary in her overcoat and straight-legged pants, the authors gave a lengthy description of her career and noted that in any other country her work during the Civil War "would have caused her to be recognized as a heroine of the nation." But Mary had little time to relish such accolades. Her attention was drawn to national matters as she studied the ongoing government actions in relation to Hawai'i and became increasing distressed by what she learned. In December she returned to Washington. If the last few years had been a mishmash of legal wranglings, she was about to regain a sense of commitment and control over her activism through one of her most notable battles—against the imperialist activities of the United States government.[47]

CHAPTER 12

Anti-Imperialism and the World Stage

Mary's return to Washington in January 1898 was covered by the city's major newspapers, which now hailed her as "a remarkable woman" whose work was not yet completed. It took only a matter of days for political circles in the city to recognize that she had come with the intent to challenge the United States' annexation of Hawai'i. Although the U.S. government had immersed itself in Hawai'i's economy and politics for decades, it advanced its efforts at domination in 1893 when the military helped depose Queen Lili'uokalani and put a U.S.-aligned oligarchy in place on July 4, 1894, with Sanford B. Dole as president. Dole was instrumental in the Hawaiian legislature's forced adoption of the Bayonet Constitution that granted voting rights based on wealth and greatly diminished the power of the monarchy. The U.S. government's actions were even more brutal and blatant in 1897–1898 when it moved to annex Hawai'i, claiming it needed to use the islands as a base to protect against "abandonment to Asia." To Mary, these imperialistic activities were in absolute contradiction to the values of her country. Her first action was to invite each member of the Senate Committee on Territories to attend her lecture on why Hawai'i should not be annexed. No senator appeared. In earlier days, such an event would have been used to mock her efforts, but the political climate was changing; one of the reporters who attended the lecture saw the legislators' absence as "proof of the degeneration of the United States Senate . . . that not a single senator availed himself of this opportunity to acquire much useful information."[1]

Mary immediately sought an audience with Queen Lili'uokalani. They met in the Queen's rooms at the Shoreham Hotel in Washington. Little is known about the content of their discussion, except that Mary expressed her sympathy with Hawai'i's political situation and that, when the meeting was over, she bowed before the Queen and kissed her hand to demonstrate respect for the position of royalty that was due her. Mary followed the meeting by submitting a lengthy letter to the editor of the *Washington Post* in which she detailed her reasons for opposing annexation. Discrediting a recent claim that every argument against annexing Hawai'i had also been used in opposition to the United States' "annexing" of Louisiana, Florida, and Alaska, she argued that "no rulers were dethroned" and peaceable negotiations were involved in those processes. While she proclaimed there was "no usurpation of Texas, as nine-tenths of the people asked for annexation," she noted correctly that "21,000 of the Hawaiians have a petition in the United States Senate that is but another way of voting against annexation." Nor was an oligarchy established in the earlier territories, she reminded the *Post*'s readers. Equally abominable was the way in which the Hawaiian ruler "was placed in durance vile and threatened with death if an abdication paper was not signed." Mary explicitly criticized the power given to the Dole family, which profited extraordinarily from its control of the Hawaiian economy. That the Dole government was using U.S. men-of-war "to enforce the Dole tribe acts" was unconscionable. The precedent established in the government's actions most concerned her: "'annexation' means departing from republican justice to a small sister nation with which we were at peace." The Dole government, which she accused of "highway robbery of the islands," called loudly for annexation because "they have found that the brave people are not so easy to deal with in oligarchy as was expected with the sham republic reality."[2]

In early February when President McKinley hosted a White House reception for President Dole, Mary asked for an invitation based on her war record, and it was granted. Concerns surfaced as to whether or not she would raise the issue of annexation at the reception, but Mary was a model of decorum, knowing that her presence made annexation the unacknowledged elephant in the room. In fact, it was her conversation with the Chinese minister that drew the attention of the press. The minister, Wu Tingfang, asked Mary why she wore pants. Politely but pointedly, she replied, "Why do you wear a gown, or dress?" "Because it is the custom of my country," he replied; Mary countered, "Well, I wear trousers because this is a free country, and people are not handicapped by custom." In an account of his trip to America published several years later, he recalled that leaders walking in the streets of England and the United States demonstrated a remarkably "unrestrained liberty and equality" as represented by Dr. Mary Walker.[3]

In the meantime, she worked the halls of Congress week after week, talking with congressmen about why they should vote against the annexation of Hawai'i. Legislators and reporters alike listened to Mary's arguments, often noting that she was there without pay, not as a lobbyist for a corporation, and she was acting out of a sincere respect for Queen Lili'uokalani, whom she saw as "a grand and worthy specimen of her sex." Mary extended her argument to include the assertion that to annex the islands would lead to the end of the U.S. republic. "There is a clause in the constitution," she reminded the nation, "which forbids any citizen to meddle with or interfere in the affairs of a foreign nation with which we are at peace. And hence it is proposed that the government itself shall go and violate the constitution." She repeatedly used the title of Queen in her references to the Hawaiian sovereign; annexationists and many among the press used denigrating nicknames for her such as "Lil." Annexationists adamantly denied accusations that Hawai'i had been colonized as "a white man's republic," but Mary insisted on articulating the realities of what had happened in the island nation. She charged the U.S. government with making its citizens complicit in criminal acts: Queen Lili'uokalani "was so cruelly cheated out of her dominion. That was a crime committed in the name of the people of the United States. Now we are asked to receive stolen property. Oh, it is a shame, a burning shame!" It was Mary at her best, using logic, patriotism, and pathos to work for a cause rooted in questions of American justice.[4]

She published one of her most important writings of the 1890s, *Isonomy*, when she first arrived in Washington that winter, and she distributed it widely in the early months of 1898. *Isonomy* as a title was significant. Defined as equality before the law, including equal distribution of rights and privileges, the concept had been used from ancient times to assert democratic concepts of sovereignty and citizenship—and of governance without violence. Apparently self-published, the ten-page pamphlet's cover was a sketch of Iolani Palace where the Queen was held prisoner for eight months. Although the text was signed at the end, the first page read, "By One of America's Sovereigns, to the Servants of the People," and the document was addressed to legislators. *Isonomy* was a blend of blindness and acuity. Among Mary's neighbors when she was in her teens were Fannie and John Bishop, the parents of Artemus Bishop; it was from the Bishops that she initially learned about the history and sovereignty of Hawai'i and about their son's missionary work in that nation. Perhaps because of this personal association, Mary was surprisingly silent in *Isonomy* and elsewhere about the role of missionaries like Reverend Bishop as participants in the processes of imperialism. About the government, however, she was intrepid. Hawaiians were fully capable of determining for themselves whom they wished to have as a ruler, she declared, and arguments from annexationists that controlling Hawai'i was the only means of preventing "abandonment to Asia" constituted pure sophistry. Further, for the government to act in this unconstitutional manner was an "annihilation of the foundation principles of our dear and glorious republic." Her argument specifically employed the gendered nature of U.S. politics:

> Never, all time, and countries, have there been so many and various wrongs to civilized women, by the gentlemen, as since a great government has sanctioned and abetted the high-handed robbery of a Queen! This, by its physical strength and bravado, and hid behind sophistry too contemptible for a school-boy, too weak for the smallest court to entertain, and the Supreme Court of the United States ought to defend, and of right will do so, if matters are carried where necessity compels such an appeal.

Citing sections of the Constitution that banned the use of any U.S. vessel for another country to commit hostilities against its people, she insisted that the president, cabinet members, and congressmen who backed the use of a man-of-war in support of the Dole government should be deemed "guilty of high misdemeanor . . . and fined not more than ten thousand dollars and imprisoned not more than three years," as the Constitution demanded. It was incumbent upon the Congress of the United States, she argued, to act with justice, but its members' greed over the business advantages that the islands offered led them to act in concert with President Dole: "Woe to America when the great deliberative body loses the respect of the people, for that means that respect for their laws will be etherized. As a sovereign in this country I deplore such an event." She called on the government to restore the Queen to her throne and protect *her* with the man-of-war. Do not be taken in, she commanded, by the "Dole-ful sound" of a cry for protection from the very people responsible for usurping the Queen's throne.[5]

It was many years since Mary had participated in an NAWSA convention, but as the group was set to meet in Washington this year, she decided to attend. She continued to have a following among suffragists, although it was smaller than in the heyday of the 1870s. Susan B. Anthony's commitment to the association and its predecessor, the NWSA, now numbered fifty years. But she and Mary were more intractable than ever. After a congressional hearing in the morning, the convention opened on February 15 with Anthony presenting to a large audience the pioneers of the movement, who had been invited to be seated on the stage. Mary was not among the group nor invited to the convention. She came in the afternoon when the regular meeting was being chaired by Carrie Chapman Catt. At one point Mary rose from her seat and attempted to attract Catt's attention, but Catt instead called on a Mrs. Harrison from Missouri. Both Mary and Harrison began to speak at once; Catt immediately commented that she had recognized Mrs. Harrison. "I was on my feet first and addressed the chair first, and I am entitled to the floor," Mary responded. In spite of Catt encouraging Harrison to continue, the latter declined in favor of letting Mary have the floor. Mary's first comments were about her pride in the movement, but then she remarked that it was not being well directed and offered suggestions for improvement. When Catt stopped her by saying the topic was press work for the organization, Mary insisted that she was addressing press work and other means by which the NAWSA could improve its practices. Attempting to speak over Catt's pounding gavel, Mary's voice failed, and Catt won the day. The following day, Mary arrived while a work conference was in session and the doors locked; she waited in the lobby and when attendees came out for a break, she spoke with many of them. When the chair refused again that afternoon to recognize her, she took a seat in the back of the hall and made no attempt to interject her comments. When one of the officers was asked in the evening about the refusal to allow Mary to speak, the officer used the old line that free speech was not allowed at the convention.[6]

A few days later, Mary spoke to a group of participants during a break in convention proceedings and was volubly critical of Anthony. "Sue Anthony doesn't want suffrage for the women at all, for when they get it her occupation, like Othello's will be gone," she declared. When the women were shocked at such a declaration, she replied, "You need not look so astonished for I know all about Sue Anthony. I have been through her with a lighted candle. The love of power is the keynote of her character." One woman cautioned Mary that Anthony might hear her. "Let her hear," Mary stated defiantly; not without irony, she added, "If they had conducted this campaign with any common sense, if they hadn't spent so much time trying to suppress me, if they had done as I wanted them to do, women would have been voting for the last fifteen years." When a man in the group said he did not understand the basis of her disagreement, she spoke fully on her opinions of how to work through the legislature for acknowledgement of women's right to vote as citizens of the United States. A woman reporter for the *St. Louis Globe-Democrat* listened to the conversation and remarked that "with her diminutive form drawn up to its full height, her eyes flashing and her face lit up with enthusiasm, [Mary] gave reasons for the faith within in her, making the best argument for women suffrage that I have heard." The reporter said she forgot about women's inferiority, forgot that women should not dress in men's clothing, "forgot everything but Doctor Walker's eloquence, and at the conclusion of her speech I went and shook hands with her and patted her on the back."[7]

It was a month of rebuffs, however. After the suffragists silenced her, so, too, did the Daughters of the American Revolution. Mary could trace her family's history to the Revolution, and she decided that she wanted to become a member of the D.A.R. Her patriotism was an essential trait of her character, but the highly conservative D.A.R. was otherwise an unlikely association for her. Mary's appearance at the convention on February 23 created a stir among its delegates. That evening the D.A.R.'s National Board of Management issued a statement acknowledging that Mary had submitted necessary paperwork for admittance some months earlier. There was no question about her qualifications; rather, "The board decided that this society, being one composed of women, could not consider the candidate as eligible or acceptable, she having repudiated the recognized apparel of women. Both papers and money were returned to the applicant." Mary made no disturbance at the convention; only the D.A.R. itself made her presence an issue, and the focus of newspaper accounts of the convention was thus on their refusal of her application. One more rebuff came Mary's way soon thereafter. In spite of earlier positive reports, she was again turned down for an increase in her pension. Assistant Secretary of the Interior Webster Davis, who was actively revising pension rulings, questioned whether her heart and lung diseases or her lameness were related to her military service; the only health issue that could be considered was her eyesight, and he insisted that she was not qualified under the act of July 14, 1892, which granted a pension rate of $50 to veterans.[8]

But the tide of rebuffs was about to change, as reflected in an editorial that appeared in the *Washington Post* on February 27, 1898. Albert Johnson was editor of the *Post* for only one year, but he became keenly interested in Mary's political commentaries and maintained a commitment to her right to express them. In "Persecuting Dr. Mary Walker," the *Post* took exception to the attempts by several organizations to suppress—with "superfluous severity"—her free expression. It was only natural that she should wish to speak, the account asserted: "seeing earnest audiences ready for the absorption of true eloquence," what was more natural than to "have sought to improve the shining hour?" The *Post* questioned what appeared to be a "concerted action" and thought such suppression deserved interrogation: "Dr. Mary Walker is a speaker, a student, a publicist, a faithful worker in the vineyard of moral and material advancement. Why has she been muzzled so callously and so persistently?" It should matter less that she was a member than that she had something of interest and importance to convey to those in attendance:

> Why did the Presidents General, and the eminent high potentates, and the rest of the authorities in charge at different times and places refuse, with such significant unanimity to let Dr. Mary Walker uncork the vials of her information and empty them upon an anxious world?
>
> We have received a painful impression from this incident, or rather series of incidents. We receive the impression of an unkind and intolerant conspiracy against one of the most gifted and willing teachers of the age.

When the charge of conspiracy came from the *Washington Post*, it carried a new potency.[9]

Mary used her moment of support from the *Post* to its fullest advantage. She appeared in Equity Court No. 1 on February 24. After waiting for a pause in the proceedings, she moved to the front of the court where she could address presiding Judge Cox. Reading from a prepared statement, she asked that the judge call for a stay on the annexation of Hawai'i "for the purpose of having verbal sworn testimony taken before the Committee on Foreign Affairs or before the committee of the whole. I most respectfully set forth to your honor that as one of the sovereign people I have a right to ask that illegal acts by the Senate of the United States be stayed, since said Senate is proceeding without verbal sworn testimony, and has refused in a previous sitting to hear a deposed Queen whose relations with the United States were peaceable and who was unconstitutionally deposed by the United States citizens and the United States man-of-war named the Boston." Repeatedly in her commentaries about Hawai'i, Mary invoked the rights of the people—both of the United States and especially of Hawai'i—to be heard in the processes being advocated by the U.S. Senate. The Senate "should, according to the usage of just bodies, hear verbal sworn testimony where aggrieved parties are in jeopardy in person and property, and where so grave a subject as the annexation of midocean territory against the expressed wishes of the people, owners thereof, are concerned, and also against the large petitions of American sovereign people. Anarchy in the United States Senate should have a stay since United States Senators have declared 'Law or no law, we shall annex Hawaii to the United States.'" Judge Cox listened quietly until she had completed her statement, then asked, "What do you want me to do?" She requested that her lawyer, Judge John A. Clarke, be allowed to make an argument before the court, adding, "Had the United States Senate heard testimony from the ex-Queen and others we would not now be in the trouble regarding Cuba." Mary asked Cox to deliver an opinion as to whether or not he had the jurisdiction to stay the Senate in this matter. Cox quickly announced that he did not have such jurisdiction. Mary thanked him, said that she would appeal his decision, and left a copy of the statement with the clerk but did not pay the fee to have it placed in the record.[10]

Immediately thereafter she met with a *Post* reporter to explain her procedures: "No one could know better than myself that Justice Cox had no jurisdiction, and my sole object in asking for a hearing was for the purpose of getting the opinion." The equity court held an important resonance, as Mary knew; it was the court in which equity could trump law. She explained that if she had gone directly to Congress, she would have gotten nowhere with her call for a stay on the joint resolution, but once she could demonstrate that an unsuccessful attempt had been made in the courts to have such action taken, a bill could be introduced to that effect. "We are a great people with unusual contingencies staring us in the face," she declared, "and national life must have the preventive treatment. Every conceivable safeguard should be had against the possible, and not wait for the storm to burst before any preparation is made. We must not forget that 'governments derive their just powers from the consent of the governed' and that force can not keep us together, and that with all the isms and nationalities, diversities of interests, we require greater safeguards than in the primitive days." Her ultimate goal was to have the Supreme Court rather than Congress determine the constitutionality of the government's present actions. "Absolute power should not be tolerated under a republican form of government," she concluded. It was a losing battle, but not one that Mary would soon concede.[11]

As spring came to the capital, Mary worked on several fronts, national and personal. She renewed her interest in building a hospital, home, and school for consumptives on her Oswego property, and she sent letters seeking support for the project to several prominent people. She also continued her efforts to gain membership in the D.A.R., believing it was due recognition to her ancestors. She had surprising support from across the country for her claim. One Midwestern newspaper acknowledged that Mary had made the necessary proof of her eligibility and thus asked what right the D.A.R. had to reject her because of her clothing: "What is recognized apparel of woman? Is it golfer's uniform, the tailor-made garment or the shirt waist and short skirt of the summer girl? If Dr. Mary Walker prefers to wear the golfer's coat and the bicycler's trousers as a regular costume, does that make her any the less a patriotic daughter of the revolution?" The paper captured the changing culture of the New Woman's physical activity and clothing appropriate to that change. Popular culture now referred to women's trousers as "Mary Walkers," and articles about her life in trousers were published from Boston to Los Angeles.[12]

In March, the *Boston Globe* printed a long interview with Mary about her clothing choices and her activism. The article began by noting that she was a woman who wore trousers but "doesn't wish she were a man." As new "scientific" arguments emerged about "sexual inversion" (Havelock Ellis's derogatory term for lesbianism), articles often compared cross-dressing women with Mary. But her insistence on identifying herself as a woman and rejecting a liminal sense of gender, even as she performed the undoing of gender norms in her appearance and comments, cast her into a realm that fit none of the contemporary sexual "isms." In the *Globe* interview, she used precisely this mixture of tactics to deny an easy category of sexual identity. In addition to identifying herself as a woman, she recalled that when she had worn her overcoat in the post-war years, "I looked every inch the man, and I am sure I acted it, for I was the only woman who has been granted a medal by congress for active military duty." At the same time she lamented "the brazen effrontery" with which some young women flirted with her; she assumed they thought she was a man. She acknowledged still having to face ignorance about her choices but asserted that it had significantly diminished and was only proffered by "ill-bred people.... You would be surprised to find how little trouble I really have. And then think what a relief it is, when one arrives in a strange city, to be able to pick up one's grip and walk up the street without bothering anybody, and without having some soft-spoken fellow come up with a smirk and 'Is there anything I can do for you, miss?' O, I tell you, trousers are a great thing." She also revealed that Chinese Minister Wu's wife had been a patient of hers while the couple was in the country and delightedly noted that Madame Wu wore "broadcloth pants and tunic. She was dressed just about as I am.... I don't see why they should be called men's clothes when they answer just as well for women." Mary added, "I don't pretend to be a dude, and I don't care very much about following the latest styles.... All I ask is that they look well and fit comfortably." When the influential editor Mrs. Frank Leslie spoke out in favor of women dressing appropriately for the new occupations they were undertaking and for pleasures such as bicycling, she sought a comment from Mary, in spite of the fact that Leslie had called explicitly for "feminine—never mannish" attire. Mary's reply was succinct: "Business women should dress like business men. Doll women, like dolls."[13]

Such interviews interested Mary less than did her work against U.S. imperialism. She increased her efforts in April when President McKinley enacted a blockade of Cuban ports. She spoke in the lobby of the Capitol, hopefully but erroneously declaring that there would be no war: "The whole matter will be decided by arbitration. In fact, it must be so decided. I am here to talk about it and will show the explosion of the *Maine* was not due to Spanish treachery, as has been claimed. The charge is a false one, and I have the evidence in my pocket to prove that fact." She claimed instead that U.S. government officials had been in league with the insurgents. She went so far as to threaten to communicate the details of the conspiracy to the Spanish government if Congress did not back off from war. In spite of a growing anti-imperialist sentiment among a segment of the population, the destruction of the man-of-war was a rallying point for Americans to support war. Reflecting the spirit of a country that embraced the cry of "Remember the *Maine!*" the *Chicago Tribune* charged her with "treasonable talk," although nothing came of such accusations, and she did not back down. Shortly thereafter Mary created a disturbance in the gallery of the Senate. Reacting to proceedings on the floor of the Senate through gestures from the gallery was a tactic she had used many times. In this instance she waved her handkerchief in favor of anti-annexation speeches; in spite of a warning, she repeated the gesture the following day and was ordered by a guard to leave. She rose and moved to the door, but in a final act of defiance, waved her handkerchief one last time as she exited. Her action had the desired effect: reporters followed her as she moved to the halls of the Navy Department, where she held a press conference. She insisted that the U.S. shift toward war was unnecessary because Spain was willing to accede to America's demands. This was true in part. Spain had agreed to McKinley's demand for a halt to its brutal movement of Cubans into camps and to armistice, although it did not agree on the important point of Cuban independence. Two days after receiving Spain's agreement, the president sent a request to Congress seeking authority to go to war against Spain. Mary was waging a losing battle, but she was not alone. A small group of aging activists that included Carl Schurz, Edward Atkinson, George F. Hoar, and Andrew Carnegie spoke out against the war and U.S. empire-building. In May a group of New Englanders formed the Anti-Imperialist League. As the League grew to a membership of nearly 50,000 over the next few years, it would count as its members William James, Mark Twain, Jane Addams, Samuel Gompers, and many progressive reformers. No record is extant of Mary's membership in the League, perhaps because she disagreed with those League members who asserted that "tropical people" were incapable of "self-government." But peace activism was not to be heard in these months as the country moved further into war.[14]

Foregoing her usual trip to Oswego, Mary stayed in Washington for the summer. After nearly thirty years of effort, she was notified that her pension had been raised to $20 a month for life. It was a small triumph, since it still did not match pensions for men who held the same position during the Civil War. In spite of her anti-war stance, many Americans expressed agreement with the raise in her pension and understood it was long overdue.[15]

Mary was seated in the gallery in July when the U. S. War Senate met. The other forty-one people in the gallery included Queen Lili'uokalani, representatives from Cuba, Brazil, Japan, Peru, and elsewhere around the world, and distinguished Americans such as Hon. William Jennings Bryan. The battle against annexation was lost when the Senate adopted the Hawaiian annexation resolution by a vote of 42 to 21. Although the action had to be confirmed by the Hawaiian legislature, its control by American interests assured a speedy confirmation. Perhaps even more important in terms of Mary's efforts was the acknowledgment that many who opposed McKinley's actions were now silent. She continued to protest in the Senate with the wave of her handkerchief, but the result was once again her ejection from the Senate gallery. She and Queen Lili'uokalani met at least once again in August for what was described as an earnest conversation.[16]

One clue survives as to the psychological methods Mary used to maintain the courage to speak openly according to her principles in the face of the onslaught of criticism she received. She maintained a collection of quotes gathered from newspaper commentaries over the years, and a few that she may have written herself. The notes included proclamations such as, "No one can talk so plainly on social questions and command such close attention and profound respect, as Dr. Mary E. Walker" and "Dr. Mary E. Walker will sometime be missed, as no American will be for a hundred years to come" and "Dr. Mary E. Walker's worth as a woman, with her ability to maintain her exponency of principles through science, regardless of bigotry, has placed her on the pinnacle of enduring fame." Envisioning her place in history became the staff that supported her in these volatile years.[17]

By August 12, the Spanish-American War was over. Although the U.S. government had initially advocated independence for Cuba, official policy quickly changed and Cuba, Hawai'i, the Philippines, Puerto Rico, and Guam were either part of the treaty negotiations with Spain or annexed. In spite of Mary's distress at the government's rampant leap toward empire-building, she returned to her work for women's rights. In mid-February she attended the National Council of Women's convention in the city. The NCW was founded as an umbrella organization for national women's organizations in 1888 by Frances Willard, Susan B. Anthony, and May Wright Sewall. On the last day of the session, the NCW presented a wide-ranging list of resolutions. Some of the proposals concerned organizational policies; others were directed at national political issues, including a denouncement of war, support for the czar of Russia's call for gradual disarmament of all nations, and a request to President McKinley to halt bullfighting in Cuba as an animal rights issue. All of these resolutions were presented with unanimous support. However, differences arose over the matter of U.S. Representative Brigham H. Roberts from Utah. The majority of attendees wanted a resolution passed that said any person who was not a law-abiding citizen—in this instance, did not support monogamy—should not be able to hold national office. Mormon women delegates fought the resolution, arguing that none of the other proposals had been directed at an individual. Late in the afternoon Susan B. Anthony spoke against the resolution; there were numerous men in Congress who broke family laws, she observed, thus why was it necessary to go to Utah to find such a man to punish? The debate continued, the charges against Mormons increasingly virulent. Finally, one of the Mormon women, Susan Young Gates, spoke: "If you want the women of my people to accept your views, why not treat us with gladness?" Mary entered the room as Gates spoke, and she walked down the aisle, kissed Gates' cheek, and then took her seat. In spite of Mary's and Anthony's objections, the resolution passed. At the end of the year, Mary followed up with a petition in support of Roberts' right to hold a seat in Congress as a duly elected representative chosen by the people of Utah.[18]

In February Mary also attended the Mother's Congress and the Daughters of the American Revolution convention. At both gatherings she merely observed the proceedings. She had much more fun participating in an extravagant bicycle show at the Armory. An enormous crowd appeared, the lights were glittering, and colors swirled through the arena as hundreds of wheels whirled on display. The special attraction was Mary's lecture on the first evening of the show. She was greeted with a resounding ovation of clapping and handshaking. Fifteen hundred people attended that day, the largest crowd of the event. She spoke on dress reform for bicycling, noting that safety and comfort demanded short skirts, and she advocated the use of the pedal locomotor for all women. Although she had to compete with band music and a multitude of bicycles, her lecture was a grand success.[19]

That summer an interview she granted S. W. McGovern of the *Home Magazine* created a sensation when she revealed that she had a picture taken of herself in a coffin to see how she would appear when she was dead. She was clearly delighted with such an antic, lying in quiet repose in the makeshift coffin with flowers scattered across her torso. She also observed that she had a much stronger following in the West now than the East, because women of the West were embracing dress reform much more fully than her Eastern sisters. The coffin aspect of the interview made headline news around the country; several newspapers reprinted the photograph, and the *Toledo Bee* declared that Mary had started a new craze in photography. In spite of the fact that the custom had been around for decades, she was perfectly willing to accept the suggestion that she originated the idea.[20]

In the early fall, Mary granted an interview to an *Oswego Times* reporter. The Dreyfus Affair, Admiral Dewey, U.S. imperialism—all were part of her commentary. With the opening declaration that "[t]he condemnation of Dreyfus is one of the most outrageous occurrences of the century," she expressed her political views in unequivocal terms. The publication of Émile Zola's "J'accuse!" a few months earlier had ignited the international community, radicals and conservatives alike. Alfred Dreyfus, a French military officer, was found guilty of high treason in 1894 and condemned to life imprisonment in complete isolation on Devil's Island. Zola's text exposed the government cover-up and the anti-Semitism integral to the false accusations against Dreyfus. The French president pardoned Dreyfus in September, although he would not be fully exonerated until 1906. The affair brought to the forefront issues of nationalism, imperialism, and human rights integral to the arguments Mary had been making about the U.S. government's military actions and the direction in which the nation's political landscape was moving.[21]

In this context, she condemned Admiral George Dewey as an American traitor. At the moment Mary made her charges against Dewey, he was being hailed as an American hero for his success at the Battle of Manila Bay. In addition to his hero's welcome when he returned to the States, Dewey was granted unprecedented recognition by Congress when he was made Admiral of the Navy. In part, Mary's charges against Dewey—and, surprisingly, every soldier who participated in the war in the Philippines—were rooted in her belief that the actions of the U.S. government were a crime and thus anyone who supported them was also acting in a criminal manner. Yet her "J'accuse!" went much further in terms of Dewey himself. Initially Dewey worked closely with the Filipino freedom fighter Emilio Aguinaldo; but when the U.S. government moved away from independence for the Philippine nation in early 1899, relations broke down and Dewey threatened to bombard Aguinaldo's forces if he did not allow U.S. troops to land at Manila. Mary's charges were specific: "When [Dewey] was in Manila he sent word to the Filipinos—poor innocent people ignorant of American ways and knowing nothing of bombardment—that if they did not remove the women and children within a specific time, he would shell the place with them in it. A fine specimen of the humane American, that!" Although the reporter challenged Mary's assertions, she continued, "Two hours before the time set for the bombardment when sick women and helpless children were still in the city, when the poor Filipinos had no thought of an attack, he shelled the place. Disgraceful! Villainous! A blot on the fair name of this government!" She cited the Constitution to support her charges of treason for U.S. interference with a foreign government, much as she had in her arguments against the annexation of Hawai'i. McKinley's administration itself was treasonous for this reason, she declared; it had undermined the entire system of government. She concluded, "We are fighting the Filipinos to extermination. We are committing a great national sin from which this government can never be absolved." Whether or not the United States committed atrocities in the Philippines was being hotly debated at the time Mary made her statements. When the Anti-Imperialist League published *Soldiers' Letters: Being Materials for the History of a War of Criminal Aggression* the following year, not only were the atrocities made evident but the blatant racism of many soldiers was also revealed. It was later exposed that the U.S. Army had committed extraordinary atrocities in the Philippines, with nearly 600,000 Filipino deaths during the war.[22]

In December 1899 Mary traveled to Cortland, New York, to visit her longtime friend Dr. Lydia Strowbridge. The trip was meant to offer rest after her arduous efforts in Washington, but she soon turned her attention to a murder case that was garnering headlines in New York. Circumstantial evidence was at issue in the trial of Robert B. Molineux, a chemist accused of poisoning Katherine J. Adams. Molineux was a member of the Knickerbocker Athletic Club, and Harry S. Cornish, a relative of Adams, was its athletic director. The two men had been involved in several disputes relating to athletic prowess and social standing. Mary was interested in the trial as a means of making an anti-capital punishment argument, efforts that she would continue in the new century.[23]

Mary believed that there was insufficient evidence to convict Molineux. By mid-February she was in Albany to support Assemblyman John Maher's bill to abolish the death penalty. Initially the codes committee intended to table the bill rather than present an adverse report, but both Mary and Maher worked the press to bring public pressure, and they succeeded in forcing the committee to consider the bill. Mary was granted a hearing to speak on its behalf before the committee. Chairman John Weeks noted when he introduced Mary that it was highly unusual to allow a citizen to speak before the committee but that he had succumbed to her persuasions. The audience was filled with women who had come to hear her speak, some standing on chairs in order to see her. Mary argued against execution in any form, including the current New York State practice of electrocution, and in favor of life sentences without parole. She noted that much of the case against Molineux was rooted in questionable testimony, such as that of the young woman who supposedly sold the silver goblet in which the poison was served to Mrs. Adams, but who could not assert beyond reasonable doubt that it was Molineux who bought it. Further, Mary called Cornish a liar; in his testimony against Molineux, he claimed to have taken a swallow of the poison-laced seltzer before it was given to his aunt. If he had done so, Mary observed, he would have died on the spot or after a painful struggle against death. But she was not there merely to detail a specific case before the committee; she was interested in the larger question and argued that "[m]urderers, at the time of the commission of crime, are in a trench of insanity, or in a never properly balanced condition, and should be the pitiable wards of state protection, instead of candidates for a chair of state electrocution." She further observed that eight people were on death row in New York State for murder and thus execution obviously did not deter future criminals. "I think it high time that, with the civilization of the age and boasted intelligence of the State, judicial murder should cease. If there be members of the Legislature who have not been convinced that calm judicial murder is worse than individual murder, let them amend the statute so that no one shall be electrocuted whose conviction has been obtained on circumstantial evidence." After the speech, even newspapers typically critical of Mary remarked that she had made "a telling speech against the barbarous method of punishment in cases of conviction of murder." Yet, as predicted, the bill never reached the full assembly.[24]

After meeting with the committee, Mary left immediately for Washington, acting on two separate goals simultaneously—one to abolish the death penalty, the other to gain financial support to establish a sanitarium for tubercular patients on her property. While Molineux awaited execution in Sing Sing, Mary continued her efforts to have his sentence commuted to life in prison. She prepared a petition for the governor of New York and sent it to the *New York Times* requesting that individuals clip it out of the paper, sign it, and forward it to the governor or directly to her in Washington. She preceded the petition with a reminder that Americans had rallied on behalf of Dreyfus and asked them not to be silent when it came to one of their own citizens who was to be electrocuted within the month. The petition reiterated her charges that Cornish's testimony was false, and it asked the governor to pardon Molineux for a crime he did not commit. Although Molineux spent twenty months on death row, he was granted another trial in 1902 on the basis that hearsay evidence was admitted at the first trial. Mary and other death penalty opponents were heartened when Molineux was acquitted of the crime at his second trial.[25]

Her second goal was less successful. She spoke before the Senate Finance Committee on February 22 in favor of a bill seeking to establish a tuberculosis sanitarium in the Adirondacks. When the bill did not pass, she issued a broadside, *Consumptive School Sanitarium*, in which she explained the need for a sanitarium and her own qualifications to run such an institution. The broadside was similar to the one she issued five years earlier for the New Woman Colony in that it explained how her property would be a beneficial site "with freedom from fogs, away from city noises and smoke . . . where there is natural lime-water, vegetables right out of the ground, and from stalks, vines and bushes; fruit also fresh vines, trees and bushes; milk fresh from individual cows; eggs newly laid; clothes dried in sunshine; growing fruits, and flowers to watch and tend." This time, however, she was much more direct about the need for funding: her property offered "a combination of all the excellences desirable, but personally I am unable to carry out building projects, from lack of funds, therefore, I make an appeal for money to erect and furnish suitable buildings, where patients may have a home during treatment, and get the advantage of schooling in preventive methods of the disease." She wanted no boards to be named to fund the project, since the salaries for its members could better be spent on the building projects, and she openly noted that she could better select persons who would have the knowledge and experience to handle the realities of running a medical institution. She wanted "luxurious pay apartments" to be built as well so patients used to "esthetic homes" and financially able to pay for such accommodations would do so, which would help the institution provide for other patients unable to pay for their care. But, she cautioned, she would not accept funds that would require poor patients to be placed in undesirable rooms; everyone must have "the comforts and attractions essential to treatment and education of consumptives." She promised that wealthy patrons' suggestions would be seriously considered if she was allowed to direct the sanitarium without a board of overseers.[26]

Mary also included an extensive section on her fitness to direct a sanitarium. In addition to practicing medicine successfully for forty-five years, she revealed that at one time while living in Washington, she suffered from tuberculosis and, as her own patient, recovered fully. Her goal was an institution in which she "could teach young doctors at the bedside of patients, in all stages of consumption, the methods of cure and prevention as well." She was soon to return to Oswego, and she invited wealthy humanitarians interested in supporting this worthy cause to visit the property and to learn more about the great work their money could endow. Mary never received the financial support she hoped to garner, in spite of contacting everyone from Mrs. Astor to the czar of Russia. Eventually, however, she was able to accomplish her goal on a very small scale. For many years she used her farm as a retreat for tuberculosis patients, and classes on prevention of the disease were occasionally offered, based on a model of treatment she had devised.[27]

Recognition came that spring for Mary's years of work on behalf of numerous reform causes. Congressman Charles Foster of Ohio called for the creation of a pantheon of illustrious American women. Mary was included in the list of potential honorees, along with Martha Washington, Dolley Madison, Susan B. Anthony, Maria Mitchell, Clara Barton, Harriet Beecher Stowe, Julia Ward Howe, Mary Wilkins Freeman, Sarah Orne Jewett, and others. Public sentiment toward Mary had turned to tolerance and, for some, admiration.[28]

Soon Mary had to return to Oswego, a trip precipitated by the tragic death of her sister Aurora. The seventy-five-year-old widow's body was found in her home, lying in a pool of blood, on May 13. The coroner determined the death was due to a hemorrhaged lung. While Mary loved all of her sisters, Aurora had been her greatest companion; when she was in Oswego, she saw Aurora on a daily basis, and the abiding love between the two sisters had been marked from childhood. Aurora's marriage to a wealthy farmer seemed to cast her as a conventional woman, but she was as nontraditional in her own way as was Mary. They had many interests in common, from farming to phrenology. Mary spent a quiet summer, recovering from her loss.[29]

Mary's abhorrence of President McKinley's abuses of power ignited her efforts during the fall presidential campaign, especially when Admiral Dewey announced his candidacy for the presidency on the Democratic ticket. Dewey conducted his campaign so ineptly, however, that he undermined his own tide of popularity. Acknowledgment that he had never voted in a presidential campaign and his talk of America's "next war" soon diminished his chances. William Jennings Bryan again stepped forward as the Democratic candidate. Mary began her political activities this year at a Democratic county convention in her home state. She had long known the three major Democratic Party leaders in the region: Judge Charles N. Bulger, James R. O'Gorman, and A. Salladin, Jr. While these men often used Mary's ability to draw large crowds, they would not go so far as to award her a county political office as she sought in September. Her goal was to be appointed county coroner, both for the opportunity such a position would allow in making inroads toward women's enfranchisement and to have a legal voice in determining causes of death. If the local Democrats tried to ignore her influence, Bryan did not. As Mildred Sherman, reporter for the *Syracuse Evening Telegram* reported in October, Bulger and others tried to draw Bryan away from hearing Mary's private comments while he was in Syracuse, but he and Mary had known each other for many years. "I want to hear what this lady has to say," he told them, insisting he be given five minutes alone with her to hear her opinions. To her dismay, McKinley was reelected.[30]

In January 1901 Mary set out by train for Syracuse, where she planned to spend a few days. She offered a free lecture on the timely subject of "Influenza, Improperly Called the Grip," in the assembly room of the Yates Hotel on the evening of January 19. In spite of bitterly cold weather, the lecture drew seventy-five people. She offered her audience sensible advice on preventing colds, and she insisted that she would have died years before from tuberculosis if she had dressed as other women do. She once again rejected germ theory, insisting that influenza, diphtheria, and pneumonia were not contagious, as some doctors were then arguing, and she answered questions afterward, during which she admonished the decision to bury Murray Hall in female clothing. Hall's death had created a sensation a few days earlier when it was discovered that the Tammany Hall politician who lived for thirty years as Murray Hall had been born Mary Anderson. Mary declared, "It was an outrage not to bury that woman Hall . . . in man's clothes. When she'd lived in them for more than thirty years, she was entitled to them in her grave."[31]

Mary spent the next two months in the Albany area, after which she settled in Brooklyn at 79 Willoughby Avenue for an extended stay. She scheduled several lectures, including a benefit for the Fulton Street mission and a women's anti-vice society. As the *Brooklyn Eagle* observed, she was always "doing good where she can." In one such endeavor, Mary was appalled by her experience of visiting the Raymond Street Jail. Her purpose was to check on Dr. Everson, a woman physician who was incarcerated for practicing without the now-required state license; since Everson had practiced for years, Mary thought it an "outrage" that the woman was jailed. She spent two hours talking with Everson; but it was some of the other women prisoners who most distressed her. "The prisons were not overcrowded," she acknowledged, "but the women—oh! the women! I did not believe there were such women in the world. The things they said to me were simply awful." She attempted to meet with Assistant District Attorney Robert H. Elder the next day to discuss the need for a new women's prison, but the city had no interest in such an investment.[32]

On a happier note, she enjoyed the theater, attending a performance of "The Butterflies" at the Park Theater and being hosted by the manager to a backstage tour. During this time there was also a flurry of book publishing that reviewed the past century's great events, and in many of them Mary was either castigated or praised for her work as a physician and reformer. While numerous reviews of *Gail Hamilton's Life and Letters* picked up on Hamilton's disparaging description of Mary "in her infernal old trousers" as the only white woman among African Americans who mourned the death of Charles Sumner, other publications were appreciative in nature. W. F. Beyer and O. F. Keydel's *Deeds of Valor* detailed her Civil War accomplishments and included an illustration of her treating a wounded soldier on the battlefield, and Harriet Fontanges's *Les Femmes Docteurs en Mèdicine* examined the changes in women's place in the profession on an international basis, acknowledging Mary as one of the important U.S. women physicians of the nineteenth century.[33]

Mary returned to Oswego late in the summer. Within weeks the nation was stunned by the assassination of President McKinley. He had traveled to Buffalo for the Pan American Exposition, and on the afternoon of September 6, as he received visitors in the auditorium of the Temple of Music, Leon Franz Czolgosz shot him. After lingering for several days, McKinley died on September 14. An assassin would naturally evoke the rage of people who had seen their leader murdered, but as the son of Polish immigrants and an avowed anarchist, Czolgosz touched a wellspring of anti-immigration and postwar political conservatism that enflamed the public response. Czolgosz confessed, leaving the only possible defense that of mental defect. His counsel did not raise the issue until closing arguments, however, and after a notably short trial, the jurors took only thirty minutes to find the defendant guilty.[34]

Immediately a story spread that Mary had pronounced in a public setting that the "State of New York if it electrocutes the assassin of McKinley is just as great a murderer as he is. President McKinley was a murderer, because he killed the poor Filipinos." National outrage followed, spreading out across the country over the next two months. She was purportedly at a New York train station when she made the remarks. A group of laborers in the vicinity surrounded her; one raised his hand to strike her, but then stopped because she was a woman. Others suggested she be lynched or cast verbal attacks at her, insisting she was "in the same class as Carrie Nation and Emma Goldman. You all ought to be put out of the way." (To put someone "out of the way" was a colloquial phrase for incarceration in an insane asylum.) Eventually she was allowed to board the train and leave. The story was repeated from New York to California.[35]

Mary immediately wrote letters to the editors of the *Oswego Palladium* and the *Oswego Times* to clarify her remarks: she never asserted that Theodore Roosevelt was behind the assassination, as some papers reported, and she did not want to be aligned with Nation and Goldman because she believed in "law and order" and had been working for years within the legislative system to attempt to eradicate capital punishment. Nor was there a crowd of workingmen surrounding her—there were three men with dinner pails, and she was in no way hindered from boarding the train. She did not "hurriedly leave the depot," as reported: "I am not such a base coward as to be afraid to express my sentiments when they are of the best of human life, and if they had been a part of the New York State laws, and judicial murder struck from the Codes, and life imprisonment substituted, the assassin in Buffalo might sometime tell who was back of him that are not considered nihilists." She added in one letter, "What I did say at the railroad station, was that I do not believe in murder of any kind—either by assassination, hanging or electrocuting, in the United States, the Philippine Islands or anywhere else." Her rebuttals were not reprinted in the national press, however, and she was branded a traitor. Calls were made for a congressional investigation into her loyalty and for the rescinding of her military pension; the U.S. marshal was dispatched to New York to investigate the situation; and state suffragists barred her from their convention in October. As the tide swelled against her, she had an attorney, Samuel Daull of Elmira, New York, make public notice of her denial that she said McKinley was as great a murderer as Czolgosz. Commissioner of Pensions Evans reluctantly announced that he had no authority to rescind her pension, although he added that Congress could do so if it wished. Finally, a few voices began to challenge the calls to punish Mary for her comments. Some were little better than the damnation itself. The *Rochester Post-Express*, for instance, ran an editorial in which it asserted that her comments were "foolish" and that as a woman she deserved "chivalry . . . to protect her from any serious consequences of a criticism not likely to do harm," but they added, "Wide tolerance of hostile opinion is much more becoming in the American people than narrow intolerance, especially toward an unbalanced woman." Certainly most surprising, a long interview with Judge Lewis Shepard of Chattanooga was published in the *Atlanta Constitution*. Shepard was one of the Confederates who had known Mary during her captivity. He did not specifically mention her comments on McKinley, but he praised her work during the Civil War, recalling a previously unreported commission she had undertaken in 1863 to cross into Confederate territory to deliver much-needed medicine to Union prisoners. It was a successful "mission of mercy and humanity," the judge declared.[36]

In spite of the extraordinary level of nationwide criticism she faced in these weeks, Mary continued her efforts to halt the scheduled execution of Czolgosz. She drafted a petition seeking executive clemency from Governor Odell that would allow for a life sentence with the contingency that Czolgosz would name his accomplices. She was unsuccessful in gathering signatures on the petition, however, and Odell was unwilling to consider clemency. Czolgosz was executed on October 29. In spite of the heated rhetoric of the fall, within a few months Mary was again being praised along with congressmen and justices as one of the prominent figures in Washington politics. In part this was to her credit for refusing to back down, but perhaps even more so, it reflected the changing political culture of the new century.[37]

CHAPTER 13

The Age of Alienation

As the new century advanced, Mary maintained her medical practice and her commitments to suffrage and dress reform, but the law was increasingly important to her activism on both personal and national issues. She mended fences with the remaining Greenwich relatives and was granted power of attorney for the sale of Mary and Vashti Walker's home. But it was constitutional and criminal law to which she turned her attention in early 1902. She was again dividing her time between Oswego, New York City, and Washington. In New York she attended several trials, including Florence Burns's trial for the murder of her lover; Mary sat at the reporters' table and closely followed the case. When the prosecutor asserted that men in the courtroom were affected by the defendant's comeliness and facetiously remarked that if the situation continued it would be necessary to have an all-female jury, Mary applauded.[1]

She also relished the national progress in dress reform. Fashions were clearly moving in a direction closer to Mary's ideas of healthy attire, and her thoughts on the latest trends were published in newspapers from Boston to Los Angeles. That summer she was invited to publish a lengthy article on men's attire in the *Washington Times*. Mary had learned a lot about the publishing world over the years, and she copyrighted the article in her own name so reprints, which appeared in the *Chicago Tribune* and elsewhere, would be to her financial benefit. "Dr. Mary Walker's Views Regarding Proper Masculine Attire" began by acknowledging that she had "always held what have been termed radical views on the subject of woman's dress" but now those ideas were "adopted by women in nearly all respects in a somewhat modified form." That point, however, was "a twice-told tale," so she wished to focus on men's attire because she held equally "radical, so-called, views as to their apparel." For warm weather, she advocated the new waist shirts that buttoned to men's pants, eliminating the need for a belt that would hinder blood circulation; the suit could be completed by black alpaca trousers and attractive suspenders. If men insisted on wearing a coat, she recommended a black alpaca sack coat without a lining and a Wu Tingfang vest to cover the sack coat for cooler days. Healthy attire for dress occasions was also described. She advocated Revolutionary-era style lace collars cut with a v-neck rather than stifling buttoned collars and cuffs in hot weather, though she recognized it was unlikely to become common attire as "it requires a high order of moral courage to do differently from the masses." She did not shy away from observing her own courage in donning the Prince Albert coat, a neck pin, and other alternatives to normative styles as a conclusion to her essay.[2]

In April 1903 Mary traveled to St. Louis where her lecture was the major attraction at the Exposition Carnival. Introduced by Sergeant John McDonald, Mary stepped onto the stage in her usual attire but with an American flag "draped gracefully about her shoulders." The crowd broke into vigorous cheering. Stirringly patriotic in her remarks, she was received with enthusiasm. She returned to Oswego and in the summer was welcomed at the local society circus. The circus had a long tradition in the city, and over the years many famous Oswegonians had their first opportunities to speak publicly at the event. Mary was given the pedestal of honor from which she lectured on the opening night on "Women's Dress in Relation to Strong Men" and the second night on "Human Electricity." She particularly enjoyed such events, as they gave her a forum for speaking to large audiences and to people who would not normally attend formal lectures on dress reform or popular medical issues. She was soon immersed in local political debates as well. Her nephew, Byron Worden, was running on the Republican ticket for town supervisor with an anti-ring platform. Mary delivered a long speech in his favor at the Oswego Town caucus, in which she impeached the "party boss" system that supported "ring" candidates. Worden trounced his opponent and became the town's new supervisor.[3]

In the fall, Mary attended the Medical Women's National Association's convention in Washington, and the next day she went to Dr. Mary D. Rushmore's surgical clinic to observe a laporotomy (the removal of fallopian tubes and ovaries). Mary was deeply moved by Rushmore's skill and the possibilities of such surgery. At the same time she was receiving praise from diverse quarters. Her longtime friend Susan Fowler was celebrated in the *Philadelphia Inquirer* for her eightieth birthday; Fowler was commended for her long and healthy lifestyle, her work for dress reform, and for being well read and "a brilliant conversationalist," but she shifted the laudatory comments to her lifelong admiration of Mary. At this time Washington photographer Barnett McFee Clinedinst also created a photographic collage of forty-seven individuals prominent in Washington politics. Amidst the cabinet members, congressmen, and Supreme Court justices depicted in "The Special Session of Congress" was Dr. Mary Walker, walking with them up the steps of the Capitol. Accolades were welcomed, but Mary had a new focus for her activism—resistance to Theodore Roosevelt's presidency because of his pro-imperialism advocacy and the "strenuous life" hyper-masculinity that he embodied. Several months earlier, the *New York Herald* had satirized nontraditional women such as Mary and the actress Marie Dressler with grotesque caricatures; they depicted Mary with an oversized head and a very large medal on her breast, standing in front of a "No Smoking" sign, and described her as "Inventor of the strenuous life for women." Indeed, she did advocate rigorous physical and political activism for women; but she and Roosevelt could not have been more opposed in their political views of what constituted the best direction for the United States at the beginning of the twentieth century. In January 1903, when the editor of the People's Column of the *Boston Globe* skeptically asked readers if they believed Roosevelt could be beaten in his bid for reelection, Mary responded. "I answer 'yes,' he 'can,' and will be 'beaten,'" using McKinley's assassination as the basis for her belief. "The American people are slow to remember, but here and there, all over the country the question was asked when he was 'hunted up in the Adirondacks after poor McKinley's death,' why was he the 'only person in all our broad land who excluded himself from telegraph or telephone communication.'" There were many people with axes to grind in relation to Roosevelt, she concluded, and they would not forget his absence at a moment of national crisis. With the campaign season seeming to be an apt moment to argue once again before Congress for sufficient pensions for widows of Civil War veterans, she headed back to Washington in late February.[4]

Soon Mary was speaking out against the Panama Canal treaty. The treaty was crafted by President Roosevelt in the fervor of the successful empire-building of the Spanish-American War; it required Great Britain to agree to rescind the 1850 Clayton-Bulwer Treaty that assured neither nation would assert control over the Isthmus of Panama. When Colombia sought to increase its financial gains from the building of the canal, the United States helped organize an uprising that led to Panamanian independence and the American government's ability to negotiate directly with the new nation. Mary met with several senators, asking them to oppose the "atrocious" treaty's ratification and promising to work for their reelection campaigns in each of their states if they did so. Other issues drew her attention as well. Although a lifelong temperance advocate, she did not support the Hepburn-Dolliver bill, which would ban packages of liquor from being delivered in Prohibition states. She explained to the House Judiciary Committee, "I have been a temperance advocate; I have written temperance articles; I believe in total abstinence. . . . But it seems to me, Mr. Chairman, that there is only one question before your committee, and that is, if you undertake to pass such a law, can you enforce it?" She also went to several federal departments and introduced herself to new officials, noting she had known their predecessors since the era of Grant's administration, and attended hearings of the Senate Committee on Privileges and Elections in the Smoot case. Senator Reed Smoot was fighting to retain his seat against anti-Mormon factions in the Senate and the country at large. Smoot's serving as a Mormon apostle at the same time he held his Senate position had outraged some Americans, but as his attorney observed during the hearings, no laws or social conditions in Utah had changed since Smoot's election in 1902 or since Utah had been admitted as a state, and Mary supported his right to serve in Congress because his constituents had elected him. While in the city, she also continued to offer lectures on how to combat tuberculosis.[5]

In mid-April, Mary returned to Oswego. As usual, her return attracted a local reporter to seek her opinions on current events, and she used the opportunity to continue her disparagement of President Roosevelt. "Not since the war of '61, nor during the war, has the country been in such a deplorable condition as at the present time," she declared. "There are men in the House and Senate who are in their dotage and do not realize what they are saying and doing, and as to the President—well, he is not entitled to a passing notice." She had a great deal to say about the need for political change. It was not a party issue, but a national issue, she declared: "All this Philippine and Panama controversy has been outrageous, and no one short of that Teddy would have promoted or tolerated such proceedings. The Smoot investigation is a perfect farce. Far worse things have been approved of by the present Administration." Within days she also announced once again that she would found a consumptives' hospital in the coming summer. While some regional papers mocked the idea, the *Syracuse Evening Telegram* asserted that she had "done more kind acts in her life than any of the people who make fun of her." Even if she is "an oddity," they noted, "she is kind hearted and generous and in the course of her long career has often deprived herself of luxuries that others less fortunate might have the necessities of life." It was a fitting tribute, perhaps aided by the sense of her advanced age. By June she announced her intention to attend the Democratic convention in St. Louis. Even attending was insufficient—she once again called for a mass meeting at which a woman delegate would be elected to attend the convention. She telephoned the local newspapers so the notice would appear broadly, invited men to attend, and announced she would offer an address at the meeting. The newspapers predicted a large attendance and Mary, not surprisingly, as the chosen delegate. But only twelve people attended, including five reporters. In spite of the low attendance and reporters' jibes, Mary presented her speech. She would not commit to a particular Democratic candidate, but she was clear in her rejection of Roosevelt, whom she blamed in large part for the Spanish-American War.[6]

She was in St. Louis as the Democratic convention opened in early July, vociferously espousing her anti-Roosevelt positions and seeking to be seated as a "regularly elected" delegate by the Oswego Democrats. She also sought New York Congressman M. Z. Haven's support for giving a speech at the convention; Haven expected Judge Charles Bulger, "our mutual friend," to support her request, but Bulger would not do so. Although she met with the credentials committee and indicated she would contest the failure to seat her as a delegate, she was unsuccessful. She did succeed at garnering considerable press for herself and for the need to have women delegates as part of the Democratic Party. "I came here to do what I can for women," she announced at Democratic headquarters. "We are entitled to as much consideration in politics as in business." Her attendance at the committee on credentials' hearings to seek the seating of women delegates fit with the year's controversies over who would constitute the Democratic Party's representatives. After long debates, the Democrats awarded votes for the first time to delegations from the Philippines and Puerto Rico; but no woman was seated as a delegate. Mary then turned her attention to trying to have a woman's suffrage plank included in the platform of the convention, but no Democrat was willing to offer such a plank. The convention closed without women's participation being addressed.[7]

By fall Mary was again in the news. Her activities were always discussed with each new political season in Washington, but now she was also increasingly included in retrospectives that looked at the accomplishments of pioneer suffragists. One notable assessment came in a lengthy article in the *Washington Post* that recognized Mary as a regular among the radical thinkers who were longtime visitors or residents of Vineland, New Jersey. Vineland was founded in 1861 by Philadelphia lawyer Charles K. Landis; it was known for its ethnic diversity and receptive attitudes toward radical thinkers and new "isms." Vineland was particularly accepting of dress reform, and Mary had often visited her friends Susan Fowler and Mary Tillotson there over the years, as the city was a haven from the constant criticism and observation she faced elsewhere. With Fowler over eighty and Tillotson's recent death, Mary found herself among the distinct few surviving dress reform pioneers. One sad event of 1904 was the death of her last surviving sibling, Vesta. Mary outlived her entire family, and she knew that the time was short to effect the goals she had envisioned for a lifetime.[8]

While Mary did hold a continuing place within Washington politics, her own sense of her importance sometimes exceeded reality, as demonstrated in a letter she sent to Czar Nicholas II of Russia in the fall. She had been in contact with the czar years earlier, and her call for the czar to seek peaceful resolutions with Japan was well-intentioned. But the self-aggrandizing claim that her advice had been instrumental in effectuating the birth of the czar's son ("But for my professional advice you would not now be the father of a son heir") also exposed her ever more extremist personal and medical views. At times her thinking reflected a modern sensibility—describing, for instance, a preventative method in relation to heart failure that was like the twentieth-century's CPR methods or recognizing the health dangers of smoking—but many of her medical commentaries were now outside the bounds of modern medicine. Yet in terms of political activism, she was as decisive and committed as ever. She began in the fall, therefore, to stump on behalf of Alton Brooks Parker, the Democratic presidential candidate; her support of Parker was news that was reported throughout the States. She spoke on his behalf across the Northeast—not because she felt strongly about Parker but because she adamantly opposed Roosevelt's reelection. Parker stood little chance, however, and the president's popularity led to a landslide victory in November.[9]

As 1905 progressed, Mary's activism followed its usual course—state and national politics, suffrage, dress reform, and anti-capital punishment arguments.

For the latter, she attended the Henry Manzer murder trial in Auburn, New York. Manzer was convicted of the murder of Cora Sweet and executed on September 12, 1905. Mary again claimed insanity as a reason to oppose the man's execution, since she believed anyone who committed murder was insane at the moment the crime was committed. For the first time, she also spoke out briefly on the issue of lynching. The level of public agitation over the murder reached feverish pitch and talk of lynching Manzer circulated throughout the region. Mary admitted she found the details of the crime wrenching ("I couldn't read it without weeping"), but she abhorred the talk of lynching: "That would be the greatest outrage and we don't want anything like that to happen in this country. It may be all right for the South, but not for here." While the comment was meant to assert pride in the North, which she had privileged since the Civil War, it was a surprisingly casual, indeed dismissive, reference to Southern lynching for someone who had so long supported racial equality. Her anti-capital punishment commentaries were widely published, but she never took the opportunity across the decades to openly condemn lynching.[10]

A new phase of her activism now emerged; she began to offer support to women who faced public examination over their gender identification. On the one hand, she aligned herself with their right to dress and act as they chose; on the other hand, she never clearly addressed what was often a transgendered choice that went far beyond donning so-called masculine attire. Frank Williams, born Frances Lamouche, for instance, lived as a male for many years while working at a Cincinnati hotel until hospitalization revealed his sex. While many letters were addressed to "Frances" condemning her for disgracing her sex, Mary offered Frances a place to stay at her sanitarium and to pay her transportation from Ohio. "You need not be afraid to wear boys' clothing here," Mary wrote. "We dress to suit our inclinations, and the fact that you have discarded the horribly conventional clothing of women shows you to be a woman of more than ordinary intelligence, and consequently worthy of championship." Near death, Frank revealed that he had lived as a male since a child and that doing so allowed him an education and a chance at self-employment, though he struggled to achieve a living wage even then. Although no response to Mary from Williams is extant, Professor Randolph Milbourne of Ohio sought her legal advice on the issue of cross-dressing. Milbourne lived publicly as a man but he had desired to be a woman from the time he was a child. At home he dressed and lived as a female and in the spring of 1905 began to take strolls in his neighborhood in female attire. When he was arrested, he decided to challenge the courts. The Ohio attorney general refused to advise him, so Milbourne contacted Mary because her experience in contesting her arrests was well known. She replied that it was the issue of disguise that must be considered, yet she also enclosed a picture of herself to demonstrate her own lack of disguise. Newspaper reports noted the different philosophies of "becoming" another sex and "playing" that role, as they viewed Milbourne and Mary respectively. Mary did not invite Milbourne to live at her home in Oswego, but she often invited both men and women to do so. In addition to Susan Fowler, Frances Lamouche, and individuals who were to be treated for tuberculosis, she took in troubled Civil War veterans such as Harry Horan, whom she had met during the war. In spite of her vocal opposition to alcohol, she sympathized with the elderly veteran who struggled with alcoholism; she offered him work on her farm and a place to stay. When he was arrested for public intoxication and appeared in police court, expressing penitence for his "fall," Mary accepted him back at her Bunker Hill home. Her home was a temporary refuge for many people in these years.[11]

In the late summer and fall of 1905 Mary enjoyed a wide variety of activities that revealed her continuing interest in the New Woman movement she had helped to shape. She published an essay in the *Washington Post*, "Punching the Bag Makes Pale Cheeks All Abloom," advocating many indoor sports in which women could participate as winter neared. Using a punching bag engaged "every muscle in the body," Mary explained, and she advocated exercise as varied as walking, bowling, skating, skiing, and tobogganing not only for women's physical health but also to dispel "the blues," since rigorous exercise required exhilarating mental effort. She also introduced two bills at the Albany legislature. One focused on having the name of any woman whose property was assessed for taxation added to the registry of eligible voters; the second argued that a woman's style of dress should be insufficient cause for arrest and any police officer making such an arrest should be guilty of a misdemeanor and fined or imprisoned for his actions. Although the legislature refused to pass either bill, she would annually present them to that body over the next several years in order to keep the issues before the public and the lawmakers.[12]

In January Mary returned to Albany to support what had now become an annual bill for the abolition of capital punishment. She herself was coming under scrutiny by the new science's obsession with "sexual inversion." One such notable publication, *Human Sexuality: A Medico-Literary Treatise on the Laws, Anomalies, and Relations of Sex with especial reference to Contrary Sexual Desire*, was written by a former acting assistant surgeon in the Union army, Joseph Parke, who revealed his distaste for the actions of the woman who had held the same medical position as he. Discussing Mary in a section on "Delusional Masculinity," he declared it "regrettable" that no medico-psychologist had researched "the case of Dr. Mary Walker." For Parke, clothing style equaled sexual desire. In many ways, the pseudo-scientific emphasis on sexual inversion of this era reflected the success of gender-challenging changes in female clothing and the fear such success raised in some individuals, but its intent was to reorient U.S. culture to normative ideals of femininity and motherhood precisely as the New Woman movement was thriving. Thus Mary became one of the targets of New Woman opponents. A common charge beyond her "masculinity" was that speaking publicly on political issues was not "dignified." The rarer comments of support often offered details of how Mary administered medical assistance to strangers who had been injured in the streets of Boston, Washington, or New York, but these accounts did little to soften the harsher attacks that focused on her sexuality. In the midst of such charges, Mary was rushed to Sibley Memorial Hospital in Washington with severe respiratory problems. She had fought chronic bronchitis since her imprisonment during the Civil War, and as she aged the disease often debilitated her. Even though she felt the need for hospital rest, she insisted that she be recognized as her own physician. "All I want is a room here in the hospital until I get well," she declared. Even her ability to care for herself was ascribed generally as a "masculine trait." The nurses remarked that she would not let them tend to her, but they liked the small, aging woman; as one noted, "she is just as good a woman as any of us." Before editors could begin to pen eulogies for the ailing doctor, however, she recovered and was back at work.[13]

That summer Mary turned her attention to a new avenue of dealing with imprisoned Americans. Recognizing that so-called rehabilitation in the present prison system was ineffectual, she offered to turn over her residence and acreage in Oswego if the county would legalize the method for reforming young prisoners that she advocated. She felt that her fight for better sanitarium facilities in the state had been successful, even if not built on her own property as she had hoped; her new practice had been to forego admitting charity cases to her sanitarium but rather to pay for their transportation to the state institutions. Thus her property would now be available for transfer to the county. She explained her ideas: "My latest desire is again to try to better humanity. Our penal institutions for old and young are, in my judgment, worthy of the days of the rack and the stake." Whatever a young man has done, he has some good in him, she declared, and the present system destroys rather than nourishes that aspect of his nature. At the Bunker Hill institution, each inmate "should be compelled to work a certain number of hours each day in the fields, and the remainder of his day should be spent in classrooms under the direction of the best teachers. Good clothes, neat linen, wholesome food, and plenty of it should be furnished. The young man should be taken when he enters and educated from the beginning to the end." In addition, she offered to donate $10,000 of her own money to help rebuild the place into an appropriate facility and to work to raise additional funds. Although the county considered her offer, they ultimately did not accept it, and she continued to use her home as a sanitarium for the occasional patient.[14]

Another, more audacious proposal she offered at the end of the year was also refused. Theodore Roosevelt was awarded the Nobel Peace Prize for his role in negotiating the Treaty of Portsmouth to end the Russo-Japanese war in 1905. She declared in an open letter to the public that she should have been a co-recipient of the prize because she "was the first person to make an effort to secure peace between Russia and Japan. When there were naval battles with great loss I wrote the Czarina to tell the Czar that I asked that the harbor [Port Arthur] be given to the Japanese government and that the war would cease, and also the Russian people be given what they asked." Mary insisted, "I fully believe that Roosevelt took his 'cue' from me in interesting himself in the peace measures. That Russia did give the harbor in question to Japan in the peace negotiations, and that she has since given her subjects extended liberties never before accorded, are facts too well known to need mention, only as explanation of the part taken in peace measures by myself." While this incident represented Mary's self-aggrandizement, she was often accorded a status equal to America's leading politicians. For instance, as plans developed the following year for Utica's centennial celebration, she was listed along with President Roosevelt, the governor and senators as "notables" to be invited to the event—the only woman to be so honored.[15]

Infamous trials still attracted Mary, and none more so than the "trial of the century,"—although it was only 1907—that of millionaire Harry K. Thaw. The murder case involved sex, notoriety among its prominent participants, and a locale nothing less than the rooftop of Madison Square Garden. It would again pit Mary against the ardently conservative, anti-women's rights activist Anthony Comstock, who supported Thaw. The story was not uncommon, but the identity of its players brought attention to the murder. Although only sixteen years old, Gibson Girl model Evelyn Nesbit had led a provocative life. In June 1906 she married millionaire Thaw, but then was "debauched" by the renowned New York architect Stanford White. On the evening of June 25, Thaw sought his revenge; entering a party attended by his wife and White, he shot and killed White. Two trials ensued, each fodder for sensationalized newspaper reports of the participants' lives. The first resulted in a hung jury. Mary became part of the sensational commentary surrounding the trials, as it was the perfect opportunity to articulate her ideas about insanity and capital punishment. In April 1907, a Syracuse reporter traveled to her home at Bunker Hill to ask her opinion of the case. Mary predicted that Thaw would eventually be released. He was insane at the moment of the crime, as are all murderers, she explained, but added that his mind was now cleared. The second jury agreed in part—Thaw was declared insane at the time of the crime and committed to a state mental hospital for six years.[16]

At this time, Mary was delighted to receive a replacement Medal of Honor. Congress reissued the medal and sent the new version to recipients. She proudly displayed the new medal—along with the original—on her lapel every day for the rest of her life. With the reissuance, Brigadier General H. M. Duffield of the U.S. Volunteers published a two-volume retrospective of Medal of Honor recipients, in which he included an admiring narrative of Mary's battlefield endeavors.[17]

As the next generation of suffragists, led by Carrie Chapman Catt and others, offered a reinvigorated challenge to the country on behalf of woman's suffrage, Mary reissued an expanded and contentious version of the *Crowning Constitutional Argument*. At times powerful, at times petulant, Mary's argument reflected her continuing support of suffrage but her frustration at not being embraced as a pioneer by the new generation of suffragists. With Susan B. Anthony's death the previous year, Mary was one of the last of her generation, but her refusal to consider a constitutional amendment, her commitment to dress reform (most of the new generation of suffragists wore traditionally feminine attire), and her outspokenness against sister activists with differing opinions alienated her from the mainstream suffrage movement in the early twentieth century. The new *Crowning* began with a powerful epigraph: "Franchise was not a creation of the United States Constitution, any more than it was a creation of the soil of the United States. It expressed the Ideal of Birthright." Indeed, franchise was "a *conceded part*" of the Constitution, without reference to a citizen's sex, and every state was banned from creating laws that challenged that concession: "As a house is a protection against the possibilities, as well as the probables, so is the United States Constitution, and our glorious ancestors saw such a house as a necessity at the time and for the great future." She noted that naturalization laws were equally accepting of women as citizens: a woman from another country who married a U.S. citizen was granted citizenship, and if a man seeking naturalization died before his paperwork was completed, the law read "'his widow and children shall be considered as citizens of the United States. . . . ' This does not say, *boys*, but '*children*.'" Since citizenship entitled one to "all the rights and privileges," universal suffrage was built into the Constitution. How ironic, Mary noted, that the current legislation should put a "native born woman" in the position of wishing "to be born again, and that outside of the United States" so she, too, might benefit by naturalization laws. If "the *colored women*" and "the naturalized women and their *daughters*" have the right of suffrage as citizens, then so must all native-born women. Mary appealed to women whom she believed held the right to vote to do so: "*lose no time* in your exercise of the 'rights, privileges and amenities' guaranteed to you, since the *protection of such rights* is guaranteed you as well." She called for women of all nationalities to join the cause of making the United States a "true Republic."[18]

Had she stopped there, her argument would have been powerful and persuasive. But Mary's anger at Stanton, Anthony, and Rev. Anna Shaw was unabated and the new *Crowning* continued her diatribes against them. She recalled how they tried to block her from attending the 1898 convention after many years' absence. They were afraid of the power of her *Crowning* argument, Mary insisted, and that it would sway suffragists away from the idea of an amendment. Had those blocking her died earlier, she asserted, "every woman in these United States who wanted to vote, would have been voting. The wheels of progress have been held back by them . . . because their brains did not originate the CROWNING CONSTITUTIONAL ARGUMENT. We as women are not *beggars* for our own rights, but *demanders*." To Mary's mind that was the crux of her differences with amendment suffragists— they were pleading for the right to vote whereas she felt the right was inherent and should be demanded at the polls. But the tide had shifted in favor of an amendment, and personal attacks did nothing to aid the cause. Not all activists drew Mary's ire, however. She liked the work of Carrie Nation, although not always her tactics. As Nation aged, Mary extended her increasingly common offer of a home for life to the temperance reformer, if she wished to come to Oswego. Mary faced a disparate response from sister activists in these years—outrage and banishment from many, support and admiration from a smaller, enduring but aging group.[19]

Often these days, reminiscences of the Civil War were the primary means by which Mary's accomplishments were recalled. Aging Civil War nurses continued to maintain contact with the woman who had helped insure they received a pension, and many veterans published newspaper reminiscences of her medical work on the battlefield. So, too, did Mary promote such recollections. She recalled her meeting with President Lincoln after she had been freed from Castle Thunder in a long essay published in March 1909. A few months later, the president of London's Royal College of Surgeons recalled seeing Mary at St. Bartholomew's in 1866—but this time his reminiscences were before a banquet of medical *women* in England. If the source of her influence on the national stage seemed to be shifting to that of nostalgia, she was still well regarded in her home state. She was often referred to in local newspapers as "Our Mary." As the Oneida County Agricultural Society planned its annual fair in August, the committee sought two notables for lectures: the lieutenant governor, and Mary. She was asked to speak on the agricultural interests of the state. Delighted to accept, she attracted a large crowd for the address. She also used the opportunity of traveling to Oneida County to attend the Blue and Gray reunion the following day. The entire event was a rejuvenating experience, and she stopped on the way in Rome, where she stayed with Mrs. Charlotte Ward and met with several old friends. She was so pleased with her renewed acquaintance with the city in which she had begun her medical practice that she declared she would have her cremated body buried in Rome when she died. She and Ward advanced the idea, suggesting that Ward's house on Dominick Street could be purchased by the city and used as a small hospital and crematory; if Romans wanted to erect a monument in her memory, Mary remarked, they could name the facility the Dr. Mary E. Walker Crematory. For all of Mary's plans, this was her last visit to Rome.[20]

She returned to Washington with the desire to participate again in suffrage meetings, and she began by attending a meeting of the House Judiciary Committee. Although not on the program of speakers, she was granted an opportunity to address the committee. Instead of speaking about suffrage itself, however, she condemned Rev. Anna Shaw (current president of the NAWSA), the wealthy Alva Vanderbilt Belmont (who held suffrage meetings at her "Newport palace"), and others who made running suffrage associations their *business*. Mary argued (as she had about Anthony) that if leaders profited from the movement, they would not truly seek passage of a suffrage bill. Her lengthy speech, which was published in the Judiciary Committee's records, addressed the "methods taken to suppress the Crowning Constitutional Argument by women who have aimed to defer the exercise of franchise because of *Graft*." It was not her attire that they disdained, she declared, in spite of their claims to that effect: "I here and now make it plain that *dress* has nothing to do with the matter; but some women are made to believe that it does have, so as to still keep the 'Amendment' graft uppermost." Newspapers, always eager to exploit differences within the movement, headlined her comments across the country.[21]

In spite of her alienating commentaries on NAWSA leaders, Mary was embraced by other suffragists. Mary Eleanor O'Donnell's "Suffragettes of Yesterday and Today," for example, appeared in the *Chicago Tribune* in May 1910, illustrated with ten portraits, including those of Mary, Anthony, Lockwood, and Stanton. Mary also sought to remind citizens of the history of calls for independence, which she aligned with woman's suffrage. Thus that summer when she was invited to speak at Oswego's Fourth of July celebration, her topic was the Mecklenberg Declaration of Independence. The declaration, signed by citizens in Mecklenberg County, North Carolina, on May 20, 1775, called for independence from Britain more than a year before the 1776 Declaration of Independence. The topic blended Mary's love of history and her patriotic belief in universal independence and suffrage. Yet as she lectured throughout the year, she did not forego her brash criticisms of amendment suffragists, calling them "grafters" and "fools" and their amendment bills "silly rubbish." As the decade closed, much of her significant work for suffrage was overshadowed by her self-imposed alienation from the next generation of activists.[22]

CHAPTER 14

The Pioneer Embraced

During an "Old Home Week" celebration in Oswego, Mary was asked to contribute to the festivities. She penned "Welcome Home," a tribute to "Vesta, Aurora, and Luna; the Walker Sisters, who were Educators nearly sixty years since." Proud of her sisters and of "Oswego—dear old native land," Mary honored the innovative education fostered by her parents and continued by her sisters. But America itself was equally Mary's "dear old native land." While her last decade would see an acceptance of pants for women, an honoring of her many contributions to women's rights, and recognition of her role as one of the pioneering women physicians, it would also be as contentious and labor-intensive a period as any of her life.[1]

"It's a vindication," she happily declared in early 1911 when Paris fashions embraced harem trousers for women. She lectured on behalf of the healthfulness of her style throughout the coming years, with more appreciative audiences as women's pants became increasingly accepted in American culture. But amendment suffragists were not among her champions. In February suffragists and anti-suffragists descended upon Albany as the joint judiciary committees of the senate and the assembly heard arguments on the subject. Mary's longtime supporter Assemblyman Sweet put forth an alternative suffrage bill that proclaimed any law denying women equal privileges with men would be deemed unconstitutional. In March Mary presented a long argument before an assembly committee and answered a series of questions about the bill. She concluded her remarks by proclaiming that New Yorkers would do well to make her a senator because *she* had read the Constitution.[2]

In May Mary's lifelong friend Susan Fowler died. A teacher, author, actress, businesswoman, and farmer, Fowler exemplified the New Woman. As the public recognized, with Fowler's death, Mary was the lone survivor of the original "bloomer brigade." During the summer, Mary was involved in another controversial event. In August Mrs. Reginald Waldorf advertised for a "living right index finger," offering to pay anyone who was willing to offer their finger as a replacement for her own digit, lost in an accident. Waldorf declared she was independently wealthy and willing to pay almost any price if the finger suited her. Mary immediately wrote to Waldorf, seeing an opportunity to earn the funds she needed to build a sanitarium. "Will you give me enough to erect a consumptive ward on my estate?" she asked Waldorf. "I have saved hopeless cases, [but] because I declare consumption is not contagious, money is not forthcoming to erect a ward." She offered to travel to Waldorf's home if her transportation costs were covered. The news of Mary's willingness to sell a finger exploded nationwide across newspaper banners. Reporters mocked the seventy-nine-year-old physician for thinking a younger woman would want her finger, although no comment was made against Waldorf for seeking to purchase a body part. Eventually, Waldorf's surgeon announced that Mary's finger would not be appropriate, as Waldorf was a musician who needed dexterity and Mary was "altogether too old for our purposes." Once again, the hope of a sanitarium was foiled and Mary was left the subject of much ridicule.[3]

Ignoring the responses as much as possible, she spent the remainder of the summer attending veteran reunions and fairs around the state. When Isabelle Kingsbury Hart took guests on a ride out to see the famous Dr. Walker's home, she was surprised to be cordially invited in—and even more surprised to be asked to sign a visitors' register. She seemed to "regard herself more as an institution than as a private citizen," Hart noted. Indeed, Mary's accomplishments were being recognized more widely. The *Washington Post* ran a long article about her in the fall, "Dr. Mary Walker's Reforms Finally Win Recognition." She dressed as she did out of conviction, not notoriety, the paper asserted, and she was "willing to pay the cost." In many ways the tide of criticism had turned; the *Post* even lauded her in retrospect for attempting to sell her finger, as it represented her long commitment to treating tuberculosis.[4]

In the fall, Mary traveled to Syracuse to be one of two keynote speakers, the other being Anna Shaw, at a coalition meeting held during the state fair. The meeting drew women from the temperance unions, Lady Maccabees, suffragists, Women's Relief Corps, and other groups. Mary garnered the headlines and a larger audience than Shaw, which undoubtedly pleased her, and she was awarded first prize for best dressed woman at the fair in recognition of her role as the major force in American dress reform for the past half century. She determined to build on this moment of recognition to advance several of her political concerns by leaving for Washington at the end of the year in time to attend President Taft's New Year's reception, which she knew from past experience would garner newspaper coverage of her attendance and thus announce her return to the capital. A few days later she lectured on tuberculosis at the Leader Theater and demonstrated her CPR-like process to aid someone suffering a heart attack. She also had a photograph taken at this time with two lifelong friends and coworkers in women's rights, Rev. Susanna Harris and Belva Lockwood. The intent was to capture the "pioneers"—of religion, law, and medicine as well as suffrage. Belva always carried the newspaper photo with her, labeling the three friends as the "triumvirate of woman's suffrage." She and Mary were about to reinvigorate their efforts on behalf of suffrage and unite once again, as they had not since the 1870s.⁵

On February 14, Mary spoke before the U.S. House Judiciary Committee on women's enfranchisement. Aspects of *Crowning* were incorporated into the speech, but she also revealed her discussions with constitutional lawyers and her reasons for studying law in the 1860s. She insisted that when she first presented the idea of women's constitutional right to vote, it was so new a concept that legislators needed time to absorb the idea. When the chair of the committee, Henry D. Clayton of Alabama, interrupted her to ask if she believed states had the right to "confer suffrage upon women without any amendment to the Constitution," she quickly replied, "Not the power to confer suffrage, because it is already conferred by the Constitution." But just as she was gaining her point, she shifted to charging Shaw and other amendment suffrage leaders with graft, while insisting that she had "never been given a dime in the interest of women's franchise." If she were financially able, she would take her argument to the Supreme Court. Clayton suggested she read *Williams v. The State of Mississippi* before she wasted her energies; Mary thanked him for the reference, but added: "The Supreme Bench had not then read the Crowning Constitutional Argument . . . there can no new ideas be given that will do away with what I state in this Argument. It can not be done. Truths are immortal and all the quibbles can not do away with truths."⁶

A few days later Mary E. Carrell hosted a dinner in Mary's honor which was attended by sixteen women and men activists in Washington. Violin selections offered a melodic backdrop and patriotic emblems decorated the table. It was a lovely evening, one that demonstrated support for Mary's views. In mid-March she traveled to Albany for suffrage hearings and to New York City for a lecture on behalf of the Betterment League on the Prevention of Disease, an organization she helped found. But on arrival at the New York train station, she was suddenly taken ill; she had contracted a cold while in Albany that developed into bronchitis, necessitating her hospitalization. Once again she insisted on doctoring herself, asking only that she be allowed a bed in which to rest until she was well enough to leave. Physicians at Presbyterian Hospital wanted to treat her with drugs to be sure she avoided pneumonia, but Mary still held to her eclectic medical philosophy and refused. An old Central New York friend, Mrs. Nellie B. Van Slingerland, arrived to check on Mary, and after two days in the hospital Mary moved to Slingerland's rooms at the Hotel Gerard, from which she issued a statement that the newspapers should not waste time writing her obituary as she was "not dead yet." Van Slingerland, a novelist who wrote under the penname "Neile Bevans," was secretary of the Betterment League on the Prevention of Disease and founder of the Jeanne d'Arc Suffrage League. She also opposed capital punishment for murder, and although she wore traditionally feminine clothing, she and Mary were supportive of one another's endeavors. The suffrage league's *Joan of Arc Magazine*, edited by Van Slingerland, had devoted its April 1910 issue almost exclusively to articles about Mary's activities. Although Mary could not lecture, she dictated an address in support of world peace from her sick bed. As Van Slingerland declared, "Dr. Walker's mind is as keen and alert as ever and she is watching her own progress with intelligence and with professional discrimination. Thus far she has proved the power of mind over medicine." Letters from well wishers, including Belva Lockwood, poured in, and Mary soon improved.[7]

By mid-April Mary was well enough to return to Oswego. As newspapers noted, it was "sheer force of will" that aided her recovery. As much as her strength of will led Mary to a grand egotism, it was equally the source of her achievements. Among those sending well wishes to Mary was Princess Frederika Nicholas. She wrote when Mary first became ill, apologizing that her own illness was the only thing that kept her from coming from Rutland, Vermont, to her "Dear Friend and sister." Their paths would cross again. As soon as Mary was recovered, she undertook another lecturing tour around the Northeast.[8]

As election-year party debates geared up, Mary continued her support of the Democrats and her opposition to Roosevelt. Although Woodrow Wilson was not a woman's suffrage supporter, and Theodore Roosevelt came out in support during the campaign, she stumped for Wilson and was happy when he defeated Roosevelt. But party politics were put aside by newspapers across the country on November 26 to recognize Mary's eightieth birthday. After a brief celebration, she set out on a lecture tour to Chicago, arriving on December 1. She would remain in the city for nearly four months, staying with relatives, Mr. and Mrs. F. L. Hunt and their daughter Dorothy. She was soon immersed in local political debates about suffrage and the upcoming election. Although she was invited to attend the state suffrage association meeting, she was ignored by the leaders when she appeared; shortly before the meeting began, she had criticized Jane Addams' support of Roosevelt. Yet a number of suffragists agreed with her perspective, and the newly formed Human Rights Party invited her to speak at their first meeting and warmly accepted her constitutional arguments. So, too, did she receive recognition in the tome published by Mrs. John A. Logan this year, *The Part Taken by Women in American History*. Mary Cunningham Logan was a powerful force in Washington social and political circles and a lecturer on many topics, including labor advances of African Americans. Noting Mary's prominence in several reform movements, Logan asserted that it was only "people of narrow minds" who would ridicule her many accomplishments.[9]

The larger suffrage movement itself was once again facing a split in loyalties and vision. After more than sixty years of seeking equality, suffragists' frustrations were causing implosion. Alice Paul, who wanted to engage in the more militant tactics employed by some British suffragists, founded the Congressional Union (later the National Women's Party); as a result, she and her followers were expelled from the NAWSA. It would take another four years before the groups would work closely together to push for an amendment. The splintering granted Mary a new albeit small audience of disaffected suffragists who appreciated her idea that men had no right to "grant" women rights they already held. It also allowed her to voice her opposition to militant tactics, which she did vociferously; women peace activists resisted such tactics—as Lockwood asserted, they were "not our ways." But Chicago held its challenges for Mary as well. In spite of the general change in attitudes about women's attire, she was arrested once again because of her clothing, and, as usual, released after being taken to the police station. The arrest had its benefit, however, as her acquaintance was sought out by the well-known gynecologist, Dr. Bertha Van Hoosen, who read about the policeman's actions. Van Hoosen was a professor of medicine at the University of Illinois, with wide-ranging influence in the women's medical community of Chicago and beyond; in 1915 she would found the American Women's Medical Association. She had followed Mary's career for thirty years and was delighted with the woman she met. Describing Mary as having a manner "astonishing for its reserve and quietness" and a face that "showed intelligence and character," Van Hoosen immediately became a friend. She offered to drive Mary wherever she might want to go in her new electric car, which delighted Mary. On their drives, they had long discussions about their lives as women physicians, the changes that had occurred in the profession and American culture in general. On one of their drives, Van Hoosen recalled, Mary "leaned forward and looked into my eyes with that dreamy far away expression like a small Peter Pan and said, shaking her head: 'It is a great thing to have lived from punk [dried wood used for tinder] to electricity.'"[10]

Van Hoosen wanted Mary to meet other medical women in the city, so she hosted a dinner in her honor at the Fine Arts Building. When she arrived to pick up the honoree, Van Hoosen discovered her friend "in a beautiful swallow-tail evening suit, three glittering diamonds in her shirt front, her tall silk hat with the thin slightly curly hair showing beneath it, and over all a wonderful cape that gave the air of a foreign potentate." She was "more charming and more attractive than any one else at that dinner," Van Hoosen declared, and she captured Mary's ability to transcend generations when she concluded that the physicians in attendance "that evening felt that they had had a glimpse backward into the past and a glimpse forward into the future."[11]

Mary had fallen shortly after the dinner in her honor and had been briefly hospitalized, delaying her return to Washington until April. Thus she was not in the city for the suffrage march on March 3 lead by Alice Paul. But she wasted little time in expressing her disdain for the march because its purpose was to support an amendment. In opposition she scheduled a free lecture at Moore's Garden Theater. There, and later at the NAWSA headquarters, she advised women to use a different kind of march: "March to the polls in numbers at the next election and cast your votes." She was returning to a battle with other suffragists that was a repetition of the 1870s, going so far this time as to assert that English suffragists should be brought to the States and tried for criminal actions. Not surprisingly, such comments alienated her even further from mainstream activists. Yet her status in the movement was still strong enough to garner a place in the legislative hearings held in April. Even with the split within suffrage ranks evident at hearings before the U.S. Congress later in the month—with one day designated for the NAWSA, two hours the following day for the National Association for Equal Suffrage, and twenty minutes for Mary—the mood of the country was changing, and the push for suffrage would not stop until the goal was achieved less than seven years hence. In mid-June Mary headed back to Chicago to participate in the city's parade celebrating the granting of the vote to women in Illinois. Although Mary did not approve of parades to demand suffrage, this parade in celebration of achieved rights had her strong approval. It was a glorious day for suffragists as women from around the country joined dozens of state organization leaders. Mary rode in an automobile, standing throughout the entire procession, waving an American flag.[12]

She returned to Oswego, looking forward to her usual summer of rest and regional lecturing, but within a few days she was called to Rutland, Vermont, where Princess Nicholas had fallen ill while on a tour of the States. Nicholas insisted on being treated by Mary, noting that she had cured her of a similar illness several years earlier. After examining the Princess, Mary determined she would need several weeks' treatment and took the Princess to her home-sanitarium at Bunker Hill, where she now also rented out rooms. Their mutual friend Lorrie Jenkins wrote Mary a letter of encouragement when Mary's patience with the demanding patient was waning; Jenkins cautioned Mary to be sympathetic and not blame the patient for her ill-temper as "[s]he may not be with us long." But no repair of Mary and the Princess's relations could be achieved. Nicholas left Bunker Hill, went to a neighboring farm, and demanded a local constable serve a warrant for Mary's arrest for what she claimed was ill treatment—primarily, that Mary had insisted she arise during the night and attempt to walk. Later Mary explained that the Princess could walk a little with the use of a chair, but she refused for safety reasons to let the patient walk down a set of stairs in order to sit on the front lawn; when the patient continued to attempt the stairs, Mary removed the key from her door. The constable refused to serve papers, however, noting that there were two other doors through which Nicholas could have access to the outside of the house. It was just the fodder the press needed to make Mary once again headline news, insisting she had "imprisoned" the Princess. Mary responded by exposing the dubious nature of the Princess's claim to royalty. The two women met during the Civil War when Eleanor Bishop served as a nurse; Bishop later married a man named Nicholas who claimed to be a Greek prince, but worked in Rutland at a hotel.[13]

Equally strange was a story that emerged in October. A group of youthful marauders, the story went, came to Mary's home and yelled that the house was on fire so that when she emerged they could tar and feather her. It was reported that Mary escaped back into the house and called the justice of the peace, who rushed to her home. By then the mob had dispersed. Mary asserted that the attack had undoubtedly been instigated by the Princess. Suddenly the tide turned, and Mary was heroic for foiling the miscreants. Years later she insisted no such event ever occurred; whether or not it did, it made very good copy at the time for the newspapers. A real experience from that winter may have been less dramatic, but it offered Mary important insights into international politics. She met Assistant Secretary of the Navy Franklin Roosevelt at a New York State Historical Association meeting, and they had the opportunity to discuss the war with Mexico, Japan, suffrage, and many other timely topics.[14]

On January 5, 1914, Mary returned to the New York stage, giving lectures twice a day on women's rights at Hammerstein's Victoria Theater and drawing large crowds. She originally said she was going to lecture against the militant actions of Emmeline Pankhurst, but she apparently determined to focus on her own views and other current events. At the same time she continued her interest in the peace movement by asserting that President Wilson's special envoy to Mexico, John Lind, was the wrong choice at this crucial moment. "I think that President Wilson should send me to Mexico as a special peace envoy," she asserted. "Something should be done at once to relieve the situation there. The killing and wounding of the Mexicans is disgraceful," she added, arguing that President Huerta was in danger of being assassinated if peace negotiations were not established immediately. After the assassination of Mexico's president and vice president in February of the previous year, which included U.S. ambassador Henry Wilson in the plot, Lind was selected by President Wilson as an envoy to Mexico. Lind's temper was infamous, and Mary had a foundation for her concerns; within a few months, tensions would culminate in the Tampico Incident in which Huerta marched U.S. sailors through the streets, threatening war between the two countries. As these events were developing in January, Mary attended a gathering of the Women's National Democratic League, where she supported Democratic Senator Charles S. Thomas's call for equal suffrage and his peace efforts after the "period of dissipation" under Roosevelt's administration. Mary encouraged women to push for peace and for admittance to organizations that would allow them to express their political opinions. On the last day of the WNDL's meeting, Mary attempted to put forth a resolution "conveying the sympathy of the league to the women of Mexico and requesting the latter to exert every influence in establishing peace in their republic," but she was quickly ruled out of order.[15]

Shortly thereafter Mary was again successful in having a bill presented to the Judiciary Committee that claimed seeking an amendment "to give women existing rights is simply tautology" and, with the support of the District Suffrage Association, she presented a lecture on the subject that drew several hundred people. At meeting after meeting over the next months, she set forth the principles of the *Crowning Constitutional Argument*, with another version published in the Congressional Record. As president of what was now termed the American

Constitutional Association, she left a memorandum expressing the ACA's views with President Wilson's office. The ACA's membership was drawn primarily from her supporters in the District Suffrage Association. Its formulation was a necessary political move, as she had not been allowed to speak at some events over the last decade because she did not represent an organization. When Wilson later met with a delegation of working women suffragists, however, he gave them no hope of support for the cause.[16]

Several unionist groups recognized Mary's longstanding support of labor, and invited her to join them at the International Cutters' Association banquet. Tables were set up so that the famous attendees could sign autographs, and the *Washington Post* reported that of the four hundred autographs signed that night, three hundred were sought from Mary. Thoroughly enjoying the attention she was receiving in the capital, she lectured on many aspects of women's rights, arguing that dress reform was for health, divorce was "as respectable as marriage" but trial marriages would diminish the need for divorce, and the institution of marriage was "essential to the Government, but at the same time it is a lottery. You take a chance. Love and courtship should be frank." Temperance also remained an important aspect of her lectures. At a meeting of the Sons of Jonadab, whose members were recovering alcoholics, her comments were hailed when she clarified that she did not advocate temperance but rather complete abstinence. In another lecture, she again challenged Anthony Comstock's moralistic rantings—this time he had charged that nudity in art was immoral. Mary countered that young children could be taught about their bodies by the use of art statues made into toys. The nude figure of woman was beautiful, she declared; it was only the way in which some art figures were draped that made them vulgar. She had more fun when she demonstrated how a change in clothing style would allow women more freedom to participate in modern dances. The depiction of Mary's demonstration of a step she created—the "Dress Reform Dip"—as she danced with a beautiful young woman who was the stenographer in her Washington office was reprinted throughout the country. It was the culmination of two of her great loves—dress reform and dancing. She also attended to more grave women's rights issues when she introduced a legislative bill that would require the government to pay a pension to a woman who divorced her veteran husband on the grounds of cruelty, just as they would if he died. Although the bill was defeated, it demonstrated the precarious financial status of women in abusive marriages. The various discussions of marriage and divorce led Mary to reiterate the story of President Arthur's proposal to her. She explained that his tobacco smoking was the key separating point, but she added, "I would not lose my identity in his. As his wife I would have been the first lady in the land for a few years and then would have been nobody as his widow. I will always be somebody." This was the core of Mary's life actions: to "be somebody," independent of associative identities as a wife or as a member of a group. It was both her strength as well as the core of her inability to gain broad support for her goals of running an organization or leading the suffrage movement.[17]

At the end of March she joined many longtime associates in honoring Rev. Olympia Browne, president of the Women's Federal Suffrage Association. Belva Lockwood, Dr. Clara McNoughton of the District Woman Suffrage Association, Dr. Cora Smith-King and Dr. Elnora Folkmar, Washington activists, Ida Husted Harper, who would later write the first major biography of Susan B. Anthony, and many other Washington suffragists joined in the celebration. Mary herself was recognized a few days later at a meeting at the WFSA headquarters. Newspaperman John B. McCarthy recalled the early days of the suffrage movement in Washington, regaling his audience with stories about the actions of Mary, Lockwood, Sara Spencer, and others. McNoughton added a report on the many reforms secured by women in the District over the past decades. Mary also found an unexpected supporter in comedienne Etta Hastings who was performing in Syracuse at the time. Laugh as people will at Mary's attire, Hastings asserted, after sloshing through mud she herself feels "like lifting my voice in a hallelujah of praise for Dr. Walker. . . . let's hope for real dress emancipation sometime in the near future."[18]

After the exhausting but fulfilling months in Washington, Mary took a much needed rest for the summer in Oswego, although "rest" always included participating in county and state fairs. She traveled only on brief jaunts to nearby cities to lecture, preferring to express her opinions in letters to local editors on everything from electric lights in the city to a welcome for participants in the State Grange's annual meeting. In the latter she detailed the history of her beloved Oswego, noting the historical sites in the city that the visitors might enjoy. Outlining the city's many accomplishments, such as the development of the Normal school and its role in the underground railroad, she concluded that "an Oswego woman" had here cast the first vote and penned the *Crowning Constitutional Argument*.[19]

With the advent of World War I, it became evident that women's support was essential to the country's economic and moral stability. Numerous articles appeared that recalled Mary working "shoulder to shoulder with men" during the Civil War as an action to be emulated by the current generation of women. Accounts of her years of activism and support of suffrage appeared as well. When the largest suffrage parade in history was organized in New York City in October 1915, scheduled to precede the November elections, Mary set aside her disparagement of suffrage parades and joined in because it was an inclusive parade, allowing those of every view to participate. Alberta Hill, head of the Women's Political Union, was the grand marshal, and "Dr. Anna Howard Shaw, Dr. Mary Walker, Mrs. Herbert Carpenter, Mrs. Norman De R. Whitehouse, Miss Rosalie Jones, Mrs. Carrie Chapman Catt, and Miss Fola La Follette were among the scores of women who head[ed] various sections." Thirty thousand women from twenty nations marched in the four-hour parade from Washington Square to Central Park. From the 1860s reigniting of the suffrage movement to that day, the world had never seen such a demand for equality.[20]

After the excitement of the New York gathering, Mary returned to Washington. When Clara Colby organized an East Coast peace meeting to coincide with the closing ceremonies of the Panama-Pacific Exposition in San Francisco, both Mary and Belva Lockwood attended and supported the call for a League of Nations. In the first week of December 1915 they joined other suffragists as parade marshals to welcome Western suffragists who had driven across the country to present a petition with 500,000 names in support of women's enfranchisement at the White House. In mid-December, in spite of their differences in approach, five hundred women representing numerous suffrage groups again joined the NAWSA in meetings to demonstrate unification, and Mary was one of the speakers. As the younger women of the National College Equal Suffrage League declared, "Make friends, not enemies" was the new goal. Although strains in the fabric of this national coalition would continue to be evident, the sense that success was nearing was a strong motivator for women to be a part of the momentous occasion. Mary certainly continued to argue her views, but she abandoned the personal attacks that had distinguished her remarks for so long.[21]

Mary used a time-honored argument of women peace activists when speaking before the House Committee on Naval Affairs on January 25, 1916: instead of increasing funds for the Navy, Congress should send fifty women to meet with Japanese women as the most expedient means of forwarding peace between the nations. She lectured on these issues and attended meetings for such diverse groups as the Secular League and the First Spiritualist Church. Two years earlier a Midwestern chapter of the DAR had accepted Mary's membership application, and she attended the national convention in the city with no objections this time. When asked by a reporter if she was a delegate to the April congress, she smilingly replied, "No; I am a high private in the rear ranks." She also had the pleasure of seeing females, from society ladies to women lawyers, embracing the new style of short hair for women. In a widely published article by the author Mrs. Wilson Woodrow, her efforts on behalf of dress reform were acknowledged as pathbreaking. With these successes, she returned to Oswego in the summer to again call a Democratic convention in order to be elected a delegate to the national convention scheduled for St. Louis in June. One of the city's aldermen was selected chair, speeches were made about her qualifications, and she was given credentials as the convention's delegate. She correctly asserted that Wilson would be reelected.[22]

By mid-January 1917 Mary was back in Washington, attending hearings over corruption in the U.S. House Rules Committee and working for the election of James Beauchamp Clark (who had lost the nomination to Wilson) as the next Speaker of the House. She also resisted the practice of "silent sentinels" in which a group of suffragists picketed outside the White House. "I do not believe the suffragists will ever be able to gain their point until they cease such tactics," she explained, outlining her ideas about preferable suffrage tactics before the Secular League and other groups. There was an increasing urgency to every gesture Mary made in these months; at eighty-four, she was aware of the short time she had left to enact her goals. She began to plan for the distribution of her property, offering it to the New York State Historical Association after her death. The property included items that she kept under lock and key and called her "Chamber of Horrors"—corsets, hoop skirts, and other items that had been a part of women's oppressive clothing throughout her lifetime, as well as the cap worn by Guiteau, a braid from Lincoln's coffin, items she had kept from her visit to Paris in 1867 and from her travels around the States for nearly sixty years. The Historical Association declined the offer, citing insufficient funds to maintain the property. The various artifacts she gathered over her lifetime would largely be discarded by her nephew Byron Worden at her death.[23]

At this time, Mary and 911 male recipients of the Medal of Honor received word that their medals were being rescinded under new regulations that required "actual combat with an enemy . . . above and beyond the call of duty." She wrote a statement of protest, requesting reconsideration; when it was denied, she simply refused to return the Medal and wore it for the rest of her life. As World War I continued, Mary announced that she would take an active part in Red Cross work. But she had not abandoned her hope of a peaceful solution, and once again sought to intervene in international politics. In April she sent a cable to Kaiser Wilhelm in which she invited him and European leaders to her home to discuss terms of peace. No response was forthcoming, but the letter supported the call among activists to negotiate for peace. Mary's work for the Red Cross was thwarted in the early summer when she fell on the Capitol steps. The injuries were severe; her nose was broken, and one knee and hand were badly sprained. The trauma of the fall forced her to return to Bunker Hill for bed rest. A celebration of her eighty-fifth birthday was held at her home, but Mary was far more interested in writing, and the ideas poured forth. She sent a public letter to President Wilson in which she lamented "outrages to health, and particularly the people who are or will be suffering from tuberculosis," because of wheat flour being sent overseas instead of being available for Americans' use. She traced the extraordinary usage of sugar (a precious commodity during the war) in the manufacturing of tobacco as a means of covering the "poison of nicotine." She also advocated a new method of commuting sentences of inmates on death row. With a potential national coal strike threatening to shut down mines for the summer and perhaps into the fall, she argued that governors should commute electric chair sentences in favor of putting the convicts to work in the coal mines.[24]

After months of being confined to her house, Mary was able to travel into Oswego. Frail but determined, she presented the city with a poem she had written about her hometown, "Home to the World," and was welcomed by old friends in the city. Although she hoped to work with the American Women's Hospitals in the war effort, her health failed. She tried to remain at home, but in early August was taken by ambulance to the U.S. General Hospital at Fort Ontario. Her status as a veteran allowed her admittance, and she improved in the atmosphere of the old veterans who knew the history of her Civil War service. After being hospitalized for over a month, she insisted on being allowed to return home. Hospital officials indicated it was necessary for her to have live-in care if she did so. Such details did not interest Mary—if she must die, she declared, she wanted to pass away amidst the beauty of Bunker Hill and in her own home. On October 1, several Oswego veterans submitted a letter to the town board requesting $500 be given for a nurse to care for Mary. It was appropriate that one of the last gestures of support came from her Civil War compatriots, but it was certainly not the only gesture of support. Letters of condolence and support poured in from friends, relatives, and strangers. The accolades were personal and political. Lorrie Jenkins and Mary's nieces Dorothy Hay and Aurora Parkhurst sent their love, and the Woman's National Democratic League sent a note signed, "Often in our thoughts / Always in our hearts." A neighbor, Mrs. Frank Dwyer, cared for Mary in her last months and noted that "her mind was clear and active" to the end.[25]

At 8 A.M. on February 22, 1919, Dr. Mary Walker died at her beloved Bunker Hill. Family, friends, and neighbors gathered for her burial in the family plot at Rural Cemetery in Oswego Town. Newspapers throughout the country published extensive obituaries hailing her as a remarkable patriot, war hero and veteran, pioneer suffragist, women's rights crusader, wearer of masculine attire (a description she could not escape even in death), and Congressional Medal of Honor recipient. Perhaps the most fitting memorial to Mary came from Dr. Bertha Van Hoosen: "Dr. Mary's life should stand out to remind us that when people do not think as we do, do not dress as we do, and do not live as we do, that they are more than likely to be a half century ahead of their time, and that we should have for them not ridicule but reverence."[26]

Epilogue

Eighteen months after Mary's death, on August 18, 1920, the Nineteenth Amendment to the U.S. Constitution was ratified by Congress. It recognized women as citizens and granted them the right to vote.

Notes

ABBREVIATIONS

DUCOM   Papers of Lida Poynter, Acc. #026, Drexel University College of Medicine, Archives and Special Collections on Women in Medicine and Homeopathy

MEW   Dr. Mary E. Walker

NARA   Records of the War Department, Office of the Adjutant General, Record Group No. 94, The National Archives and Records Administration, Washington, D.C.

OCHS   Dr. Mary Walker Papers, Oswego County Historical Society, Oswego, New York

SUSC   Mary Edwards Walker Papers, Special Collections Research Center, Syracuse University Library

CHAPTER 1 — THE SEEDS OF RADICALISM

1. MEW, "Consumptive School Sanitarium," 1900 (broadside); J.B.R. Walker, A.M., *Memorial of the Walkers of the Old Plymouth Colony* (Northampton, MA: Metcalf & Co., 1861), 21.

2. J.B.R. Walker, *Memorial of the Walkers*, 21.

3. MEW, "Consumptive School Sanitarium"; Lida Poynter, "Dr. Mary Walker, The Forgotten Woman," 6 (unpublished manuscript, DUCOM); Charles V. Groat, *Dr. Mary Walker: A Reader* (Oswego, NY: Oswego Town Historical Society, 1994, 2000), 29, 11; J.B.R. Walker, *Memorial of the Walkers*, 247–248.

4. J.B.R. Walker, *Memorial of the Walkers*, 247; Charles McCool Snyder, *Dr. Mary Walker: The Little Lady in Pants* (North Stratford, NH: Ayer, 1962), 9–10; Groat, *Dr. Mary Walker*, 11.

5. The family home, which MEW owned after her father's death, was destroyed by fire in 1933 (Poynter, "Dr. Mary Walker," 10).

6. Charles McCool Snyder, *Oswego: From Buckskin to Bustles* (Port Washington, NY: Ira J. Friedman, 1968), 147–149; Ralph M. Faust, *The Story of Oswego County* (Oswego, NY: n.p., 1954), 40–44; Judith Wellman, *The Landmarks of Oswego County* (Syracuse, NY: Syracuse University Press, 1988), 82.

7. Faust, *Oswego County*, 41–44; "Varieties: Oswego," *Water-Cure Journal* 10 no.3 (Sept. 1850), 131.

8. Valentine poem MS, titled "She's Beautiful" (SUSC).

9. Turner to Poynter, Apr. 11, 1932 (DUCOM); Groat, *Dr. Mary Walker*, 12; Snyder, *Walker*, 11–12. Only Alvah, Jr. sided with his distant relative. In later years, he identified himself as an "Evolutionist" and "an Ingersollian agnostic" (quoted in Poynter, "Dr. Mary Walker," 11).

10. Franz Mesmer popularized Spiritualism through the use of hypnotism. Since Mesmer's hypnotic techniques were used by early physicians (see below), MEW may have encountered his work through the history of surgical practices.

11. Octavius Brooks Frothingham, *Gerrit Smith: A Biography* (New York: G. P. Putnam's Sons, 1878), 164; Snyder, *Oswego*, 154–159; Dale L. Walker, *Mary Edwards Walker: Above and Beyond* (New York: Forge Books, 2005), 25.

12. Lorrie Arden-Sebold, "Dr. Mary E. Walker," in *Oswego: Its People and Events*, ed. Anthony M. Slosek (Interlaken, NY: Heart of the Lakes Publishing, 1985), 180; undated newspaper clipping (OCHS); Linden F. Edwards, "Dr. Mary Edwards Walker (1832–1919): Charlatan or Martyr? Part I," *Ohio State Medical Journal* (Sept. 1958), 1161; Faust, *Oswego County*, 51, 91.

13. *Report of the Executive Committee of the American Temperance Union* (1844), 11.

14. Andrea Moore Kerr, *Lucy Stone: Speaking Out for Equality* (New Brunswick, NJ: Rutgers University Press, 1992), 12; "Dr. Mary Walker," *Hornellsville (NY) Weekly Tribune* (2 May, 1890), 2; Lori D. Ginzberg, *Untidy Origins: A Story of Woman's Rights in Antebellum New York* (Chapel Hill: University of North Carolina Press, 2005), 2–3; Allen D. Spiegel and Peter B. Suskind, "Mary Edwards Walker, M.D.: A Feminist Physician a Century Ahead of Her Time," *Journal of Community Health* 21no.3 (June 1996), 212; "Declaration of Sentiments," *Public Women, Public Words: A Documentary History of American Feminism*, 3 vols., ed. Dawn Keetley and John Pettegrew (Madison, WI: Madison House, 1997), 1:191.

15. "Dr. Mary Walker," *National Reformer* (9 Dec. 1866), 381–382; S. R. Charles, "The Only Self Made Man in America: A Talk with Dr. Mary Walker," *Minneapolis Sunday Tribune* (4 July 1897), n.p. (clipping SUSC; hereafter cited as "Charles interview"); "Dr. Mary E. Walker," *Penny Illustrated Press* (2 Mar. 1867), 132.

16. Most accounts of MEW's education repeat Poynter's assertion that Mary attended Falley in 1850–51 and 1851–52 (Poynter, "Dr. Mary Walker," 12), but the school catalogues for those years list her only in the second year (*General Catalogue of the Falley Seminary* [Fulton, NY: Printed at the Gazette Office, 1855], 47, 10–11).

17. *Annual Catalogue of the Falley Seminary* (Fulton, NY: n.p., 1854–55), 12; "Dr. Mary E. Walker," *Penny Illustrated Press* (2 Mar. 1867), 132; Snyder, *Walker*, 13; "Dr. Mary Walker," *Nashua (NH) Telegraph* (11 Nov. 1893), n.p. (clipping, DUCOM).

18. Allen D. Spiegel, "Mary Edwards Walker, M.D.: The only woman ever awarded the Congressional Medal of Honor," *New York State Journal of Medicine* 91 (July 1991), 298; Poynter, "Dr. Mary Walker," 26; "Dr. Mary Walker," *National Reformer* (9 Dec. 1866), 382.

19. Charles interview.

20. Alvah Walker accompanied MEW to Syracuse and joined her when she met with the Dean (*National Reformer*, 382); Alexander Wilder, M.D., *History of Medicine: A Brief Outline of Medical History* (Augusta, ME: Maine Farmer Publishing Co., 1904), 555–576; John S. Haller, Jr., *Medical Protestants: The Eclectics in American Medicine 1825–1939* (Carbondale: Southern Illinois University Press, 1994), 160.

21. "Editorial," *Physicians' and Surgeons' Investigator* 2 no.9 (15 Sept., 1881), 278; Wilder, *History of Medicine*, 581; Beatrice Levin, *Women and Medicine* (Lincoln, NE: Media Publishing, 1988), 91–92; Spiegel, "Mary Edwards Walker," 299.

22. Spiegel, "Mary Edwards Walker," 299; Poynter, "Dr. Mary Walker," 29.

23. Spiegel, Mary Edwards Walker," 299; Spiegel and Suskind, "Mary Edwards Walker," 214; Arturo Castiglioni, M.D., *A History of Medicine*, trans. E. B. Krumbhaar (New York: Knopf, 1941), 723–724.

24. Poynter, "Dr. Mary Walker," 30, 49; *National Reformer*, 381–382. Initially, MEW designed a white reform outfit, but the impracticality of that color when she was attending clinics soon became evident.

25. MEW, "Dr. Mary Walker's Love Story," *Syracuse Telegram* (26 Dec. 1900).

26. MEW's medical degree is housed at OCHS; Poynter, "Dr. Mary Walker," 32; "Commencement of Syracuse Medical College," *American Medical & Surgical Journal* 7 no.4 (Apr. 1855), 141–153.

27. Albert E. Miller, "The Liberal Thinker," *American Medical & Surgical Journal* 7 no.3 (Mar. 1855), 101–104.

28. "Commencement," 144–147.

29. Ibid., 147–148.

30. Ibid., 148–151.

31. Ibid. Potter estimated that between forty and fifty women had studied at the college, although a significant number did not complete their studies.

32. Snyder, *Walker*, 16; MEW is believed to have been the first woman doctor in Columbus (Edwards, "Dr. Mary Edwards Walker," 1160); Stockwell to MEW, May 31, [1855] (SUSC) and June 3, 1855 (NARA); *Rome City Directory*, 1857; Alvah, Jr. later married Sarah Miller (Groat, *Dr. Mary Walker*, 30).

33. Poynter offers no source for her claim that Miller did not want MEW to wear a reform dress at their wedding; but he had known MEW for more than two years, and it is unlikely they would have married if they differed on a point of such importance to her. MEW, "Sickles and Key Tragedy," *The Sibyl* (15 May, 1859), 553 (Lucy Stone and Henry Blackwell used a similar ceremony seven months earlier); Alvah Walker's will (SUSC). Although MEW did not take Albert's name, she signed her initial publications for *The Sibyl* sometimes as "Miller Walker" and other times simply "Walker."

34. *Rome City Directory*, 1857, 1859–60; Charles interview.

35. Charles interview; *National Reformer*, 382.

36. Clews to MEW, Sep. 23, 1856, and Feb. 1, 1857 (SUSC).

37. Harriet L. Harris to MEW, Apr. 1875 (DUCOM).

CHAPTER 2 — DRESS REFORM AND *THE SIBYL*

1. "Commencement" 150; Clews to MEW, Sep. 23, 1856 (SUSC).

2. This family scrapbook is housed at SUSC; handwritten manuscript (SUSC).

3. Elisabeth Griffith, *In Her Own Right: The Life of Elizabeth Cady Stanton* (New York: Oxford University Press, 1984), 91–92.

4. On dress reform in America, see Gayle V. Fischer, *Pantaloons and Power: A Nineteenth-Century Dress Reform in the United States* (Kent, OH: Kent State University Press, 2001) and Carol Mattingly, *Appropriate[ing] Dress: Women's Rhetorical Style in Nineteenth-Century America* (Carbondale: Southern Illinois University Press, 2002).

5. Nancy Isenberg, *Sex and Citizenship in Antebellum America* (Chapel Hill: University of North Carolina Press, 1998), 54; Snyder, *Walker* 21; "Dress Reform Convention," *The Sibyl* (15 July 1856), 1.

6. Robert E. Riege, "Women's Clothes and Women's Rights," *American Quarterly* 15 no.3 (Autumn 1963), 391; *The Sibyl* (1 Jan., 1857), 100.

7. Dr. Lydia Sayer Hasbrouck, "Fanny Fern," *The Sibyl* (15 Apr. 1857), 156; Fanny Fern, "Lady Doctors," *Fresh Leaves* (New York: Mason Bros., 1857), 111–112.

8. Alice Cary, "Motherhood," *The Sibyl* (1 Aug., 1856), 24; John Greenleaf Whittier, "We Shape Ourselves," *The Sibyl* (15 Dec., 1856), 89; Hasbrouck, Editorial, *The Sibyl* (1 Dec. 1856), 88; Hasbrouck, "Taxation and Representation," *The Sibyl* (15 Mar. 1857), 140.

9. Alvah Walker's diary is housed at Oswego Town Historical Society; MEW, "Incidents Connected with the Army," typescript (SUSC; unnumbered pages presented in episodic style).

10. MEW, Letter to the Editor, *The Sibyl* (1 Jan. 1857), 102; MEW, "Dress Reform Convention," *The Sibyl* (15 Jan. 1857), 108; Hasbrouck, Untitled, *The Sibyl* (15 Jan. 1857), 109.

11. MEW, "A Bloomer in the Street," *The Sibyl* (15 Jul. 1858), 398; Elizabeth Cady Stanton to Mary Morris Hamilton, reprinted in *The Sibyl* (1 Dec., 1858), 508; MEW, "Mount Vernon Association," *The Sibyl* (15 Feb. 1859), 508.

12. Mrs. Vesta Walker, "'Let Your Women Keep Silent!'" *The Sibyl* (15 Feb. 1859), 508.

13. The issue of *Frank Leslie's Illustrated Magazine* that was devoted to the Sickles-Key case, for instance, sold more than 200,000 copies (Dale Walker, *Mary Edwards Walker*, 72); Karen Halttunen, *Murder Most Foul: The Killer and The American Gothic Imagination* (Cambridge, MA: Harvard University Press, 1998), 3–6.

14. "The Homicide at Washington," *Harper's Weekly* (12 Mar., 1859), 162; "The Washington Tragedy," *Harper's Weekly* (19 Mar., 1859), 178; "Biographical Sketch of Hon. D.E. Sickles," *Harper's Weekly* (9 Apr., 1859), 225–226.

15. Quoted in Edward Van Every's *Sins of America: As "Exposed" by the Police Gazette* (New York: Frederick A. Stokes, 1931), 36–37; "A National Morality Play: The Trial of Daniel Edgar Sickles," (assumption.edu/dept/history/Hi1113net/sickles); quoted in Sam Roberts, "Sex, Politics and Murder on the Potomac," *New York Times* (1 Mar., 1992), review.

16. MEW, "Sickles and Key Tragedy," *The Sibyl* (16 May, 1859), 553–554.

17. Ibid.

18. "Married, by themselves," *The Sibyl* (1 Sept., 1858), 417; Snyder, *Walker*, 14; Lola Montez, *Lectures of Lola Montez, Including Her Autobiography* (New York: Rudd and Carleton, 1858), 89, 95, 104–107, 249–250. MEW could not have known that the "autobiography" was highly fictionalized, as it was long after Montez's death that the facts of her life were uncovered.

19. MEW, "N. York State Foundling Hospital," *The Sibyl* (1 Aug. 1859), 593.

20. Ibid., 593–595; Morantz-Sanchez, *Sympathy and Science: Women Physicians in American Medicine* (Chapel Hill: University of North Carolina Press, 1985), 189; the *National Police Gazette* sensationalized the case in its coverage of the trial, "Wonderful Trial of Caroline Lohman, alias Restell" (1847); James H. Cassedy, *Medicine and American Growth, 1800–1860* (Madison: University of Wisconsin Press, 1986), 185.

21. MEW, "N. York State Foundling Hospital," *The Sibyl* (15 Sept., 1859), 622.

22. Quoted in Allen D. Spiegel and Andrea M. Spiegel, "Civil War Doctress Mary: Only Woman to Win Congressional Medal of Honor," *Minerva* (30 Sept., 1994), 24.

23. L. J. Worden, "Utica NY March 21st 1866," (SUSC). The details of this scene are drawn from Worden's eyewitness document, which was part of the written testimony in MEW's divorce proceedings (SUSC).

24. MEW's account book (SUSC); Worden; Norma Basch, *Framing American Divorce: From the Revolutionary Generation to the Victorians* (Berkeley: University of California Press, 1999), 105; Griffith, *In Her Own Right*, 203, 103–104.

25. Poynter, "Dr. Mary Walker," 44–45; quoted in Basch, *Framing American Divorce*, 203–204 n.16; Snyder, *Walker*, 25–26; *Dubuque Herald* (27 May 1869).
26. MEW account book (SUSC); *History of Delhi County, Iowa* (Chicago, 1878).
27. *History of Delhi County*.
28. B. F. Chapman, "Abstract of Authorities on Foreign Divorces" (SUSC).
29. MEW, "Women Soldiers," *The Sibyl* (1 Sept., 1859), 110.

CHAPTER 3 — CIVIL WAR SURGEON

1. Divorce decree, September 16, 1861 (SUSC).
2. Undated MS poem in MEW's handwriting (SUSC); "Dr. Mary Walker," *National Reformer* (9 Dec. 1866), 382.
3. J. N. Green to Robert C. Wood, Nov. 5, 1861 and J. M. MacKenzie letter, Oct. 28, 1861 (NARA); MEW, "Incidents"; George Worthington Adams, *Doctors in Blue: The Medical History of the Union Army in the Civil War* (New York: H. Schuman, 1952), 48; Ira M. Rutkow, *Bleeding Blue and Gray: Civil War Surgery and the Evolution of American Medicine* (New York: Random House, 2005).
4. J. M. Mackenzie to "To Whom It May Concern," October 28, 1861 (SUSC); Walter Kidder, surgeon, to "Scottgood," undated (OCHS).
5. MEW, "Incidents"; MEW to "Brother and Sister" (Alvah Jr. and probably her sister-in-law, Sarah Walker; OCHS).
6. Terry Reimer, "Smallpox Vaccination in the Civil War" (civilwarmed.org); "Report Dr. Charles S. Tripler" (civilwarhome.com); Green to Wood, Dec. 11, 1861 (NARA); Mrs. Elizabeth Conklin to MEW, Dec. 28, 1861(SUSC).
7. MEW, "Incidents."
8. Olmsted quoted in Lisa A. Long, *Rehabilitating Bodies: Health, History, and the American Civil War* (Philadelphia: University of Pennsylvania Press, 2004), 84; Rutkow, *Bleeding Blue and Gray*, chapter 2; MEW, "Incidents."
9. MEW, "Incidents"; Adams, *Doctors in Blue*, 131; Stewart M. Brooks, *Civil War Medicine* (Springfield, IL: C. C. Thomas, 1966), 99.
10. MEW, "Incidents." In "Petition of Dr. Mary E. Walker," U.S. Senate Mis. Doc. No. 226, 51st Congress, 1st Session, August 25, 1890, MEW specifically names Capt. Elliott and T. F. Bailey, both of Pittsburgh, and T. D. Bramsby of Philadelphia as men who could confirm she had saved one of their limbs from unnecessary amputation; see also letters from veterans at SUSC.
11. Lucy Stone to MEW, Jan. 7, 1861, and Dec. 9, 1861 (SUSC); Justin Kaplan, *Walt Whitman: A Life* (New York: Simon and Schuster, 1980), 273; Snyder, *Walker*, 30; MEW, "Incidents."
12. MEW, "Incidents."
13. Ibid.
14. MEW, "What Can Women Do?" *The Sibyl* (Jan. 1862), 1011.
15. MEW, "Petition" (1890), 2.
16. Allen Mikaelian, *Medal of Honor: Profiles of America's Military Heroes* (New York: Hyperion, 2002), 7; Poynter, "Dr. Mary Walker," 18; "The Hygeio-Therapeutic College," *Herald of Health* 4 (Nov. 1864), 174; "A History of the Natural Healing Practices in America" (naturalhealthperspective.com); Dale Walker, *Mary Edwards Walker*, 105–106.
17. On Trall's medical philosophies, see Spiegel and Suskind, "Mary Edwards Walker," 213–215 and Spiegel, "Mary Edwards Walker," 299; see, for example, theses for the Female

Medical College of Pennsylvania (DUCOM); "The Hygeio-Therapeutic College," *Hygienic Teacher* 33 (May 1862), 109–110; "Extract from Dr. R. T. Trall's Herald of Health," undated newspaper clipping (University Libraries Special Collections, University of Iowa).

18. "Extract from Dr. R. T. Trall's Herald of Health"; MEW, "Letter from Dr. Mary E. Walker," *The Sibyl* 7 (Jul. 1862), 1059; Lucy Stone, Letter to the Editor, *The Sibyl* (Jul. 1857); Stanton quoted in Griffith, *In Her Own Right*, 72.

19. MEW, draft of "On Washington" (SUSC).

20. *Hutchinson's Washington and Georgetown Directory* (Washington, 1862); MEW, "Petition" (1890), 2–3; MEW, "Incidents."

21. Major General Burnside, Nov. 15, 1862 (NARA); "Battle of Fredericksburg—Lee versus Burnside" (nps.gov/frsp/fredhist.htm).

22. MEW, "Incidents"; Faust, *Oswego County*, 41–44.

23. "Battle of Fredericksburg"; MEW, "Petition" (1890), 11; Whitman quoted in Kaplan, *Walt Whitman*, 269; Mercedes Graf, *A Woman of Honor: Dr. Mary E. Walker* (Gettysburg, PA: Thomas Publications, 2001), 100 n3. Fredericksburg was one of three times MEW was fired upon during her war service.

24. The pass is among the Walker Papers at SUSC; MEW, "Incidents"; L. P. Brockett, M.D. and Mary C. Vaughn, *Women's Work in the Civil War* (Boston: Ziegler & McCurdy Co., 1867), 644; MEW, "Petition" (1890), 7.

25. NARA; U.S. Department of the Army, Board for Correction of Military Records, Proceedings in the Case of Dr. Mary E. Walker, Washington, DC, May 4, 1977 (NARA).

26. *New York Tribune*, Dec. 1862 (quoted in Graf, *A Woman of Honor*, 34); Spiegel and Suskind, "Mary Edwards Walker," 218.

27. "The National Anti-Slavery Subscription-Anniversary," *Liberator* (20 Feb. 1863), 30; "Annual Meeting of the American Anti-Slavery Society," *Liberator* (15 May 1863), 78.

28. Dale Walker, *Mary Edwards Walker*, 124; MEW, "The True Spirit; Go on Faithfully," *The Sibyl* 7 (Mar. 1863), 1123.

29. "Letter from Dr. Walker," *Oswego Commercial Times* (15 Jan. 1863), n.p. Many of the old Central New York newspapers are available online through SUNY-Oswego's Library Archives. However, newspapers' edges have worn away and page numbers are not always available or readable; as complete documentation as possible is provided hereafter. William Clawyer to MEW, Nov. 4, 1863 (SUSC); Alexander Springsteen to MEW, Nov. 12, 1863 (SUSC); Lois W. Banner, *Elizabeth Cady Stanton: A Radical for Woman's Rights* (Boston: Little, Brown, 1980), 72.

30. MEW, "Woman's Mind," *The Sibyl* 7 (Apr. 1863), 1133.

31. Quoted in Snyder, *Walker*, 39.

32. MEW, "Petition" (1890).

33. T.M.N., "Women in the Army," *New York Tribune* (18 Sept. 1863), 1; Hasbrouck, "Women in the Army," *The Sibyl* 8 (Nov. 1863), 1188; Seymour quoted in *The History of New York State*, ed. James Sullivan (usgennet.org).

34. Medal of Honor citation; see also, "Mary Edwards Walker: A North Georgia Notable" (ngeorgia.com); MEW, "Petition" (1890), 8.

35. NARA.

36. MEW, "Positions that Women ought of Right to Occupy," *The Sibyl* 8 (Dec. 1863), 1196.

37. Graf, *A Woman of Honor*, 46; MEW, "Petition" (1890), 3–4; MEW, "Incidents." Chase was the daughter of Salmon Chase, treasury secretary to President Lincoln (and later chief justice of the Supreme Court). In her early twenties, Kate Chase's renown as a hostess made

invitations to her soirees highly sought by Washington's elite. MEW, "Lodging Rooms for Homeless Women," *National Republican* (17 Dec. 1863), 3; MEW, "Women's Free Lodging Rooms," *National Republican* (21 Dec. 1863), 2.

38. MEW, "Incidents."

39. MEW, "Lodging Rooms for Homeless Women," 3; MEW, "Women's Free Lodging Rooms," 2.

40. Griffith, *In Her Own Right*, 113–115; Elizabeth Cady Stanton, *Eighty Years and More: Reminiscences 1815–1877* (1898; repr., Boston: Northeastern University Press, 1993), 180; "We Are Living, We Are Dwelling" (1850) was written by Arthur Cleveland Coxe; "Women's Relief Association," *National Republican* (29 Jan. 1864), 2.

41. NARA.

42. Ibid.

43. John Farnsworth to Wood, Feb. 30, 1864 (NARA); MEW to President Johnson, Sept. 30, 1865 (NARA); *Leicester Journal* (5 Apr. 1867).

44. Adams, *Doctors in Blue*, chapter 2; Rutkow, *Bleeding Blue and Gray*, chapter 2; Leonard, 114.

45. Quoted in Albert Castel, "Mary Walker: Samaritan or Charlatan?" *Civil War Times* 33 (May/June 1994), 42. NARA records confirm MEW's version—she was examined by Cooper's board and he reported their results to Perin on Mar. 8, 1864 (G. Thomas and G. Perin telegrams; NARA).

CHAPTER 4 — SURGEON, SPY, PRISONER OF WAR

1. MEW, Letter to the Editor, *National Republican* (20 Feb. 1864), 3; "Benefit for the Women's Relief Association," *National Republican* (8 Feb. 1864), 2; Poynter, "Dr. Mary Walker," 78.

2. Oliver Wendell Holmes, "The Stereoscope and the Stereograph," *Atlantic Monthly* 3 (June 1859); Edwin F. De Foe to MEW, Feb. 10, 1864 (SUSC).

3. MEW, "Incidents"; Thomas to Perin, Mar. 10, 1864 (NARA); quoted in Snyder, *Walker*, 41; typescript of L.A. Ross's diary, Abraham Lincoln Presidential Library, Springfield, Illinois.

4. MEW, "Incidents"; quoted in Castel, "Mary Walker," 43.

5. "A Gallant Female Soldier—Romantic History," *National Republican* (16 Mar. 1864), 2; MEW, "Incidents."

6. MEW, "Incidents"; Thurman Sensing, *Champ Ferguson Confederate Guerilla* (Nashville: Vanderbilt University Press, 1994).

7. MEW, "Incidents."

8. Ibid.

9. Quoted in D. Walker, *Mary Edwards Walker*, 138; Thomas to E. Townsend, August 20, 1864 (NARA); MEW to Stanton (NARA); Priscilla Rhoades, "The Women of Castle Thunder," *Kudzu Monthly* (kudzumonthly.com).

10. Townsend to Thomas, Aug. 19, 1864 (NARA); Senate Report 237, 46th Congress, 2nd Session, Feb. 9, 1880.

11. "Arrival of the Yankee Female M.D.," *Richmond Enquirer* (22 Apr. 1864), 4; Lyde Cullen Sizer, "Acting Her Part: Narratives of Union Women Spies," *Divided Houses: Gender and the Civil War*, eds. Catherine Clinton and Nina Silber (New York: Oxford University Press, 1992). Several Confederate soldiers claimed after the war to have been present when MEW was arrested, each with varying accounts of where it occurred.

12. Rhoades, "Women of Castle Thunder"; Frances H. Casstevens, *George W. Alexander and Castle Thunder* (Jefferson, NC: McFarland & Co., 2004), 47, 64, 72; Lonnie R. Speer,

Portals of Hell: The Military Prisons of the Civil War (Mechanicsville, PA: Stackpole Books, 1997), 94; D. Walker, *Mary Edwards Walker*, 148; MEW to unknown recipient, Dec. 14, 1864 (SUSC); *Rochester Daily Democrat* (2 Jan. 1865).

13. "Dr. Mary E. Walker," *Richmond Whig* (2 May 1864), 4; Casstevens, *George W. Alexander*, 65; quoted in Graf, *A Woman of Honor*, 66; "Letter from Dr. Mary E. Walker," *Daily Dispatch* (25 Apr. 1864), 1.

14. "Wants to Go Home," *Enquirer* (10 June 1864); Mercedes Herrera-Graf, "Stress, Suffering, and Sacrifice: Women POWs in the Civil War," *Minerva* 16 no.3-4 (1998); "Miss Walker, The Yankee Surgeoness," *Examiner* (29 June 1864), 2.

15. "Dr. Mary Walker," *National Republican* (24 June 1864), 2 (the roommate was Martha Manus; she was released much earlier than MEW); Graf, *A Woman of Honor*, 68.

16. MEW, "Incidents"; Poynter, "Dr. Mary Walker," 91.

17. "Off By Flag of Truce," *Examiner* (13 Aug. 1864), 1; "Mrs. Dr. Mary E. Walker," *Centralia [IL] Sentinel* (25 Aug. 1864), 4; quoted in Poynter, "Dr. Mary Walker," 91; "Departure of Flag-of-Truce," *Daily Dispatch* (13 Aug. 1864), 1.

18. MEW, "Hotel de Castle Thunder," *National Republican* (25 Aug. 1864), 2; "Dr. Mary E. Walker," *Penny Illustrated Press* (2 Mar. 1867), 132.

19. "Doctor Mary E. Walker," *Louisville Herald* (10 Sept. 1864); newspaper clipping (SUSC); MEW to General Sherman, Sept. 14, 1864 (OCHS); General Thomas, Sept. 15, 1864 (NARA); Spiegel, "Mary Edwards Walker," 300. The pay was for five months' duty— one month for her work at Gordon's Mills before she was taken captive and the four months she was in Castle Thunder.

20. "Contract with a Private Physician" (NARA).

21. Snyder, *Walker*, 47; MEW to Secretary of War, Oct. 25, 1864 (NARA); Snyder, *Oswego*, 177–182.

22. "Villiam," Letter to Editor, *Oswego Commercial Advertiser* (23 Oct. 1864).

23. Gibson to MEW, Dec. 29, 1863. (SUSC); J. H. Wooll to MEW, Oct. 12, 1864 (SUSC); Susan Hall to MEW, Oct. 10, 1864 (SUSC); Holt to Stanton, Oct. 30, 1865 (NARA), hereafter cited as "Holt."

24. "Contract with a Private Physician" (NARA).

25. Ibid; MEW to Colonel Hammond [Oct. 1864] (NARA).

26. MEW to Colonel Hammond and his reply, Oct. 7 and 15, 1864 (NARA); Snyder, *Walker*, 49–50; quoted in Graf, *A Woman of Honor*, 74–75; MEW to Colonel Coyle, Jan. 15, 1865 (SUSC). On Oct. 4 Colonel Hammond wrote to Wood, supporting MEW and asking that Brown be told to "stick to his own building and patients" (NARA).

27. MEW to Coyle.

28. Ibid.

29. Cary Conklin letter, July 8, 1873 (SUSC).

30. "Doc" to MEW, Jan. 31, 1865 (DUCOM)

31. MEW to Dr. Edward E. Phelps, Mar. 22, 1865 (NARA); Brown to MEW, Mar. 22, 1865 (NARA); MEW, "Petition of Dr. Mary E. Walker, Praying Compensation for Services During the Late War. Senate Mis. Doc. 226 [to accompany S.4267] August 25, 1890"; handwritten response on envelope of letter MEW sent to Phelps on Mar. 31, 1865 (SUSC); quoted in Graf, *A Woman of Honor*, 78.

32. Quoted in Poynter, "Dr. Mary Walker," 100; Harry S. Stout, *Upon the Altar of the Nation: A Moral History of the Civil War* (New York: Viking, 2006), sections "1864" and "1865"; Mary Elizabeth Massey, *Refugee Life in the Confederacy* (Baton Rouge: Louisiana State University Press, 1964), 26, 15, 111.

NOTES TO PAGES 68-79

33. Alvah Walker, Jr. to Sarah Jane Walker, Apr. 19, 1865 (OCHS).

34. Snyder, *Walker*, 51.

35. George Cooper to MEW, May 17, 1865 (NARA); Holt; Dale Walker, *Mary Edwards Walker*, 162; Poynter, "Dr. Mary Walker," 104; Snyder, *Walker*, 52-53.

36. "Woman's Right to Dress," *New York World* (14 June 1866), 8; Albert Miller to Lyman Coats, July 19, 1865 (SUSC); statement of Nelson Whittlesey, Supreme Court, County of Lewis, New York, Jan. 17, 1867 (SUSC).

37. Hasbrouck to MEW, July 27, 1865 (SUSC); Addie Hitchens to MEW, Feb. 6, 1865 (SUSC).

38. Dale Walker, *Mary Edwards Walker*, 162; Catherine Clinton, *The Other Civil War: American Women in the Nineteenth Century* (New York: Hill and Wang, 1984), 88; Josephine Griffing, letter to the editor, *Liberator* (3 Nov. 1865).

39. MEW notes on legislative acts pertaining to female nurses, dated "186?" (OCHS); MEW, "Incidents."

40. MEW, "Incidents."

41. Edwards, "Dr. Mary Edwards Walker," 1162.

42. Ann Preston to MEW, Aug. 28, 1865 (DUCOM).

43. George Morgan to MEW, Nov. 10, 1865 (SUSC); W. H. DeMott, Indiana Military Agency, and D. E. Millard, Michigan Military Agency, June 1865 (NARA); *Lady's Own Paper* (1866); President Johnson to Secretary Stanton, Aug. 24, 1865 (NARA); Holt; quoted in Graf, *A Woman of Honor*, 79.

44. Holt; Thomas to Wood, Sep. 1864 (NARA); J. Collamer to Stanton, Aug. 28, 1865 (NARA).

45. Holt.

46. *Annual Report of the Military Secretary, 1861*, U.S. War Dept., 418. Critics of MEW's receipt of the award often claim the honor was given very freely, but that had changed with the 1863 act.

47. Poynter, "Dr. Mary Walker," 110; Andrew Johnson, President, Executive Order, Nov. 11, 1865 (NARA).

CHAPTER 5 — INTERLUDE

1. "Successful Operation," *National Republican* (27 Mar. 1866), 1.

2. G. Richmond to MEW, Aug. 13, 1866 (SUSC).

3. C. B. Brockway to MEW, Jul. 16, 1866 (SUSC).

4. Frank Fuller to Jerome Tarbox, June 19, 1866 (SUSC).

5. "An Act For the relief of Mary E. Miller," State of New York, No. 623, In Assembly, March 15, 1866. The document notes that she is "commonly known as Mary E. Walker" (SUSC). Worden Testimonial, Utica, NY, Mar. 21, 1866 (SUSC).

6. MEW to "Ma & Pa," Mar. 27, 1866 (OCHS); quoted in Poynter, "Dr. Mary Walker," 113.

7. William Rice to MEW, Apr. 27, 1866 (SUSC); Griffith, *In Her Own Right*, 123-124.

8. Griffith, *In Her Own Right*, 125.

9. Lydia Strowbridge to MEW, May 6, 1866 (SUSC); Fischer, *Pantaloons & Power*, 162-164.

10. See Patricia A. Cunningham, *Reforming Women's Fashion, 1850-1920* (Kent, OH: Kent State University Press, 2003); and Catherine Smith and Cynthia Grieg, *Women in Pants: Manly Maidens, Cowgirls, and Other Renegades* (New York: Henry M. Abrams, Inc., 2003).

11. "The Dress Revolution," *Circular* (18 June 1866), 109; "News of the Day," *New York Times* (11 June 1866), 4; "Woman's Right to Dress," 8.

12. "The Dress Revolution," 110.

13. "News of the Day," 4; "The Dress Revolution," 110; quoted in "More About the Short Dresses," *Circular* (18 June 1866), 117.

14. "Woman's Right to Dress," 8; quoted in "The Dress Revolution," 110.

15. Poynter, "Dr. Mary Walker," 118–119; quoted in "The Dress Revolution," 110.

16. "Woman's Right to Dress," 8.

17. Quoted in "More About Short Dresses," 110; and "Woman's Right to Dress," 8.

18. Griffith, *In Her Own Right*, 118.

19. Ann Russo and Cheris Kramarae, eds., *The Radical Women's Press of the 1850s* (New York: Routledge, 1991), 314; Griffith, *In Her Own Right*, 118–123.

CHAPTER 6 — TOURING BRITAIN

1. D. H. Craig to "Friend Spear," Aug. 7, 1866 (DUCOM); quoted in Fischer, *Pantaloons*, 162–164.

2. Quoted in Poynter, "Dr. Mary Walker," 126; Forsyth to MEW, Oct. 2, 1866 (SUSC).

3. Lawrence Goldman, *Science, Reform, and Politics in Victorian Britain: The Social Science Association 1857–1886* (Cambridge: Cambridge University Press, 2002), 174; "Social Science Congress," *London Illustrated News* (13 Oct. 1866), 358; Poynter, "Dr. Mary Walker," 128.

4. Thomas Archer, *The Terrible Sights of London and Labours of Love in the Midst of Them* (London: Stanley Rivers and Co., 1870), 14; "Social Science Congress," *Medical Press and Circular* (17 Oct. 1866), 397; "Summary of the Morning News," *Pall Mall Gazette* (6 Oct. 1866), 7; "Infanticide," *Pall Mall Gazette* (8 Oct. 1866), 1–2; "The Week," *Court Journal* (13 Oct. 1866), 1161.

5. Sheila R. Herstein, *A Mid-Victorian Feminist, Barbara Leigh Smith Bodichon* (New Haven: Yale University Press, 1985), 160; Snyder, *Walker*, 61; "Social Science Congress," *Morning Star* (11 Oct. 1866), 2. MEW purportedly was presented to Queen Victoria while in England. A relative later referred to a photograph MEW had taken of herself with the Queen, and the OCHS owns a silk shawl that was purportedly presented to MEW by Victoria. I have been unable to locate any documentation of such a meeting; considering the extraordinary coverage of MEW's activities during her year in England, one would expect to find commentary on such a meeting if it occurred.

6. "Social Science Congress," *London Illustrated News* (13 Oct. 1866), 358; quoted in Poynter, "Dr. Mary Walker," 129–30; Sheldon Amos to MEW, Oct. 1866 (DUCOM).

7. Poynter, "Dr. Mary Walker," 129–30.

8. Sarah Cooke to MEW, Oct. 9, 1866 (DUCOM); Moncure Conway to MEW, Oct. 8 and Nov. 1, 1866 (DUCOM); George Dornbusch to MEW, Oct. 1866 (SUSC); "Vegetarian Soire," *London Times* (2 Aug. 1851); Poynter, "Dr. Mary Walker," 132.

9. Holmes Coate to MEW, Oct. 30, 1866 (SUSC); Waymouth to MEW, Oct. 30, 1866 (SUSC); "This Week," *Court Journal* (3 Nov. 1866), 1242; "Dr. Mary Walker," *Lancet*, reprinted in *Chicago Tribune* (22 Nov. 1866), 2.

10. Poynter, "Dr. Mary Walker," 133–138.

11. "The Experiences of a Female Physician in College, in Private Practice, and in the Federal Army" handbill (SUSC); Poynter, "Dr. Mary Walker," 124; "Dr. Mary Walker's Lecture at St. James Hall," *Medical Times and Gazette* (24 Nov. 1866), 561–562; "Echoes of the Week," *London Illustrated News* (24 Nov. 1866), 514; "Dr. Mary E. Walker," *Morning Star* (21 Nov. 1866), 1, 3; "Dr. Mary Walker," *National Reformer* (9 Dec. 1866), 381–382; "Our

Courier," *Court Journal* (24 Nov. 1866), 3; "Occasional Notes," *Pall Mall Gazette* (23 Nov. 1866), 9; "Freedom of Dress," *Pall Mall Gazette* (24 Nov. 1866), 3; "Our London Letters," *Chicago Tribune* (13 Dec. 1866), 2; "M.D.," *All the Year Round* (8 Dec. 1866), 514–516.

12. "Dr. Mary Walker," *National Reformer*, 381.

13. See, for example, "Charges Against Medical Students," *Medical Times and Gazette* (1 Dec. 1866), 588; *Medical Gazette*, 561; *Court Journal*, 1312; *Medical Times* (24 Nov. 1866), 561; *All the Year Round*, 514; "Marriage Laws," *Fraser's Magazine for Town and Country* 76 (Aug. 1867), 175; *Pall Mall Gazette*, 9.

14. *Morning Star*, 1; "Dr. Mary Walker," *National Reformer* (9 Dec. 1866), 381–382; "Mary Walker," *National Reformer* (23 Dec. 1866), 1.

15. Mr. Nimmo, the manager, tried to take an unwarranted percentage of the night's income, but MEW refused; he then offered to serve as MEW's business manager while she was in Britain, which she also declined (letters Nov. 1867, SUSC).

16. P. F. André to MEW, Nov. 21, 1866 (SUSC); "Occasional Notes," *Pall Mall Gazette* (23 Nov. 1866), 9; Poynter, "Dr. Mary Walker," 149.

17. Edmund Burke, ed., "Great Reform Meeting of the Working Classes of London," *The Annual Register . . . for the Year 1866* (London: Rivingtons, 1867); James Edmunds to MEW, Jan. 10, Jan. 22, and Feb. 12, 1867 (DUCOM); Charles Denison to MEW, Nov. 20, 1866 (SUSC).

18. *London Anglo-American Times*, 2; Edmunds to MEW, Dec. 19, 1866 (SUSC); "Dr. Mary Walker," *Lady's Own Paper* 1 (1866), 1; Poynter, "Dr. Mary Walker," 134; Ann Cooper to MEW, Feb. 13, 1867 and Ellen Cooper to MEW, undated (DUCOM).

19. Gay Lankester, Dec. 17, 1866 (SUSC); Miss Cox to MEW, Jan. 1867 (SUSC); Edward M. Richards to MEW, Jan. 20, 1867 (SUSC).

20. Basch, *Framing American Divorce*, 105, 216n; Nelson Whittlesey, certified statement, Jan. 17, 1867, for the Supreme Court (SUSC).

21. "Dr. Mary Walker," *Court Journal* (16 Feb. 1867), 175; Charles Ellis to MEW, n.d. (DUCOM).

22. Quoted in Poynter, "Dr. Mary Walker," 164; "Varia," *New York Medical Journal* 1 (Jan. 1867), 315–316; "London," *Round Table* (15 Dec. 1866), 322.

23. Eugenie Bertiss to MEW, Mar. 27, 1867 (OCHS); Kirkwood to MEW, May 1, 1867 (SUSC).

24. "Affairs in England," *New York Times* (12 Mar. 1867), 1.

25. See, for example, John Bent to MEW, letters of Mar. 12, 14, 20, 1867 (DUCOM); Charlotte McCarthy to MEW, June 21, 1867 (SUSC).

26. G. W. Muir to MEW, Mar. 26, 1867 (SUSC). MEW actively negotiated with Muir as to what she would be paid per lecture. She wanted a flat £150 for the twenty-five lectures; he wanted her to follow a "half-profit" plan. In other instances, organizations acquiesced to her requirements. J. Morgan to MEW, Apr. 13, 1867 (DUCOM); see note 5.

27. Poynter, "Dr. Mary Walker," 166; "Dr. Mary E. Walker," *Queen* (24 Nov. 1866), 367; "American Women," *Queen* (12 Jan. 1867), 23; "Dr. Mary Walker," *Spectator* (6 Apr. 1867), 375; "Dr. Mary E. Walker's Professional Competence," *Queen* (6 Apr. 1867), 263. Its earlier account of MEW's St. James speech included a brief questioning of her credentials, to which readers had objected.

28. David Morgan Thomas to MEW, Apr. 15, 1867 (SUSC).

29. Joseph Mead to MEW, May 12, 1867 (DUCOM); Mrs. E. A. Farmer to MEW, Apr. 6, 1867 (SUSC); NARA; Bartholow, "Varia," *New York Medical Journal* 5 (May 1867), 167–170—unfortunately, most twentieth-century scholars also accepted this assessment,

and it has been a key source of the diminishment of MEW's accomplishments for over a century. Poynter, "Dr. Mary Walker," 159.

30. MEW, Letter to the Editor, *Spectator* (6 Apr. 1867), 386; "Dr. Mary Walker in London," *Gleaner* (Kingston, Jamaica) (20 May 1867), 2.

31. Andrew to MEW, May 11, 1867 (DUCOM); Thomas to MEW, May 9, 1867 (SUSC). Both newspapers published MEW's letter, but the *Queen*'s editor insisted on adding that *Miss* Walker was responsible if the public was skeptical of her credentials prior to her explanation; and while their charges were run as a lead article, the correction was published at the back of the periodical in a small paragraph.

32. Quoted in Poynter, "Dr. Mary Walker," 167; "Reports on Meetings," *National Reformer* (16 June 1867), 381–382.

33. Edmunds to MEW, June 18, 1867 (SUSC); Henrietta Hodges to MEW, July 4, 1867 (SUSC).

34. Arthur Chandler, "Empire of Autumn: The Paris Exposition Universelle of 1867," *World's Fair* 6 no.3 (1986, http://charon.sfsu.edu).

35. Bernard Bailyn, et.al., *The Great Republic: A History of the American People* (Boston: Little, Brown, 1977),1:475; Conway, *Autobiography: Memoires and Experiences of Moncure Daniel Conway*, 2 vols. (Boston: Hougton Mifflin and Co., 1904), 2:174–175.

36. Poynter, "Dr. Mary Walker," 172; John Bigelow, *Retrospections of a Life*, 4 vols. (New York: Doubleday, Page and Co., 1913), 3:107.

37. George Dornbusch to MEW, Aug. 3, 1867 (SUSC); MEW, Letter to Editor, *Morning Star* (12 Aug. 1867), 5. Seventeen letters written by MEW to Donaldson were purchased by Poynter from a dealer in Birmingham. He packaged them in a cardboard box and mailed them to her, but the box was lost in transit (DUCOM), leaving a significant gap in our understanding of MEW's scientific interests during this period. I am indebted to Jill Norgren's biography of Belva Lockwood for the idea of the public diary, another way in which MEW's and Lockwood's understanding of political activism coincided.

CHAPTER 7 — "A REPRESENTATIVE WOMAN"

1. "A Delegation of Democratic Members of Congress Visit the President," *Syracuse Courier* (1867–68).

2. Kerr, *Lucy Stone*, 128–129.

3. Elizabeth Cady Stanton, Susan B. Anthony, Matilda Joslyn Gage, eds., *History of Woman Suffrage*, 6 vols. (Rochester: Charles Mann, 1881), 2:433—hereafter noted as *HWS*.

4. See, for example, Report #640, House of Representatives, Committee on War Claims, Feb. 21, 1888, p.1 (NARA); Wilder, *History of Medicine*, 448–511, 666, 672–673; Castiglioni, *History of Medicine*, 762–767.

5. Poynter, "Dr. Mary Walker," 184.

6. Ibid., 198; Elizabeth Brown Pryor, *Clara Barton: Professional Angel* (Philadelphia: University of Pennsylvania Press, 1987), 61.

7. Ellen Beard Harman, "Health Convention," *Herald of Health* 5 (Jan. 1865), 8.

8. Barbara Babcock, "Belva Ann Lockwood: For Peace, Justice, and President" (stanford.edu/group/WLHP/papers/lockwood.htm); Jill Norgren, *Belva Lockwood: The Woman Who Would Be President* (New York: New York University Press, 2007), xiv; "Belva Lockwood" (law.stanford.edu/library/wlhbp/papers05/Lockwood).

9. Stephen Harrington to MEW, July 27, 1868 (DUCOM).

10. "Brief Mention," *Hartford Courant* (14 Mar. 1868), 2; Poynter, "Dr. Mary Walker," 184; Snyder, *Walker*, 78.

11. Untitled, *Baltimore Sun* (26 May 1868), 4; Jill Norgren, "Before It Was Merely Difficult: Belva Lockwood's Life in Law and Politics," *Journal of Supreme Court History* 23 no.1 (1999), 21; Allen C. Clark, "Belva Ann Lockwood," *Records of the Columbia Historical Society* (1935), 35-36: 208-209.

12. "Petition," *Independent* 20 (10 Dec. 1868), 2.

13. "Aesthetic Woman," *Eclectic Magazine of Foreign Literature* 7 (Apr. 1868), 497-500. The article was an excerpt from E[lizabeth] Lynn Linton's *Modern Women and What is Said of Them* (1868).

14. Ellen Carol DuBois, *Feminism and Suffrage: The Emergence of an Independent Women's Movement in American 1848-1869* (Ithaca: Cornell University Press, 1978), 110.

15. Ibid.

16. Poynter, "Dr. Mary Walker," 178; Mary E. Miller v. Albert E. Miller, Supreme Court, Utica, New York, January 2, 1869 (SUSC). Albert lived a varied and successful life in his post-divorce years. He remained married to his second wife until her death several years later. He settled in Needham, Massachusetts, where he continued his medical practice, primarily in the field of gynecology, and served in 1887 and 1888 in the state legislature. He died in East Orleans, Massachusetts, in 1913 (Poynter, "Dr. Mary Walker," 181-182).

17. Quoted in Richard G. Case, "They Called Her Batty," *Syracuse Herald American* (4 Feb. 1862), 12; Jean H. Baker, *Sisters: The Lives of America's Suffragists* (New York: Hill and Wang, 2005) 64-65, 75-80. A rumor circulated for several years that shortly after MEW's return from England she married a man named Brown, lived with him for only three weeks, and after an argument over who would wear the pants in the family, left him. No record of such a marriage is extant, and the story too closely echoes the typical jokes about MEW's usurpation of masculine rights by wearing pants to be given credence.

18. A. J. Coyer to MEW, Aug. 21 (probably post-1875; OCHS). Discussions of sexually transmitted diseases were common, however, among graduates of the Hygeio-Therapeutic College. Trall had published several frank studies of sexuality (e.g., *Sexual Diseases* [1857]), and his graduates followed that pattern (e.g., Eli Peck Miller's *Dyspepsia* [1870]).

19. The complexities of "undoing" gender are articulated in Judith Butler's *Undoing Gender* (New York: Routledge, 2004).

20. Quoted in Katharine Anthony, *Susan B. Anthony: Her Personal History and Her Era* (Garden City, NY: Doubleday, 1954), 251; *HWS*, 2:360-362. The highly flattering depiction of Stanton and Anthony that appears in Greenwood's account—and her erasure of disputes at the convention (see below)—is the text that was included in the *HWS*.

21. "The Woman's Rights Convention," *National Republican* (20 Jan. 1869), 4.

22. Theodore Stanton and Harriot Stanton Blatch, eds., *Elizabeth Cady Stanton as Revealed in her Letters, Diary, and Reminiscences*, 2 vols. (New York: Harper & Brothers, 1922), 2:121; 1:203; 2:122.

23. "National Woman's Suffrage Convention," *Independent* 21 (23 Jan. 1869), 1.

24. The UPS was later known as the Universal Peace Union. Norgren, *Belva Lockwood*, 155; Thomas F. Curran, *Soldiers of Peace: Civil War Pacifism and the Postwar Radical Peace Movement* (New York: Fordham University Press, 2003).

25. "Universal Peace Society," *National Republican* (27 Jan. 1869), 4; Charles Durkee to MEW, Oct. 3, 1869 (SUSC).

26. "Woman's Rights," *National Republican* (28 Jan. 1869), 3.

27. "Woman's Suffrage," *National Republican* (29 Jan. 1869), 4. In "Woman's Rights" (30 Jan. 1869), the *National Republican* reporter claimed that MEW said she was not in favor of anyone—in his words, "Negro, Indian, Hottentot, or otherwise"—gaining the vote unless

women were also granted the right. If she made such a statement, it was an uncharacteristically prejudiced remark from MEW.

28. "Woman's Rights," *Macon Weekly Telegraph* (5 Feb. 1869), 7; "The Inauguration," *Zion's Herald* (11 Mar. 1867), 120.

29. "Washington: Meeting of the Female Dress Reformers," *New York Herald* (29 Apr. 1869), 5.

30. "Woman's Dress Reform in Washington," (Buffalo) *Evening Courier and Republican* (5 May 1869), 1; "The Dress Reformers," *New York Herald* (30 Apr. 1869), 3.

31. Elizabeth Stuart Phelps, "Woman's Dress—The Morals of It," *Independent* 25 (15 May 1873), 611; Betsey Johnson, "Dress Reform," *Shaker and Shakeress Monthly* 3 (Nov. 1873), 86; Liberal Christina, "Woman's Dress Reform," *Christian Advocate* 49 (13 Aug., 1874), 263; "Dress Reform Picnic," *Herald of Health* 14 (Nov. 1869), 230; "Dress Reform," *Literary World* 5 (Dec. 1874), 100; "Community Journal," *Oneida Circular* (3 Apr. 1871), 109; M. Neale, "The Coming Wave," *Zion Herald* 51 (16 Apr. 1874), 126; Patricia Ann Palmieri, *In Adamless Eden: The Community of Women Faculty at Wellesley* (New Haven: Yale University Press, 1995), 10.

32. Quoted in Alma Lutz, *Created Equal: A Biography of Elizabeth Cady Stanton, 1815–1902* (New York: Octagon Books, 1974), 123.

33. Suzanne M. Marielly, *Woman Suffrage and the Origins of Liberal Feminism in the United States, 1820–1920* (Cambridge, MA: Harvard University Press, 1996), 72–78; Baker, *Sisters*, 42; Rosalyn Terborg-Penn, *African American Women in the Struggle for the Vote, 1850–1920* (Bloomington: Indiana University Press, 1998), 34.

34. "A Wail from Kansas," *Colman's Rural World* (22 May 1869), 331; R. Garner to MEW, June 7, 1869 (SUSC); Charles Herron to MEW, May 15, 1869 (SUSC).

35. Norgren, *Belva Lockwood*, 143; "Mrs. Dr. Mary Walker," *Davenport Daily Gazette* (26 May 1869), 1; "Mrs. Dr. Mary Walker," *Elyria Independent Democrat* (23 June 1869), 1; D.R., "Letter from Washington City," *Galveston News* (21 June 1869), 2–3.

36. "Nellie's Notes, No. 4," *Colman's Rural World* (3 July 1869), 1; "Female Suffragers," *Coshocton Democrat* (2 Nov. 1869), 2; "Bloomerism vs. Real Womanhood," *New York Herald* (21 May 1869), 6–7; crowing hens had been a denigrating image for suffragists since Seneca Falls—see Sylvia D. Hoffert, *When Hens Crow: The Woman's Rights Movement in Antebellum America* (Bloomington: Indiana University Press, 1995); "Mrs. Dr. Mary Walker," *Elyria Independent Democrat* (23 June 1869), 1; "Letter from Washington," *Baltimore Sun* (19 July 1869), 4; Ellen Harman to MEW, June 12, 1869 (SUSC).

37. "Washington," *(Davenport) Daily Gazette* (5 July 1869), 1.

38. "The National Labor Congress," *New York Herald* (19 Aug. 1869), 4; DuBois, *Feminism and Suffrage*, 126–161; S. J. Kleinberg, *Votes for Women in the United States, 1830–1945* (New Brunswick, NJ: Rutgers University Press, 1999), 105, 111; "Kate Mullaney," (pef.org).

39. Stanton, who had seven children and a husband who was often away from home, rarely made lecture tours in these years; Banner, *Elizabeth Cady Stanton*, 113; HWS, 2:765.

CHAPTER 8 — A CRUSADER'S *HIT*

1. Quoted in Poynter, "Dr. Mary Walker," 190; "Woman's Suffrage Convention," *Cincinnati Daily Gazette* (16 Sept. 1869), 3; undated clipping from the *Ladies Repository Magazine* (DUCOM).

2. Untitled, *Fulton Telegraph*, 22 Oct. 1869; Announcement, *Republican Journal* (28 Nov. 1869), 3; "Lecture," *Republican Journal* (17 Dec. 1869), 3; "Dr. Mary Walker Arrested," *Kansas City Evening Bulletin* (11 Nov. 1869).

3. Poynter, "Dr. Mary Walker," 193; "Mrs. Dr. Walker was in Leavenworth Yesterday," *Leavenworth Bulletin* (8 Nov. 1869), 1 (reprinted from the New York *Tribune*); Maria DeFord to MEW, May 1, 1873 (SUSC).

4. MEW to Mary Reed, Dec. 16, 1869 (SUSC).

5. Poynter, "Dr. Mary Walker," 200; Justin McCarthy, "Eugenie, Empress of the French," *Galaxy* 9 (Apr. 1870), 513; Justin McCarthy, "The Petticoat in the Politics of England," *Lippincott's Magazine* 6 (Jul. 1870), 16. McCarthy followed this comment by praising Taylor's "moderation, discretion and gracefulness." He also criticized MEW's attire in "American Women and English Women," *Galaxy* 10 (Jul. 1870), 25–36.

6. Quoted in Poynter, "Dr. Mary Walker," 200; Charles Furer to MEW, Jan. 20, 1870 (SUCS).

7. "Road Bandits in Louisiana—Mrs. Dr. Walker a Victim," *New Orleans Republican* (5 Feb. 1870), reprinted in *National Republican* (12 Feb. 1870), 1.

8. Josephine Wightman to MEW, Feb. 23, 1870 (SUSC); D. A. Weber to MEW, March 20, 1870 (SUSC).

9. "Personal," *National Republican* (17 Feb. 1870), 2; "Personal," *National Republican* (25 Feb. 1870), 2; Poynter, "Dr. Mary Walker," 202–204.

10. Poynter, "Dr. Mary Walker," 205–208.

11. Stanton lectured in Texas shortly after MEW, but weather conditions curtailed her speaking engagements. Eric Foner, *A Short History of Reconstruction* (New York: Harper & Row, 1990), 195–196; B. F. Luce to MEW, April 26, 1870 (SUSC); Henry Latimer to MEW, May 12, 1870 (SUSC); Snyder, *Walker*, 81; "Miss Dr. Mary Walker," *San Antonio Express* (17 May 1870), 3; "Hotel Arrivals," *Flake's Bulletin* (25 May 1870), 8.

12. "Varieties," *Appleton's Journal* 3 (28 May 1870), 615; "Dr. Mary Walker and her Three Very Sick Patients," (Port Jervis, NY) *Evening Gazette* (20 Jan. 1870), 2.

13. The *Revolution* continued for eighteen months under the editorship of Laura Curtis Bullard. Harper, *Susan B. Anthony*, 348–49; Terborg-Penn, *African American Women*, 24.

14. "Dr. Mary E. Walker's Exposure of President Grant's Drunkenness," *New York Sun* (10 Oct. 1870), 1; "A Queen Pullet," *Pomeroy's Democrat* (16 Nov. 1870), 1; "Adventures of a Bloomer in Wall Street," *San Francisco Bulletin* (22 Oct. 1870), 4; quoted in Carolyn L. Karcher, *The First Woman in the Republic: A Cultural Biography of Lydia Maria Child* (Durham, NC: Duke University Press, 1994), 544.

15. Quoted in *HWS*, 813.

16. Poynter, "Dr. Mary Walker," 212–13.

17. A copy of the petition is housed at OCHS.

18. Glenn V. Sherwood, *A Labor of Love: The Life and Art of Vinnie Ream* (Hygiene, CO: SunShine Press, 1997), chapter 4.

19. Stanton and Blatch, *Elizabeth Cady Stanton*, 2:122.

20. See, for example, J. R. Beden, "A 'Hard Hit' Returned," *The Sibyl* 3.6 (15 Sept. 1958), 426; Mary E. Walker, M.D., *Hit* (New York: American News Co., 1871), dedications.

21. *Hit*, 7–9, 14.

22. Ibid., 18, 20–22.

23. Ibid., 39.

24. Ibid., 108, 114–115, 117, 121.

25. Ibid., 136, 141.

26. Ibid., 143.

27. Ibid., 147, 151, 152.

28. Ibid., 166–167.

29. Ibid., 174

30. "List of Books Recently Published in the United States," *American Literary Gazette and Publishers' Circular* (1 Apr. 1871), 237; "New Publications," *Albion* (27 May 1871), 329; Winfried to Melvin Haster, undated (SUSC).

CHAPTER 9 — WOMEN'S RIGHTS UNMASKED

1. Quoted in Snyder, *Walker*, 105. "Black Friday" or the Fisk-Gould scandal culminated on September 24, 1869, when James Fisk's and Jay Gould's attempt to corner the gold market left many investors financially ruined. Fisk and Gould used Grant's brother-in-law to influence Grant's appointment of General Daniel Butterfield as assistant treasurer. Butterfield then passed information to Fisk and Gould.

2. Snyder, *Walker*, 105; Groat, *Dr. Mary Walker*, 21.

3. Snyder, *Walker*, 94; *Evening Star* (3 Mar. 1871), 1.

4. "Want to Vote," *Evening Star* (11 Apr. 1871), 4; "Determined to Vote," *Prairie Farmer* (22 Apr. 1871), 125; "Lovely Woman," *Oswego Palladium* (19 Apr. 1871), 4 (reprinted from *Washington Sunday Gazette* of April 16, 1871—few issues of the *Gazette* are extant); "News of the Week," *Every Saturday* (6 May 1871), 415; "Raid on the Registry," *Elyria Independent Democrat* (19 Apr. 1871), 2; "The Anniversaries," *New York Times* (12 May 1871), 8.

5. Lockwood to MEW, July 29, 1871 (SUSC).

6. Clipping, July 1870, Walker Family Scrapbook (DUCOM); "Dr. Mary Walker at the Oswego Fair," *Oswego Palladium* (29 Aug. 1871), 4. The items representing women's history and MEW's reform clothing were viewed as inconsequential when she died and were sold or given away (Ella Carrier to Lida Poynter, 12 Mar. 1930, DUCOM). Clipping, Sept. 1871, Walker Family Scrapbook (DUCOM). Two family scrapbooks survive—one at SUSC and the other at DUCOM.

7. "Personal," *Oswego Palladium* (2 Aug. 1871); Lockwood to MEW, Sept. 28, 1871 (SUSC); MEW, Letter to Editor, *Oswego Palladium* (29 Aug. 1871), 4.

8. "Editor's Historical Record," *Harper's New Monthly Magazine* 44 (Mar. 1872), 633. Anthony and Stanton's support of or resistance to Woodhull shifted over the next several years from convention to convention. "The Suffragists," *National Republican* (11 Jan. 1872), 1; "Wanted—Our Rights," *Daily Patriot* (11 Jan. 1872), 4.

9. Quoted in "The Woman's Raid," *Daily Patriot* (13 Jan. 1872), 4; Woman Suffrage," *New York Times* (13 Jan. 1872), 4; *Elizabeth Cady Stanton as Revealed in Her Letters*, 2:137, 3:474.

10. *Selected Papers of Elizabeth Cady Stanton and Susan B. Anthony*, Ann D. Gordon, ed. (New Brunswick, NJ: Rutgers University Press, 1997) 3:474.

11. MEW to Benjamin Alvord, Paymaster General, Jan. 23, 1872 (OCHS); E. B. French to MEW, undated (OCHS); Mrs. H. E. Speare to MEW, Feb. 16, 1872, Sarah Carson to MEW, Apr. 9, 1872, Julia Wheelock to MEW, Feb. 16, 1872, and Mary Gaine to MEW, undated (OCHS); *Journal of the House of Representatives of the United States, 1871–1872* (24 Jan. 1872), 210; MEW Memorial to The Honorable Senate and House of Representatives (OCHS).

12. "The Women in Congress," *Daily Patriot* (25 Jan. 1872), 1; "Washington," *Chicago Tribune* (25 Jan. 1872), 1; *HWS*, 2:488–489.

13. Dance card (SUSC).

14. U.S. House of Representatives Bill No. 2058, 42nd Congress, March 25, 1872; *Journal of the House of Representatives of the United States, 1871–1872* (5 Apr. 1872), 641.

15. "Editorial," *Hartford Courant* (12 June 1872), 2; "Washington News," *Prairie City Index* (21 June 1872), 1; Williams to MEW, Apr. 17, 1872 (SUSC).

16. Quoted in Griffith *In Her Own Right*, 153; Baker, *Sisters*, 81.
17. *Selected Papers of Elizabeth Cady Stanton and Susan B. Anthony*, 2:584 n.1, 2:585.
18. "Woman Suffrage," *National Republican* (17 Jan. 1873), 4; "Woman Suffrage," *National Republican* (18 Jan. 1873), 4; "Woman Suffrage," *Morning Chronicle* (18 Jan. 1873), 4; "Woman Suffrage," *Evening Star* (17 Jan. 1873), 4.
19. MEW, *Crowning Constitutional Argument*, broadside (1873); *Selected Papers of Elizabeth Cady Stanton and Susan B. Anthony*, 2:597.
20. *Charles Sumner, His Complete Works*, 20 vols. (Boston, 1900): 14:229.
21. Preston Day to MEW, Feb. 18, 1873 (SUSC).
22. MEW, "Smallpox and Dress," *National Republican* (14 Jan. 1873), 4; see, for example, William Morgan, M.D., *Diabetes Mellitus* (New York: Homeopathic Publishing, 1877), 118.
23. Cary Conklin to "To whomsoever it may concern," Jul. 8, 1873 (SUSC). On attitudes toward the White House, see William Roscoe Thayer, *Theodore Roosevelt: An Intimate Biography* (Boston, 1919). Untitled, *Hartford Courant* (11 Jul. 1873), 2.
24. This event was reported across the country—see, for instance, "From New York," *Hartford Courant* (21 July 1873), 2, and Davenport's *Daily Gazette* (19 July 1873), 1; quoted in Snyder, *Walker*, 113-114.
25. Untitled, *Fitchburg Sentinel* (23 July 1873), 4; "Dr. Mary Walker in Baltimore," *Herald and Torch Light* (6 Aug. 1873), 1; "Dr. Mary Walker and the Police Commissioners," *Baltimore Sun* (25 July 1873), 1.
26. Edward P. Mitchell, editor of the *New York Sun*, said the best woman reporter he knew was Middy Morgan of the *Tribune* and a close second was Dr. Mary Walker (*Memoirs of an Editor. Fifty Years of American Journalism* [New York, 1924], 262); B. M. Reese to MEW, Aug. 9, 1873 (SUSC).
27. "Woman Suffrage," *Evening Star* (16 Jan. 1874), 4. Dr. Hannah Tyler Wilcox (1838-1909), a St. Louis physician, had been educated at a female seminary in Rome, New York. "Women," *Washington Chronicle* (16 Jan. 1874), 5.
28. Quoted in Snyder, *Walker*, 99.
29. *Gail Hamilton's Life in Letters*, ed. H. Augusta Dodge (Boston: Lee and Shepard, 1901), 2:744-745. The letter was dated March 13, 1874.
30. Poynter, "Dr. Mary Walker," 237.
31. Griffith, *In Her Own Right*, 158, 165.
32. "Women and the Ballot," *Evening Star* (15 Jan. 1875), 4; "Down-Trodden Women," *National Republican* (16 Jan. 1875), 4.
33. *Selected Papers of Elizabeth Cady Stanton and Susan B. Anthony*, 3:144.
34. MEW, *Washington Sunday Gazette* (28 Feb. 1875).
35. "Dr. Mary Walker," *Owyhee [ID] Avalanche* (1 Sep. 1875), 3; "Dr. Mary Walker Has a Patient," *San Francisco Bulletin* (30 Sep. 1875), 3; "General News," *Owyhee Avalanche* (30 Oct. 1875), 2; Charles interview.
36. Joan Hoff, *Law, Gender and Injustice* (New York: New York University Press, 1991), 170-174.
37. Julia Ward Howe, *Atlanta Constitution (13 January 1876)*.
38. S. Edgar Trout to Lida Poynter, June 26, 1933 (DUCOM); Banner, *Elizabeth Cady Stanton*, 139-140.
39. "Why Dr. Mary Walker Desires to Abolish the Presidency," *Decatur Republican* (15 Jan. 1877), 2; see, for example, "Musical and Dramatic Notes," *National Republican* (20 July 1877), 2; "The Women's Convention in Washington," *New York Observer and Chronicle* (1 Feb. 1877), 1.

40. "Personal," *Chicago Tribune* (23 Jan. 1877), 4. Years later, when Mary Tillotson wrote about her experiences with the NWSA, she recalled being ostracized by Stanton and others for wearing the reform dress as well. "Dr. Walker is a natural legislator, able speaker, true reformer," Tillotson told Stanton, and she deemed the NWSA's ignorance of how MEW could help the cause a major error in strategy. Mary E. Tillotson, *History of the First Thirty-Five Years of the Science Costume Movement in the United States* (Vineland, NJ: Weekly Independent & Job Office, 1885), 60–61.

41. *Great Debates in American History*, 8:343–344.

42. Bailyn, et.al., 62–64.

43. MEW to Hayes, Feb. 4, 1877 (Rutherford B. Hayes Presidential Center, Fremont, Ohio).

44. Julian had been a Liberal Republican, but corruption in the Grant administration led him to switch parties; Snyder, *Walker*, 89; "Dr. Mary Walker Bounced," *New York Sun* (23 Mar. 1877), 1; "Put Out," *Oregonian* (24 Mar. 1877), 1.

45. "Dr. Mary Walker," *Inter Ocean* (24 Mar. 1877), 3; "Social and Political," *Hartford Courant* (24 Mar. 1877), 2; "Dr. Mary Walker," *Inter Ocean* (27 Mar. 1877), 4; "Dr. Mary Walker's Wrongs," *New York Sun* (26 Mar. 1877), 5; "Dr. Mary's Mare's Nest," *New York Times* (27 Mar. 1877), 4.

46. "Dr. Mary Walker on the 'Rampage,'" *Puck* 1 no.3 (Mar. 1877), 3; untitled, *Puck* 1 no.14 (May 1877), 7; quoted in Poynter, "Dr. Mary Walker."

47. "Dr. Mary Walker on Dress," *New York Tribune* (24 May 1877), 2.

48. "The Women Suffragists," *The World* (25 May 1877), 8; "Woman's Wrongs," *New York Herald* (26 May 1877), 5.

49. "Dr. Mary Walker's Wedding," *Fitchburg Sentinel* (2 July 1877), 2.

50. "Dr. Mary Walker's Claim," *New York Times* (8 Dec. 1877), 1. On May 31, 1878, Representative Joseph J. Davis, a Democrat from North Carolina, submitted a bill to gain reimbursement for Mary's appointment at the Treasury, as it had been blocked by the assistant secretary of the Treasury, Henry F. French, in spite of earlier rulings. French was overruled by the Committee of Claims, and recommendation for payment moved forward again. See Committee of Claims, House of Representatives, 45th Congress, Report No. 896. Deed between Alvah Walker and MEW, Nov. 3, 1877; witnessed by Vesta Walker Coats and Lyman Coats (SUSC).

51. Norgren, *Belva Lockwood*, 88; Elizabeth Blackwell, M.D., *Counsel to Parents on the Moral Education of their Children* (London: H. Smyth & Son, 1878), 10, 152.

52. John D'Emilio and Estelle B. Freedman, *Intimate Matters: A History of Sexuality in America* (New York: Harper & Row, 1988); MEW, *Unmasked, or the Science of Immorality* (Philadelphia: W. H. Boyd, 1878), 2; "Dr. Mary Walker," *Chester (PA) Times* (3 Sept. 1878), 1.

53. *Unmasked*, 6, 7, 8–9, 11, 12, 14.

54. According to Alice Dreger's study of 300 commentaries on hermaphrodites published in scientific and medical literature between 1860 and 1915, all the case studies and debates were written by men (*Hermaphrodites and the Medical Invention of Sex* [Cambridge, MA: Harvard University Press, 1998], 24). *Unmasked*, 31–32.

55. *Unmasked*, 38, 49, 71–73; Clinton, *The Other Civil War*, 86.

56. *Unmasked*, 76–77, 89, 91–92, 109.

57. Ibid., 141, 145, 146.

58. "The Praying Women," *Washington Post* (11 Jan. 1878), 2; *Elizabeth Cady Stanton as Revealed in Her Letters*, 2:153.

59. *HWS*, 3:103; Mary Clemmer, "A Woman's Letter from Washington," *Independent* (24 Jan. 1878), 1; "Dr. Mary Walker and Mormonism," *Sedalia Democrat* (29 Jan. 1878), 1; "Dr. Mary E. Walker," Committee on Invalid Pensions, House of Representatives Report No. 156, February 8, 1878; Untitled, *Daily Star* (25 Feb. 1878), 1.

60. Tillotson, 46; "Dr. Mary Walker's Ambition," *Washington Post* (1 Mar. 1878), 4; "Dr. Mary's Petition," *Washington Post* (7 Mar. 1878), 1.

61. "The Police Protectorate," *Washington Post* (8 Mar. 1878), 1; clipping, undated (SUSC); "A Recent Incident," *New York Times* (20 Mar. 1878), 4 (emphasis added); Untitled, *Burlington Hawk Eye* (30 Mar. 1878), 5.

62. "Dr. Mary Walker," *Chicago Tribune* (30 June 1878), 12; "Dr. Mary Walker's Book," *Washington Post* (18 Jul. 1878), 3; MEW to Tilden, July 20, 1878 (Samuel Tilden Papers, Manuscripts and Archives Division, New York Public Library)—she termed the situation "something of a political nature."

63. "Lake Pleasant Camp-Meeting," *Fitchburg Sentinel* (24 Aug. 1878), 3; "Dr. Mary Walker," *Inter Ocean* (25 Dec. 1874), 4.

CHAPTER 10 — THE COURTROOM, THE LEGISLATURE, PARTY POLITICS

1. "Personals," *Hartford Courant* (13 Nov. 1878), 2.

2. MEW to Tilden, Nov. 11, 1898 (Samuel Tilden Papers); "Personals," *Hartford Courant* (7 Dec. 1878), 3; untitled, *Oswego Palladium* (19 Dec. 1878), 1.

3. *Hutchinson's* (1878); Gertrude F. Garland to Mrs. C. W. M. Poynter, May 2, 1931 (DUCOM); Thomas Beer's *Sins of America as "Exposed" by the Police Gazette* (New York: Frederick A. Stokes Co., 1931).

4. Beers, *Sins of America*, 203; Norman Zierold, *Little Charley Ross* (Boston: Little, Brown, 1967), 86.

5. "Charley Ross Again," *Boston Globe* (4 Dec. 1878), 1. When the governor of Pennsylvania gave Christian Ross a political appointment as harbor-master in June, the *New York Times* saw the appointment as a just gesture of sympathy, while the *Independent* argued that a position with an annual salary of $2,500 should be appointed on qualifications, not sympathy (27 June 1878). "Burglar Bill Mosher," *National Police Gazette* (19 Apr. 1879), 11. Trials MEW attended included the Oliver Cameron breach of promise case in which she was seated inside the bar, the trial of James Payton and Peter Lewis for the murder of Jacob Daym, and the Baltimore rape trial of Edward Ray, at which MEW served as the victim's chaperone while in court ("Simon's Scourge," *Chicago Tribune* [20 Mar. 1879], 6; "Two Lives for One," *Washington Post* [25 Mar. 1879], 4; and "The National Hotel Outrage," *Washington Post* [15 Apr. 1879], 2).

6. Untitled, *Nevada State Journal* (3 Apr. 1879), 1; "Dr. Mary Walker," *Oshkosh Northwestern* (23 May 1879), 2; M. J. Gage, Prospectus for *National Citizen and Ballot-Box*, 1; "Woman's Topics," from *National Citizen and Ballot-Box*, reprinted in *American Socialist* (24 July 1879), 238; J. A. Bentley to MEW, May 17, 1879 (SUSC).

7. "Subjects for articles," undated (SUSC).

8. Walker Family Scrapbook (DUCOM); Ella Carrier to Lida Poynter, Feb. 6, 1930 (DUCOM); R. S. Ould to Lida Poynter, Dec. 26, 1932 (DUCOM); "A New Party," *Washington Post* (19 Aug. 1879), 2.

9. "Those Greenbackers," *Washington Post* (10 Jan. 1880; the National Labor Party had formerly been known as the Greenback Party); Alvah H. Walker, "A Tribute," Walker Family Scrapbook (DUCOM).

10. "Congressional Notes," *Washington Post* (4 June 1880), 1; "Miss Dr. Mary Walker," Walker Family Scrapbook (DUCOM).

11. "Two Pension Cases," *Utica Herald* (20 Sept. 1880), 1; Snyder, *Walker*, 123; "A Bone of Contention," *Syracuse Courier* (10 Jan. 1881).

12. Untitled, *Oswego Times* (23 Aug. 1880), 1; "Dr. Mary Walker's Vote," *Oswego Palladium* (4 Nov. 1880), 2.

13. Untitled, *Fitchburg Sentinel* (12 Jan. 1881), 2. The extent to which their relationship was strained was evidenced in a poem Alvah, Jr. wrote in 1885 for their sister Aurora's sixtieth birthday. He indicated Aurora had *two* sisters, Vesta and Luna, but no mention was made of MEW (Walker Family Scrapbook, DUCOM). Vesta Walker had two daughters in the area—one in Oswego and the other in nearby Scriba; why their homes were not alternatives is unknown. "Minor Events at the Capitol," *New York Times* (11 Feb. 1881), 1.

14. See, for example, "The Crime Against Nature," *National Police Gazette* (21 May 1878), 14; "The Masquerade of Death," *National Police Gazette* (18 Nov. 1882), 8; "Beating Dr. Mary Walker," *National Police Gazette* 38 (13 Aug. 1881), 4.

15. "It is said," *National Police Gazette* 46 (25 Apr. 1885), 2; "Mary Walker," *National Police Gazette* 19 (Jan. 1888), 2; "Dr. Mary Walker's Visit," *National Police Gazette* 45 (17 Jan. 1885), 5.

16. *HWS*, 1:29, 2:360, 813. Ironically, Gage would also become one of the suffragists written out of the *HWS* in later volumes; see Leila R. Brammer, *Excluded from Suffrage History: Matilda Joslyn Gage, Nineteenth-Century American Feminist* (Westport, CT: Greenwood Press, 2000).

17. "A New Applicant," *New York Times* (26 June 1881), 7; "Brevities," *Oswego Express* (26 Aug. 1881).

18. "Charles Guiteau Collection," Georgetown University Library (gulib.lausun.georgetown.edu); "James A Garfield Falls Before the Assassins Bullet," *Chicago Tribune* (3 July 1881), 2; "Garfield and Guiteau," (crimelibrary.com).

19. "Garfield and Guiteau"; "At the Trial of Guiteau," Emily Edson Briggs, *The Olivia Letters* (New York: Neale Publishing Company, 1906), 439; Lucy Ozarin, M.D., M.P.H., "Activist Psychiatrist Guided Journal for Three Eventful Decades," *Psychiatric News* (4 Feb. 2005), 26.

20. "Dr. Mary Walker," *Decatur Republican* (14 Jan. 1882), 2; "Guiteau's Fate to be Sealed," *The (Olean, NY) Democrat* (20 June 1882), 2; quoted in "Guiteau," *Willimantic Chronicle* (19 Apr. 1882), 1; "New York," *Utica News* (29 June 1882), n.p.; "To Hang To-Morrow," *Washington Post* (29 June 1882), 1. The case is now considered a legal milestone in relation to capital punishment and the criminally insane.

21. Benjamin Perley Poore, *Reminiscences of Sixty Years in the National Metropolis* (Philadelphia: Hubbard Brothers, 1886), 2:456; "Dr. Mary and the Spirits," *Washington Post* (20 Feb. 1882), 4.

22. "The District in Congress," *Washington Post* (10 Mar. 1882), 1; *Congressional Record* (20 Mar. 1882): 13:pt. 1572; E. W. Morgan, Director of Pensions, Veterans Administration, to Lida Poynter, May 20, 1932 (DUCOM); "Dr. Mary in Trouble," *Daily Gazette* (16 Sept. 1882), 3.

23. "Guiteau's Sister," *National Police Gazette* (21 Oct. 1882), 7; "Scoville's Scandal," *Daily Gazette* (26 Sept. 1882), 3.

24. Untitled, *Utica Herald* (9 Sept. 1882), 1; "Guiteau's Sister," 7; "The Woman in Trousers," (Auburn, NY) *Weekly News* (19 July 1883); "The Walker in a Rage," *Los Angeles Times* (16 Sept. 1882); Snyder, *Walker*, 115–119; A. N. Fisher to MEW, postcard dated Feb. 13, 1883 (SUSC).

25. Handwritten draft of letter (SUSC); Document, Department of Interior, Pension Office, granting MEW a leave of absence from May 21, 1883, to June 19, 1883, and noting a "sickness Certificate filed" (SUSC); see, for example, "Dr. Mary Walker Discharged from a Clerkship," *Decatur Republican* (13 July 1883), 2. Charles Ransom Miller became editor on April 13, 1883, and the *Times* published much more balanced reports of MEW under his editorship. "Dr. Mary Walker Still in Office," *New York Times* (14 July 1883), 1; "Dr. Mary Walker at the Pension Office," *Washington Post* (17 July 1883), 4; "Dr. Mary Walker's Ideas," *New York Times* (17 July 1883), 1.

26. "Gone at Last," *Bismarck Tribune* (20 July 1883), 1; handwritten note, dated "June 8th 1883" (SUSC); Untitled, *Ohio Democrat* (26 July 1883), 2; "Dr. Mary Walker's Eccentricity," *Boston Globe* (15 July 1883), 6; MEW's handwritten, unpublished account of her endeavors (SUSC); "Written in 1884," unpublished (SUSC); "Washington News Notes," *Freeborn County Standard* (26 July 1883), 3.

27. "A Bill" and "A Memorial," handwritten and signed documents (SUSC).

28. "'Restore' or 'Save'?" *Washington Post* (26 Oct. 1883), 1. The donor may well have been one of her Greenwich relatives. "Dr. Mary Walker's New Departure," *Oswego Palladium* (8 Nov. 1883), 4.

29. See, for example, "Mary on Her Muscle," *Decatur Republican* (28 Aug. 1883), 2, and "Dr. Mary Walker," *Bucks Co. Gazette* (20 Mar. 1884), 2; Untitled, *Bismarck Tribune* (2 May 1884), 1(emphasis added); Untitled, *Wellsboro (Pennsylvania) Agitator* (20 Oct. 1885), 2.

30. Hale, trained as an allopath, had come to prefer homeopathic and hygienic treatments, subjects on which he often lectured, and he was recognized for his homeopathic treatments of cancer. "Dr. Mary Walker's Opinions," *Pittsburgh Dispatch*; reprinted in *Dallas Morning News* (23 Apr. 1886), 4.

31. "Dr. Mary Walker's Opinions," 4.

32. "Dr. Mary Walker's Mother" and "A Correction," *Oswego Palladium* (30 Apr. 1886). Alvah Jr. spoke at length about his mother's faith and "unorthodox" refusal to accept "eternal hell dogma."

33. United States Patent Office, Patent No. 340,837, dated April 27, 1886, filed January 31, 1884; Nancy Hoover, "Dr. Anna Easton Lake: First Lady Physician Appointed to the White House," *Journal of the American Medical Women's Association* 17 (Nov. 1962), 906–907. Lake died shortly after being appointed.

34. "National Dress Reform Convention," *Oswego Palladium* (20 June 1886); "From Advance Sheets of Punch," *Life* (2 Sep. 1886), 130; "Relative Condition of Woman under Pagan and Christian Civilization," *American Catholic Quarterly Review* 11 (Oct. 1886), 658.

35. Charlotte Perkins Gilman, *The Abridged Diaries of Charlotte Perkins Gilman*, ed. Denise D. Knight (Charlottesville: University of Virginia Press, 1998), 97.

36. "Dr. Mary in a Museum," *Washington Post* (12 May 1885), 1; "Dr. Mary Walker's New Role," *New York Times* (8 Mar. 1887), 1; M. S. Robinson to MEW, 13 December 1887 (SUSC).

37. Flyer, Wonderland Musee, Theatre, and Art Gallery, October 21, 1889 (SUSC).

38. "Protest against the Unjust Interpretation of the Constitution, Presented on Behalf of the Women of the United States by the Officers of the National Woman's Suffrage Association . . . September 17th, 1887," Matilda Joslyn Gage Website (pinn.net); C. W. Moulton, *Queries and Answers* (Buffalo: C. L. Sherrill, 1886), 67.

39. "New Year Calls at the White House," *New York Tribune*; repr. *Herald and Torch Light* (5 Jan. 1888), 2; "The Prohibition Hearing," *Washington Post* (19 Feb. 1888), 2; "Big Week

for the Women," *Chicago Tribune* (28 Mar. 1888), 2; "Dr. Mary Walker Denied a Hearing Before the Judiciary," *Decatur Kennebec Journal* (26 Mar. 1888), 1; Ethel Ingalls, "A Congress of Famous Women," *Cosmopolitan* 5 (May 1888), 217–218.

40. Indeed, the "pioneers" were very selectively acknowledged—some of the founders of the UFA were included, for instance, but not Lockwood, who had become estranged from Anthony. MEW, "Crowning Constitutional Argument," *National Free Press* (8 Apr. 1888), 2.

41. "Mrs. Belva Lockwood," *Davenport Tribune* (25 Sept. 1888), 4; "The Rival Emancipation Day Celebration," *Washington Post* (17 Apr. 1888), 1; "Dr. Mary Walker's Appeal to Women," *Newark (OH) Daily Advocate* (30 Oct. 1888), 1; "Appeal from Dr. Mary Walker," *Fitchburg Sentinel* (30 Oct. 1888), 4; "Dr. Mary Walker Proclaims," *Hartford Courant* (30 Oct. 1888), 1. 42. "Mary Walker in the Speaker's Stand," *Lima Democratic Times* (7 Mar. 1889), 1. MEW tried a similar tactic when arguing for nurses' pensions during a recess of Senate proceedings in 1872 but was unsuccessful in ascending to the Senate Speaker's desk ("Congressional Senate," *Chicago Tribune* [11 June 1872]), 1).

43. Untitled, *Oswego Palladium* (21 Mar. 1889); "Dr. Mary Walker Tonight," *Boston Globe* (31 Mar. 1889), 3; "Lives on Atmospheric Electricity," *Chicago Tribune* (5 Apr. 1889), 9; "Who Took the Cold Potato," *Boston Globe* (9 Apr. 1889), 8; "Players and Minstrels," *Boston Globe* (14 Apr. 1889), 10.

CHAPTER 11 — A PRAGMATIC UTOPIA

1. Quoted in "How It Happened," *Oswego Palladium* (20 Apr. 1890), 1.

2. "News and Notes," *New Oxford (PA) Item* (11 July 1890), 2; "Scope: Chester Alan Arthur Papers," McKeldin Library, University of Maryland (www.lib.umd.edu).

3. Untitled, *Oswego Times* (20 May 1890); "For the Relief of Dr. Mary Walker," *Washington Post* (25 July 1890), 7; "Dr. Mary Walker Recovers," (Decatur) *Review* (10 Jan. 1891), 1; MEW, *Petition of Dr. Mary E. Walker*, (U.S. Senate Mis. Doc. No. 226, August 25, 1890).

4. Quoted in "Dr. Mary Becomes Ironical," *Chicago Tribune* (13 Sep. 1890), 6 (emphasis added).

5. "Dr. Mary Walker for Congress," *Fitchburg Sentinel* (10 Oct. 1890), 3; "Dr. Mary Walker Nominated for Congress," *New Hampshire Register* (10 Oct. 1890), 1; "Dr. Mary Walker," *Inter Ocean* (13 Oct. 1890),4; "Dr. Mary Walker on Her Death-Bed," *Chicago Tribune* (2 Dec. 1890), 2; "Dr. Mary Walker Dying," *Washington Post* (2 Dec. 1890), 4; "Dr. Mary Walker Very Ill," *New York Times* (3 Dec. 1890), 4; "Kind Words for Dr. Mary Walker," *Philadelphia Record*, repr. *Oswego Palladium* (3 Dec. 1890), 5; "Dr. Mary Walker Better," (Decatur) *Review* (4 Dec. 1890), 6.

6. MEW, "A Compliment to Newspapers," *Philadelphia Inquirer* (29 Dec. 1890), 2.

7. Elizabeth Urban Alexander, *Notorious Woman: The Celebrated Case of Myra Clark Gaines* (Baton Rouge: Louisiana State University Press, 2001); Norgren, *Belva Lockwood*, 199; "Mary Walker," *Brooklyn Eagle* (23 Mar. 1891), 6; "Dr. Mary Walker on the Stand," *Oswego Times* (25 Mar. 1891), 2.

8. "A Young Woman Murdered," *New York Times* (19 July 1891), 1.

9. "Dr. Mary Walker's Fad," *Oswego Times* (5 Oct. 1893), 5; MEW, "Almy Reward Argument," 5 (SUSC). Three documents (c. 1894) written by MEW were prepared in an attempt to receive part of the reward money for Almy's arrest. There are two drafts of the "Almy Reward Argument," which is addressed to the justices of the New Hampshire Supreme Court. All references to "Almy Reward Argument" will refer to the revised 34-page version.

The third typescript is the "Report" written in response to the New Hampshire attorney general's requirement that applicants for the reward prove their cases in writing. "The Real Almy," *Daily People and Patriot* (19 May 1893), (clipping, SUSC); MEW, "Report," 3.

10. "Almy Reward Argument," 10–11.

11. "Police Would Not Bite," *Boston Globe* (1 Oct. 1891), 2; "The Real Almy;" "Almy Reward Argument," 11–12.

12. "Dr. Mary Walker in Town," *Boston Globe* (4 Oct. 1891), 4; "Almy Reward Argument," 5, 2.

13. *Ball v. United States*, 140 U.S. 118, 129 (1891); John Phillip Reid, "Almost a Hobby," *Virginia Law Review* 49 no.1 (1963), 58–72.

14. Untitled, *Oswego Times* (3 Feb. 1892) (clipping, SUSC); "She Knew Norcross," *Chicago Tribune* (13 Mar. 1892), 4; "Mr. Sage at the Coroner's," *New York Times* (13 Mar. 1892), 1.

15. "After the Big Convention," *New York Times* (1 June 1892), 2 (no woman volunteered to be the Republican candidate); "Dr. Mary Walker," *Oswego Palladium* (15 June 1892), 5.

16. MEW, "City Hall," *Oswego Palladium* (13 June 1892), 1; Snyder, *Walker*, 106; "Ante-Convention Notes," *Davenport Leader* (21 June 1892), 9; "Convention Gossip," *Duluth News-Tribune* (22 June 1892), 1; "The Names Presented," *New York Times* (23 June 1892), 2; "Uproar Over Abbett's Speech," *Chicago Tribune* (23 June 1892), 3; "Dr. Mary Walker Disgruntled," *Chicago Tribune* (24 June 1892), 9.

17. "The World's Fair," *Oswego Palladium* (27 June 1892), 1; R. E. A. Dorr, "The Exposition of 1893," *Arthur's Home Magazine* 62 (July 1892), 599–600; "Dr. Mary Walker," *Oswego Times* (16 Aug. 1892), 4.

18. "Spunky Dr. Walker," *Oswego Palladium* (7 Dec. 1892), 5; "Women as Jurors," *Oswego Times* (1 Feb. 1893), 4; "Not Ashamed of Her Age," *New York Times* (1 Feb. 1893), 1; "Did Not Steal the Dog," *Oswego Times* (13 Mar. 1893), 8.

19. "Dr. Mary Saw The Show," *The World* (5 Feb. 1893), 1; "Godey's Fashions," *Godey's* 135 (Oct. 1897), 428ff.; "Dr. Mary Walker Talks," *Oswego Times* (22 Feb. 1893), 4.

20. MEW, "Why Women Should Wear Trousers," *Home Circle* (clipping, c.1890s, SUSC).

21. "Dr. Mary Walker," *Oswego Palladium* (26 Apr. 1893), 5; "Dr. Mary Walker," *Fitchburg Sentinel* (17 May 1893), 8; "Almy Hanged at Concord," *Hartford Courant* (17 May 1893), 1. The original "Mistaken Identity" document is no longer extant.

22. "Almy Hanged at Concord," 1.

23. "The Real Almy," *Daily People and Patriot* (19 May 1893), 1 (partial clipping, SUSC); "Dr. Mary Walker," *Oswego Palladium* (18 May 1893), 5. In "Almy Reward Argument," MEW says that Grandpa Flint's belief that the wrong man had been arrested was also partially based on the fact that Almy had a serious case of varicose veins but Abbott did not (9). "Dr. Mary Walker Charges Murder," *New York Times* (5 Oct. 1893), 9; "Dr. Mary Walker's Fad," 5.

24. "Dr. Mary Walker in New Hampshire," *Macon Weekly Telegraph* (8 June 1893), 6.

25. "A Big Sensation," *Oswego Palladium* (5 Oct. 1893), 4; "Queer Dr. Mary Walker," *Boston Globe* (5 Oct. 1893), 1; "Dr. Mary Earth [sic] Walker," *Oswego Times* (10 Oct. 1893); "Dr. Mary Walker in Court," *Washington Post* (18 Nov. 1893), 1.

26. "Dr. Mary Walker," *Nashua Telegraph* (11 Nov. 1893).

27. "Dr. Mary's Plan," *Oswego Palladium* (8 Jan. 1894), 2; "Mary Walker's Latest," *Oswego Times* (9 Jan. 1894), 5.

28. Quoted in "Dr. Mary's Answer," *Syracuse Courier* (22 Jan. 1894), 4.

29. "Snoad Versus Walker," *Syracuse Journal*, undated clipping (SUSC); "Six Cents for Snoad," *Philadelphia Inquirer* (4 Feb. 1894), 7.

30. In 1890 the National and American Woman Suffrage Associations merged; the NAWSA soon was dominated by conservatives, causing several longtime leaders to found competitive suffrage associations. Quoted in Poynter, "Dr. Mary Walker," 319; Carl E. Kreische, "Dress Reform," *Locomotive Firemen's Magazine* (Mar. 1894), 273.

31. "The Almy Reward," *Oswego Palladium* (20 June 1894), 8; "The Almy Reward," *Fitchburg Sentinel* (21 June 1894), 3. During this time MEW served as legal counsel for Margaret Ewer, who had been charged with public drunkenness and misconduct; MEW was successful in seeing the complaint reduced to a "simple drunk" with no jail time ("Dr. Mary Walker Won," *Lowell Sun* [20 July 1894], 1; "Dr. Mary Walker Won," *Boston Globe* [20 July 1894], 5).

32. Untitled, *Fitchburg Sentinel* (28 Sept. 1894), 5.

33. "Stafford Springs," *Hartford Courant* (15 Sept. 1894), 8; "World's Food Fair," *Boston Globe* (19 Oct. 1894), 5; "Dr. Mary Walker's Pants," *Atlanta Constitution* (31 Aug. 1895), 5; Sara Williamson, "To Mary," 27 Oct. 1894 (SUSC); "Carey Named," *Boston Globe* (19 Jul. 1894), 1; "Sec. Scott Vindicated," *Boston Globe* (4 Dec. 1894), 4; "Capital Punishment," *Boston Globe* (5 Nov. 1894), 5.

34. "The Almy Reward Divided," *New York Times* (7 Jul. 1895), 5; Charlotte Story Perkinson, "Never-To-Be-Forgotten Memories of Famed Murder," *New Hampshire Sunday News* (15 Apr. 1951), 16.

35. *Journals of the Honorable Senate and House of Representatives of the State of New Hampshire, January Session, 1895* (Concord, NH: Edward N. Pearson, 1895), 532; *State v. Oscar J. Comery* 78 N.H. 6 (1915), citing Laws 1903, c.114, s.1; "Connecticut Death Apparatus Is Used in New Hampshire," *Hartford Courant* (9 Jan. 1917), 12.

36. The will is housed at SUSC. "Dr. Mary Walker Again," *Evening Democrat* (4 Apr. 1895), 1; Dorris Moore Lawson, "Dr. Mary E. Walker: A Biographical Sketch" (M.A. Thesis, Syracuse University, 1954), 104–105. Vashti Walker died on Nov. 15, 1895.

37. MEW, *A Colony for New Women*, broadside (OCHS).

38. Ibid.

39. Ibid.

40. Poynter, "Dr. Mary Walker," 322; "American Notes," (Brisbane) *Queenslander* (30 Nov. 1895), clipping (SUSC); "Eden Without Adam," *Chicago Tribune* (5 Oct5. 1895), 16; "A New Woman Factory," *Trenton Evening Times* (30 Sept. 1895), 3; "A Garden of Eden," 3; W. D. Inslee, "Dr. Mary Walker's Colony of One," *Metropolitan Magazine* (clipping, SUSC).

41. "Bill Nye Gets a Poem," *Boston Globe* (27 Oct. 1895), 30.

42. "Dr. Mary Walker Spends Sunday in Monson," (Palmer, MA) *Journal* (7 Feb. 1896), "Dr. Mary E. Walker," *Rome Sentinel* (Jan.? 1896), and "'Capt. Jack' at Kernwood," (Palmer, MA) *Journal* (clippings, SUSC).

43. Untitled, Boston *Standard* (29 Feb. 1896), clipping (SUSC); "Dr. Mary's Reminiscences," *Boston Globe* (10 Feb. 1896), 6; Untitled, Boston *Standard* (31 Mar. 1896), clipping (SUSC).

44. Untitled, *Journal* (29 Feb. 1896), clipping (SUSC); "New York State Topics," *Buffalo Express* (12 Jul. 1896), 11; James T. Patterson, "How Do We Write the History of Disease?" *Health and History* 1 (1998): 8–28; Morantz-Sanchez, *Sympathy and Science*, 242.

45. "Cayuga," *Rochester Democrat* (10 Aug. 1896), 4; untitled, *Utica Press* (15 Sept. 1896); quoted in Snyder, *Walker*, 107; see, for example, letter of Mary B. Bryan to MEW, Feb. 4, 1897 (SUSC); "Mason Has a Busy Day," *Chicago Tribune* (1 Feb. 1897), 7.

46. "Mrs. Booth Describes Her Work to Mothers," *Philadelphia Inquirer* (19 Feb. 1897), 5; "Mothers' Last Words," *Washington Post* (20 Feb. 1897), 3; "Let Her Wear a Bonnet," *Chicago Tribune* (20 Feb. 1897), 3; "Dr. Mary Walker's Progress in Clothes," *Chicago Tribune* (2 Jul. 1897), 13; Charles interview.

47. "Walker (Dr. Mary)," *People of the Period*, 2 vol. (London, 1897), 2:470; Frances E. Willard and Mary L. Livermore, *American Women*, rev. ed. (New York: Mast, Crowell & Kirkpatrick, 1897), 738.

CHAPTER 12 — ANTI-IMPERIALISM AND THE WORLD STAGE

1. "Dr. Mary Walker in Town," *Washington Post* (4 Jan. 1898), 5; Noenoe K. Silva, "I Kū Mau Mau: How Kānaka Maoli Tried to Sustain National Identity Within the United States Political System," *American Studies* 45 (Fall 2004), 9; "Notes and Comments," *Hartford Courant* (12 Jan. 1898), 8.

2. "Notes and Comments," 8; Doctor Mary and Queen Lil," *Oswego Palladium* (15 Feb. 1898), 8; "Dr. Mary Walker's Views," *Washington Post* (26 Jan. 1898), 9.

3. "White House Reception," *Landmark* (7 Feb. 1898); "National Capital Topics," *New York Times* (6 Feb. 1898), 13; "Dr. Mary Walker's Repartee," *Washington Post* (13 Feb. 1898), 25; Wu Tingfang, *America Through the Spectacles of an Oriental Diplomat* (1914), 43, 49.

4. "Works for Queen Lil," *North Adams (MA) Transcript* (12 Feb. 1898), 4; "President Dole of Hawaii," *New York Times* (6 Feb. 1898), 1.

5. MEW, *Isonomy* (1898), 4–5, 6, 8. Her preference for self-publication was to control all rights as well as content. No record of sales for her books exist, but the *Omaha World Herald* reported in 1899 that she had "a private income" based on earning "large sums from her writings" (6 Aug. 1899, p. 10); this is probably an exaggeration, but her books appear to have been profitable.

6. "Women's Voices Heard," *Washington Post* (16 Feb. 1898), 2; "She Wanted to Talk," *Washington Post* (18 Feb. 1898), 8.

7. "Dr. Mary Walker's Little Speech," *Oswego Palladium* (23 Feb. 1898), 3.

8. "Doctor Mary Not a Daughter," *Washington Post* (24 Feb. 1898), 2; "Dr. Mary Walker's Pension," *Washington Post* (20 Feb. 1898), 6; "Her Claim Rejected," *Evening Star* (21 Feb. 1898), 1.

9. "Persecuting Dr. Mary Walker," *Washington Post* (27 Feb. 1898), 6.

10. This may have been Judge Walter Cox, whom MEW knew from the Guiteau trial; "Dr. Mary Walker's Protest," *Washington Post* (25 Feb. 1898), 9.

11. "Dr. Mary Walker's Protest," 9; see also "Dr. Mary and 'Lil,'" *Oswego Times* (28 Feb. 1898), 7.

12. Untitled, (Humeston, Iowa) *New Era* (16 Mar. 1898), 2; Richard A. Spears, *Slang and Euphemism* (Ann Arbor: University of Michigan Press, 1981), 247.

13. "30 Years in Trousers," *Boston Globe* (20 Mar. 1898), 36; "The Dress of Business Women," *Davenport Republican* (9 Oct. 1898), 3.

14. Untitled, *Hawaiian Gazette* (29 Mar. 1898), 5; "Cubans to Help the Blockade," *Chicago Tribune* (22 Apr. 1898), 9; "Sherman to Resign His Office," *Chicago Tribune* (24 Apr. 1898), A11; "Dr. Mary Walker Again Out of Order," *Mexico (NY) Independent* (c. 25 Apr. 1898); "Dr. Mary Walker," *Oswego Palladium* (27 Apr. 1898), 4; Bailyn, et al, *Great Republic*, 2:261; Stephen Bender, "Recalling the Anti-Imperialist League" (antiwar.com).

15. "Mary E. Walker," *Congressional Record*, Fifty-fifth Congress, Second Session, July 4, 1898, pp. 7443–7445, H.R. 9732; "Dr. Mary Walker's Pension," *New York Tribune* (22 June 1898), 7.

16. Joseph Benson Foraker, *Notes on a Busy Life* (London: Foraker, 1916), 43; "Nurses Now and Then," *Fort Wayne News* (17 June 1898), 6; "Remember the Maine," *Arizona Weekly Journal-Miner* (13 Jul. 1898), 2; "Creates a Sensation," *Lima News* (14 Jul. 1898), 7; "Dr. Mary Walker Sits Like a Woman," *Daily Northwestern* (11 Aug. 1898), 2.

17. MEW, undated handwritten notes (SUSC).

18. A Protocol of Peace between the United States and Spain was signed in Washington on August 12, 1898, and the formal peace treaty was signed in Paris on December 10. "Clash Over Roberts," *Washington Post* (19 Feb. 1899), 2; "Upholds Roberts," *Oswego Times* (30 Dec. 1899), 3; "Dr. Mary's Petition," *Oswego Times* (3 Jan. 1900), 4.

19. "Dr. Mary Walker at the Mothers' Congress," *Chicago Tribune* (20 Feb. 1899), 1; "Gives Historic Edifice," *Chicago Tribune* (26 Feb. 1899), 5; "Crowds at Big Show," *Washington Post* (2 Mar. 1899), 2.

20. "Dresses Like a Man but Acts Like an Idiot this Eccentric Dr. Mary Walker," *Morning Herald* (17 Jul. 1899), 5; "Dr. Mary Walker Has Started an Uncanny Craze," *Toledo Bee* (16 Jul. 1899), 15.

21. "Dr. Walker's Views," *Oswego Times* (12 Sep. 1899), 4.

22. Ibid.; *Soldiers' Letters* (SUSC); Howard Zinn, "Put Away the Flags: Nationalism Blinds Us With Arrogance," *Hartford Courant* (30 June 2005), A13.

23. "Dr. Mary's Petition," *Oswego Times* (3 Jan. 1900), 4; Poynter, "Dr. Mary Walker," 362.

24. "The Capital Punishment Bill," *Rochester Democrat* (20 Feb. 1900), 2; "Defends Molineux," *Boston Globe* (21 Feb. 1900), 3; "Abducted Dr. Mary's Attention," *Portsmouth (NH) Herald* (7 Mar. 1900), 4; "State Capitol Notes," *Evening Herald* (20 Feb. 1900), 2; "Dr. Mary Walker to Talk to Legislators," *Post Standard* (20 Feb. 1900), 6; "'Dock' Walker in Albany," *Oswego Palladium* (20 Feb. 1900), 4; untitled, *Rochester Democrat* (21 Feb. 1900), 6.

25. "Petition for Molineux," *New York Times* (12 Mar. 1900), 10.

26. "Legislative Notes," *New York Times* (23 Feb. 1900), 4; MEW, *Consumptive School Sanitarium*, May 10, 1900; broadside (OCHS).

27. *Consumptive School Sanitarium*; Francis D. Culkin to Mrs. C. W. M. Poynter, Feb. 7, 1933 (DUCOM). Culkin was a law clerk in Oswego whom MEW hired to prepare many of her legal documents, including the letter to the Russian czar (Culkin later became a Representative to the U.S. Congress). R. Cronan, *Woman Triumphant* (New York: R. Cronan, 1919), 190.

28. "The Women's Pantheon," *Chicago Tribune* (28 Apr. 1900), 14.

29. "Dr. Mary Walker's Sister Passes Away," (Syracuse) *Post Standard* (14 May 1900), 10; Jackie Klippenstein, "Mary Walker's Sister was a Maverick, Too," *Oswego History* (Aug. 1983), clipping (OCHS).

30. "She Talked to Bryan," *Oswego Palladium* (20 Oct. 1900), 8.

31. "Men's Clothes Should Have Been Her Burial Garb," *Post Standard* (19 Jan. 1901), 18.

32. "Legislative Reception a Success," *Albany Journal* (30 Jan. 1901), 1; "Dr. Mary Walker at City Hall," *Brooklyn Eagle* (6 Mar. 1901), 1; "Dr. Mary Walker Visits Mayor," *New York Tribune* (7 Mar. 1901), 7; "Dr. Mary Walker Interested," *Brooklyn Eagle* (11 Mar. 1901), 2; untitled, (Washington, D.C.) *Evening Times* (26 Mar. 1901), 4; "Sensations for Mary Walker," *Brooklyn Eagle* (16 Apr. 1901), 20; "Dr. Mary Walker's Visit," *Brooklyn Eagle* (17 Apr. 1901), 1.

33. "Dr. Mary Walker the Guest," *Brooklyn Eagle* (14 Apr. 1901), 5; *Gail Hamilton's Life and Letters*, 2 vols. (Boston: Lee and Shepard, 1901); Walter F. Beyer and Oscar F. Keydel, *Deeds of Valor: From the Archives of the United States Government* (1901); Harriet Fontanges, *Les Femmes Docteurs en Mèdicine dans tous les pays* (Paris, 1901).

34. "Lights Out in the Great City: The Legal Aftermath of the Assassination of President McKinley," University of Buffalo Libraries (ublib.buffalo.edu); Wyatt Kingseed, "President William McKinley: Assassinated by an Anarchist," *American History* (Oct. 2001), historynet.com.

35. "Doctor Walker's Narrow Escape," *Oswego Palladium* (18 Sept. 1901), 1; see, for instance, Rebecca Harding Davis's 1870 serialized novel *Put Out of the Way*.

36. "Mary E. Walker, M.D., Defines Her Idea of Murder," *Oswego Palladium* (21 Sept. 1901), 2; "Makes a Denial," *Oswego Times* (21 Sept. 1901), 1; "Dr. Mary Walker on Rack," *Fort Wayne News* (8 Nov. 1901), 1; "May Revoke Her Pension," *Oswego Palladium* (7 Nov. 1901), 5; "Talk of Revoking Dr. Mary Walker's Pension," *Boston Globe* (9 Nov. 1901), 6; "Out With a Denial," *Oswego Times* (11 Nov. 1901), 5; "Dr. Mary Walker's Weakness," *Rochester Post-Express* reprinted in *Nebraska State Journal* (13 Nov. 1901), 4; "Judge Shepherd Tells of Joe Wheeler and Dr. Mary Walker," *Atlanta Constitution* (17 Nov. 1901), 40. The challenge to MEW's pension was pursued vigorously. The Bureau of Pensions sent a letter dated September 26, 1901, to the Oswego chief of police asking him to gather evidence "under oath, if possible" from the ticket agent at the rail station as well as provide any data available about her pension (SUSC). NARA; "Dr. Mary Walker Cannot Be Deprived of Her Pension," *New York Sun* (9 Nov. 1901), 4; "Dr. Mary Walker's Pension," *New York Times* (9 Nov. 1901), 8.

37. "Dr. Mary Walker Has Different View," *Post Standard* (26 Sept. 1901), 6.

CHAPTER 13 — THE AGE OF ALIENATION

1. *Report of the Health Officer of the District of Columbia* (Washington: Government Printing Office, 1905, 1913); see letters exchanged between George M. Gamwell and MEW from August 1901 to September 1902 (SUSC); *Standard Medical Directory of 1902* lists MEW's home address as 208 Indiana Ave., N.W., Washington, D.C.; "Dr. Mary Walker," *Hartford Courant* (7 Feb. 1902), 7; "Burns Trial," *New York Sun* (23 Mar. 1902), 1; "Burns Girl Exonerated," *Oswego Palladium* (24 Mar. 1902), 1.

2. MEW, "Dr. Mary Walker's Views Regarding Masculine Apparel," *Washington Times* (24 Aug. 1902), B3.

3. "Fair Will Close Monday Night," *Oswego Times* (18 Apr. 1903), 4; "Society Circus Well Patronized," *Oswego Times* (10 Jul. 1903), 4; "Brownell Turned Down," *Oswego Palladium* (7 Oct. 1903), 4.

4. Poynter, "Dr. Mary Walker," 377–378; "Man's Garb for Her," *Philadelphia Inquirer* (3 Nov. 1903), 3; "The Special Session of Congress," *Harper's Weekly* (14 Nov. 1903), 1822ad-1823ad (only two other women appeared in the photograph: Mrs. John Hay and Mrs. Payne Whitney, renowned Washington hostesses); "May Secure His Freedom," *Syracuse Evening Telegram* (16 Dec. 1903), 10; "He Won't Interfere," *Oswego Times* (28 Dec. 1903), 4; "Who's What and Why in America?" *New York Herald* (16 Nov. 1902); MEW, "What People Talk About," *Boston Globe* (14 Jan. 1904), 6.

5. Alan Axelrod and Charles Phillips, *What Every American Should Know About American History* (Adams Media Corp., 2003), 201–202; "It's the Panama Treaty," *Syracuse Herald* (22 Feb. 1904), 14; "Mailed Under Frank," *Washington Post* (4 Mar. 1904), 5; *Hepburn-Dolliver Bill. Full Hearings before the Committee on the Judiciary of the House of Representatives* (Washington: Government Printing Office, 1904); "A Visit from Dr. Mary Walker," *Kansas City Star* (9 Mar. 1904), 5; "Dr. Walker There," *Trenton Times* (12 Mar. 1904), 2; "Dr. Mary Walker to Lecture," *Washington Times* (5 Apr. 1904), 2.

6. "Home from Washington," *Oswego Palladium* (16 Apr. 1904), 4; "Dr. Mary Walker's Plan," *Syracuse Evening Telegram* (18 Apr. 1904), 6; "If Doctor Mary Goes to St. Louis," *Oswego Times* (28 June 1904), 5.

7. "Dr. Mary Walker Prominent as Anti-Roosevelt Boomer," *Washington Times* (6 Jul. 1904), 5; "Dr. Mary Walker Appears at New York Headquarters," *Post Standard* (6 Jul. 1904), 2; "Committee on Credentials," *Dallas Morning News* (7 Jul. 1904), 2; "Convention Quips, Likewise Some Cranks," *New York Times* (7 Jul. 1904), 5; "Dr. Mary Walker Suggests a Plank," *Fort Worth Star-Telegram* (8 Jul. 1904), 8.

8. "Vineland the Unique," *Washington Post* (11 Sep. 1904), 3; "Original Bloomer Girl is a Guest of Dr. Mary Walker," *Post Standard* (23 Sep. 1904), 11.

9. See, for example, "Quick Pictures of Washington Notables," *San Francisco Call* (14 Jan. 1900), 11, which includes photographs by Clinedinst of President McKinley, cabinet members, senators, MEW, and Secretary Hay's daughter. "Claims Credit for Heir," *Bourbon News* (13 Sep. 1904), 2; Spiegel and Suskind, "Mary Edwards Walker," 228. Her support was reported in the *Chicago Tribune* (29 Oct. 1904) and Decatur *Daily Review* (1 Nov. 1904), among others.

10. "Quick Justice for Murderer," *Post Standard* (2 and 11 June, 1905), 11, 5.

11. "Keep in Male Togs She Says to Girl," *Trenton Times* (2 Feb. 1905), 8. Katherine Vaubaugh, another such invitee, was an aged French woman who passed as a man for nearly sixty years until hospitalization revealed her sex ("Her Fellow Feeling," *Los Angeles Times* [18 Nov. 1905], I1. "A Veteran's Fall," *Oswego Palladium* (27 Jul. 1905), 5.

12. MEW, "Punching the Bag Makes Pale Cheeks All Abloom," *Washington Post* (13 Aug. 1905), EB4; untitled, *Auburn (NY) Citizen* (2 Oct. 1905).

13. "Bills in Assembly," *Syracuse Herald* (19 Jan. 1906), 19; "Two Men Attend Senate Session," *Rochester Democrat* (20 Jan. 1906), 2; Joseph Richardson Parke, Sc.B., Ph.G., M.D. (Late Acting Asst. Surgeon, U.S. Army), *Human Sexuality: A Medico-Literary Treatise on the Laws, Anomalies, and Relations of Sex with especial reference to Contrary Sexual Desire* (Philadelphia: Professional Publishing, 1906), 323–324; see, for instance, "The Argus Does Not Think Doctor Walker Dignified," *Oswego Palladium* (Jan. 1906); "Dr. Mary Walker's Aid," *Washington Post* (17 Mar. 1904), 2; "Dr. Mary Walker," *Washington Post* (6 Feb. 1906), 36; "Dr. Mary Walker is Ill," *Washington Post* (17 Feb. 1906), 1; "Fast Regains Her Health," *Washington Times* (17 Feb. 1906), 5.

14. "Dr. Mary Walker Gives Home as Humane Prison for Young," *Washington Times* (30 Jul. 1906), 5.

15. "Wants Part of the Prize," *Oakland Tribune* (29 Dec. 1906), 2; "Village Items," *Utica Dispatch-Herald* (1 June 1907), 8.

16. "Dr. Mary Walker Declares Thaw Sane," *Post Standard* (8 Apr. 1907), 8.

17. NARA; Graf, *A Woman of Honor*, 82; Brig. Gen. H. M. Duffield, U.S.V., *Deeds of Valor from the Records of the United States Government. How American Heroes Won the Medal of Honor*, 2 vol. (Detroit: Perrien-Keydel, 1907), 405–406.

18. MEW, *Crowning Constitutional Argument* (broadside, 1907).

19. Ibid.; "Disease Hides in Weed," *Washington Post* (7 Oct. 1908), 3.

20. See, for example, Kathrine L. Edwards' letter to MEW, Oct. 1908 (SUSC); "Hope for Presence of Mr. Sherman," *Utica Herald-Dispatch* (7 Aug. 1909), 5; Poynter, "Dr. Mary Walker," 385; "Dr. Mary Walker at County Fair," *Utica Herald-Dispatch* (7 Sept. 1909), 2; untitled, *Utica Herald-Dispatch* (8 Sept. 1909), 2; "Dr. Mary Walker," *Rome Sentinel* (8 Sept. 1909), 1.

21. "Dr. Mary Walker Causes Only Sign of Disorder," *Boston Globe* (10 Mar. 1910), 2; "Dr. Mary Walker Heard," *Utica Press* (16 Mar. 1910), 1; "Woman is Harsh on Suffragists," *Trenton Evening News* (18 Mar. 1910), 5; "Extract from Speech before the Judiciary Committee, of the N.Y. Assembly" (Dr. Mary Walker Papers, Library Archives, SUNY-Oswego).

22. "Doctor Walker for Sane Fourth," *Post Standard* (11 June 1910), 13; "'Such Silly Rubbish,'" *Boston Globe* (16 Mar. 1910), 3; "Criticizes Other Woman Suffragists," *Rochester Democrat* (18 Dec. 1910), 1.

CHAPTER 14 — THE PIONEER EMBRACED

1. MEW, "Welcome Home" (DUCOM). At this time, a local jeweler also negotiated with MEW to produce teaspoons with her image on them to sell to tourists (SUNY-Oswego).

2. "Dr. Walker Pleased with Paris Fashion," *Evening Post* (27 Jan. 1911), 1; "Dr. Mary Walker's Amendment," *Oswego Palladium* (22 Feb. 1911), 4; "Dr. Mary Walker May Yet Be U.S. Senator," *Sandusky Register* (11 Apr. 1911), 8.

3. "Dr. Mary Walker Offers to Sell Finger," *Chicago Tribune* (17 Aug. 1911), 6; "No Lady in Trousers Can Sell Her Finger," *Los Angeles Times* (18 Aug. 1911), I11.

4. Isabelle Kingsbury Hart to Mrs. C.W.M. Poynter, Jan. 17, 1932 (DUCOM); "Dr. Mary Walker's Reforms Finally Win Recognition," *Washington Post* (10 Sep. 1911), 13.

5. "Dr. Walker Spoke," *Syracuse Herald* (14 Sept. 1911), 5; "Dr. Mary Walker Popular," *Fulton Times* (20 Sep. 1911), 7; "Dr. Mary Gets Prize for Male Attire," *Syracuse Herald* (14 Sept. 1911), 17; "Recognition for Dress Reformer," *Los Angeles Times* (17 Sep. 1911), 11; "Dr. Mary Walker Lectures," *Washington Post* (8 Jan. 1912), 2; "American Woman's Republic," *Washington Post* (25 June 1912), 7.

6. "Statement of Dr. Mary E. Walker," *Woman Suffrage. Serial No. 1. Hearings before the Committee of the Judiciary, House of Representatives, Sixty-Second Congress, Second Session, February 14, 1912* (Washington: Government Printing Office, 1912), 6–13 (the statement notes that she is living at 602 Fifth Street NW.).

7. "Society," *Washington Post* (25 Feb. 1912), 26; "Dr. Mary Walker Ill," *New York Times* (18 Mar. 1912), 1; "Dr. Mary Walker Taken Seriously Ill on Train," *Philadelphia Inquirer* (18 Mar. 1912), 1; "Dr. Mary Walker Weaker," *New York Tribune* (19 Mar. 1912), 4; "'Don't Write Obituary Yet,'" *New York Tribune* (20 Mar. 1912), 4; Ada Patterson, "Mrs. Nellie Van Slingerland," *Idaho Statesman* (21 Mar. 1912), 4; "Doctor Walker Her Own Physician," *Kansas City Star* (22 Mar. 1912), 12; "Full of Courage," *Kennebec [Maine] Journal* (22 Mar. 1912), 1; "Dr. Walker's Strong Will," *Washington Post* (23 Mar. 1912), 2.

8. "Dr. Mary Walker Recovers," *Washington Post* (10 Apr. 1912), 4; Princess Nicholas to MEW, [March] 1912 (DUCOM); "American Woman's Republic," 7.

9. Nineteen-year-old Dorothy Hunt's photograph with MEW was published in the *Chicago News* of Dec. 2, 1912. "Mary Walker is Snubbed," *Los Angeles Times* (3 Dec. 1912), 15; "Named 'Human Rights Party,'" *Chicago Tribune* (6 Dec. 1912), 17; Mrs. John A. Logan, *The Part Taken by Women in American History* (Wilmington, DE: Perry-Nalle Publishing, 1912), 579.

10. See, for example, "Dr. Mary Walker Scolds," *Daily Northwestern* (22 Mar. 1913), 7; "Dr. Mary Walker Arrested," *Chicago Tribune* (2 Feb. 1913), 1; Norgren, *Belva Lockwood*, 219; Bertha Van Hoosen to Mrs. C. W. M. Poynter, Sep. 3, 1933 (DUCOM).

11. Van Hoosen to Poynter.

12. "Despite State Laws," *Boston Globe* (12 Apr. 1913), 9; "Babies and Votes, Too," *Washington Post* (22 Apr. 1913), 4; "Banners Greet Suffrage Parade," *Chicago Tribune* (2 Jul. 1913), 3.

13. "Doctoring a Real Princess," *Oswego Palladium* (12 Jul. 1913), 5; Lorrie Jenkins to MEW, Aug. 21, 1913 (OCHS); "Besiege by Dr. Mary Walker," *Washington Post* (3 Sep. 1913), 1; "Warrant for Dr. Mary Walker," (Watertown, NY) *Reformer* (2 Sep. 1913); Snyder, *Walker*, 131–132.

14. "Bring Tar and Feathers for Dr. Mary Walker," *Los Angeles Times* (26 Oct. 1913), I1; Poynter, "Dr. Mary Walker," 418–419. See, for example, "Tar for Dr. Mary Walker," *New York Times* (26 Oct. 1913), 1, and "Dr. Mary Walker Frustrates Plot to Tar and Feather Her," *Chicago Tribune* (26 Oct. 1913), 5.

15. "Dr. Mary Walker on Stage," *Indianapolis Star* (6 Jan. 1914), 9; "Dr. Mary as 'Envoy,'" *Washington Post* (6 Jan. 1914), 4; "Fair Hearer Hisses," *Washington Post* (8 Jan. 1914), 1, 4; "Fair Vote War Hot," *Washington Post* (Jan. 9, 1914), 1.

16. "Dr. Mary Has Bill to Insure Votes to Women," *Washington Post* (17 Jan. 1914), 4; "Women Quit Union," *Washington Post* (10 Jan. 1914), 1; "Fair Toilers Arriving," *Washington Post* (31 Jan. 1914), 4.

17. "Dr. Mary Their Guest," *Washington Post* (6 Feb. 1914), 4; "Why Men Don't Marry," *Oswego Palladium* (7 Feb. 1914), 1; "Skirts, Corsets and Cigarettes Condemned," *Oswego Palladium* (23 Feb. 1914), 1; "Knew Dr. Mary as a Girl," *Washington Post* (27 Feb. 1914), 4; "Admires Nude Figure," *Washington Post* (16 Mar. 1914), 14; "Dr. Mary Walker . . . the 'Dress Reform Dip,'" *Washington Post* (24 Mar. 1914), 4; "Dr. Mary Walker as a Maxixe Dancer," *Boston Globe* (29 Mar. 1914), 34; "Means Veterans' Pension Death," *Washington Post* (22 Mar. 1914), 4; "Whaddya Mean Your Identity?" *Lima News* (30 Mar. 1914), 1.

18. "Reception to Dr. Browne by Federal Association," *Washington Post* (25 Mar. 1914), 2; "Suffrage Fight in Sixties," *Washington Post* (1 Apr. 1914), 4; "Dr. Mary Walker has Right Idea, Says Etta," *Syracuse Herald* (9 Apr. 1914), 18.

19. "Dr. Mary Walker Did Not Tango," *Utica Press* (9 Jul. 1914), 5; "Dr. Walker's Welcome," *Oswego Palladium* (5 Feb. 1915), 4.

20. See, for example, "Many Women Are Fighting . . . ," *Duluth News-Tribune* (4 June 1915), 7; "30,000 Women March," *Washington Post* (24 Oct. 1915), 1.

21. "League of Nations Favored," *Washington Post* (5 Dec. 1915), 9; "March for Suffrage," *Washington Post* (6 Dec. 1915), 1; "Policy for Suffrage League," *Washington Post* (19 Dec. 1915), 15.

22. "Statement of Dr. Mary Walker before House Committee on Naval Affairs, Jan. 25, 1916," *U.S. House Committee on Naval Affairs* (Jan. 9, 1918), 167–195; "Cutting Costs in Navy," *Washington Post* (26 Jan. 1916), 5; "Notes of the D.A.R. Congress," *Washington Post* (18 Apr. 1916), 4; "Short Hair for Women," *Charlotte Observer* (29 Mar. 1916), 14; Mrs. Wilson Woodrow, "How the War Has Taught Women to Wear Men's Clothes," *Washington Post* (16 Jul. 1916), MT3; "Dr. Mary Walker Delegate to Democratic Convention," *Watertown Times* (13 June 1916), 10.

23. Graf, *A Woman of Honor*, 81, 92, 18; NARA. In 1977, the U.S. Congress restored MEW's Medal of Honor, and she remains the only woman recipient in U.S. history. "Critic of Suffrage Pickets," *Washington Post* (29 Jan. 1917), 7; "In Uncle Sam's Government Departments," *Washington Post* (28 Jan. 1917), AP2; "Midwinter Meeting," *Proceedings* (Albany: New York State Historical Association, 1917), 15–16.

24. "Kaiser Invited Here by Dr. Mary Walker," *Boston Globe* (8 Apr. 1917), 2; "The Danger of Handshaking," *Oswego Palladium* (13 Sep. 1917), 5. See also her letters to the *Palladium* on the need to consume less sugar in diets (8 Jan. 1918) and a letter-article on germ theory (6 Mar. 1918). "We're Surprised," *Oswego Palladium* (13 Apr. 1918), 5; "Dr. Mary Walker's Ideas," *Fulton Patriot* (12 June 1918), 3.

25. "Dr. Walker Here," *Oswego Palladium* (26 June 1918), 4; Ellen S. More, "'A Certain Restless Ambition': Women Physicians and World War I," *American Quarterly* 41 no.4 (Dec. 1989), 636–660; "Dr. Mary E. Walker Taken to Hospital," *Middletown Times Press* (7 Aug. 1918), 4; "Dr. Mary Walker Wants to Get Back to Bunker Hill," *Syracuse Herald* (15 Sep. 1918), 11.

26. John Stevenson et al., to the Town Board of the Town of Oswego, Oct. 1, 1918 (OCHS); Eva Turner to Mrs. Poynter, Mar. 31, 1932 (DUCOM); Van Hoosen to Poynter.

Index

Abbott, George, *see* Almy, Frank C.
abolition, and MEW, 8, 17, 31, 63 86, 199. *See also* African Americans; antislavery movement; race
abortion, 170; MEW on, 25, 26, 159
"Act for the relief of Mary E. Miller, An," 77
Acton, Police Commissioner, 81
Adams, Jack, 207
Adams, Katherine J., 222
Addams, Jane, 219, 244
Adirondacks, 15, 231
adultery, MEW on, 23–24, 157–158. *See also* Walker, Mary Edwards, writings: *Unmasked*
Adventists, 3
Africa, 130
African Americans: civil rights, 49, 78, 106; in Civil War, 44, 46, 63; congressmen, 140–141; education, 70; emancipation, 43, 63, 70; equality, 49; and Fifteenth Amendment, 115; and Fourteenth Amendment, 78, 79, 83, 106, 111; and labor movements, 244; and MEW, 8, 17, 31, 44, 59, 106, 111, 121, 122, 135, 140–141, 147, 153, 160, 184, 226; MEW on race organizations, 111; and presidential politics, 184; racist attitudes toward, 46, 122, 226; and Reconstruction, 141, 153; and slavery, 63; and suffrage, 78, 79, 105, 106, 110–111, 112, 115–116, 135, 152, 160. *See also* abolition; antislavery movement; Civil War: Colored Troops; miscegenation; race; suffrage movement
African Methodist Episcopal Church, 113
Agricultural Society, 136
Aguinaldo, Emilio, 222
Alabama, 160, 243

Alaska, 212
Albany, NY, 226, 235, 241, 243
Albany Assembly, *see* New York State: Assembly
Albion, The, 133
Alexander, George W., 58
Alexandra, czarina, 236
Alexandria, VA, 33, 36
allopathic medicine: and dress reform, 19; and germ theories, 208; and hygiene, 38; opposition to other medical treatments, 9, 51–52, 96, 102; use of drugs, 37, 243; and women physicians, 9, 51–52, 96. *See also* American Medical Association; medicine
All the Year Round, 88–89
Almy, Frank C., 190, 193, 197–198, 200–201
American Catholic Quarterly Review, 180
American Eclectic Medical Association, 9
American Equal Rights Association (AERA), 78, 101, 105, 106, 125; and MEW, 105
American Homeopathic Observer, 178
American Journal of Insanity, 173
American Literary Gazette, 133
American Medical & Surgical Journal, 13, 15
American Medical Association, 9, 51, 102
American National Association of the Red Cross, 187, 251
American Woman Suffrage Association (AWSA), 115–116, 118, 125, 126, 171, 278n30, and MEW, 113, 116, 126. *See also* Stone, Lucy
American Women, 209
American Women's Hospitals, 251
American Women's Medical Association, 245
Amherst College, 208
Amos, Sheldon, 86

287

288 INDEX

Amsterdam, NY, 104
anarchy, MEW on, 216
Anderson, Mary, 135
Anderson, Mary (Murray Hall), 226
Anderson, Elizabeth Garrett, *see* Garrett, Elizabeth
André, P. F., 90
Annapolis, MD, 146
Anthony, Susan B.: arrest and trial, 138, 143–144; biography, 249; and constitutional amendments, 105, 106, 115; death, 238; and dress reform, 19, 101, 142, 182; editor of *The Revolution*, 112, 115, 125; ego, 106, 149; fame, 195, 225, 240; labor activist, 117–118; lecturer, 118, 157; leadership qualities, 83, 101, 144, 147, 184; and National Council of Women, 220; and peace movement, 111; and presidential politics, 140, 141; and race, 101, 106, 111; relationship with Lucy Stone, 115, 118, 141; relationship with MEW, antagonistic, 83, 101, 106, 137–138, 141–142, 146, 151–152, 182–184, 214–215, 239; cooperative, 102, 105, 113, 117, 136, 220; relationship with Stanton, 83, 136, 147, 151; relationship with other suffragists, 107, 147–149, 166, 270n8; sexuality, 107; at suffrage conventions, 78, 106, 109, 112, 113, 136, 137–138, 141–142, 146, 147–148, 151, 182, 214–215; votes at poll, 138, 142; writings, 143–144, 171, 181
anti-immigration, 227
anti-imperialism: Hawaiian annexation, 210, 211–214, 216–217; MEW accused of treasonable talk, 219, 227–228; Panama Canal, 230–232; Santo Domingo, 134; Spanish-American War, 218–222, 225, 227–228, 231
Anti-Imperialist League, 219, 222
antislavery movement, 3, 4–5, 18, 36, 39, 43, 46, 78, 86
antitobacco, 6, 20, 30, 168, 182, 207, 251. *See also* Walker, Mary Edwards, lectures: on medical issues
Aquia Creek, 41–42
Army of the Cumberland, 52
Army of the Potomac, 40, 73
Arnold, Thomas, 94
Arthur, Chester, 169, 173–174, 186, 187, 248
Arthur's Illustrated Home Magazine, 114
Associated Press, 84
Astor, Mrs. (Caroline), 194, 224
asylums, 34
Atkinson, Edward, 219
Atlanta, GA, 57, 61, 62, 63
Atlanta Constitution, 150, 228
attorneys, female, *see* Bittenbander, Ada; Fall, Anna Christy; Lockwood, Belva; Walker, Mary Edwards

Auburn, NY, 234
Aurora, IL, 38
Austin, Harriet Jackson, M.D., 20, 79
Austin and Stone's Museum, 185, 189, 191
Austria, 98
Ayr, Scotland, 95

Bagetot, Isabella, 182
Baker, Walter R., 153
Baltimore, MD, 145–146, 179
Baptists, 3, 4, 5, 103
Barlow, Thomas, 107
Barnes, B., 188
Barnet, Scotland, 95
Barrett, Katy, 150, 191
Bartholow, Roberts, M.D., 96
Barton, Clara, 102, 103, 109–110, 182, 187, 225
Bayonet Constitution, 211
Bayou Fiche, LA, 122
Bayou Sara, LA, 122
Beard, Ellen, *see* Harman, Ellen Beard
Bedard, Josephine Marie, 185
Beecher, Henry Ward, 118
Beekman, Henry R., 194
Belmont, Alva Vanderbilt, 239
Bennett, Sallie Clay, 201
Bentley, J. A., 166–167
Bergen, Police Commissioner, 81
Bermondsey Poor Schools, 93
Bethlem Hospital for the Insane, 86
Bevans, Neile, *see* Van Slingerland, Nellie B.
Beyer, W. F., 226
Bishop, Artemus, 213
Bishop, Eleanor, *see* Nicholas, Princess Fredericka
Bishop, Fannie, 213
Bishop, John, 213
Bittenbander, Ada, 182
"Black Friday," 270n1
Blackwell, Rev. Antoinette Brown, 18, 118, 126, 149
Blackwell, Elizabeth, M.D., 10, 27, 87, 89, 156–157
Blackwell, Emily, M.D., 27
Blackwell, Henry, 106, 115, 257n33
Blaine, James G., 172
Blake, Lillie Devereux, 141–142, 151–152, 155, 181, 182
Bleak House (Dickens), 189
Bloomer, Amelia Jenkins, 15, 18, 87, 118
bloomers: clothing style, 18, 30, 80, 95, 154; dress reform activists and, 19, 30, 60, 117, 182–183, 206, 241
Bloomsburg, PA, 76
Bodichon, Barbara Smith, 85, 86
Bonheur, Rosa, 18

INDEX

Boston, MA, 69, 78, 189, 199, 202–203, 207, 217, 229
Boston Globe, 185, 192–193, 206, 218, 231
Boston University Law School, 207
Bowen Collegiate Institute, 28–29
Boyd, Belle, 59
Bracebridge, Charles, 86
Bracebridge, Selena, 86
Bradley Hubbell, Lucretia, 24, 164
Brazil, 219
Briggs, Emily, 102
Briggs, Sarah, 177
British feminists, 85–86, 244. *See also* dress reform; suffrage movement; women physicians; women's rights movement
British Medical Journal, 93
British Medical Registry, 87, 93
British newspapers, 88–89
British physicians, 85, 86–87
Brockway, C. B., 76
Brooklyn, NY, 226
Brooklyn Eagle, 226
Brown, E. O., M.D., 64–65, 262n26
Brown, Ira D., 63
Brown, John, 29–30, 42
Brown, Joseph B., 62
Brown, Sheriff, 191, 192, 198, 202
Browne, Olympia, 249
Bryan, Mary Baird, 208
Bryan, William Jennings, 208, 219, 225
Buffalo, NY, 181
Bulger, C. (Charles) N., 195, 225, 232
Bullard, Laura Curtis, 269n13
Bull Run, 31, 62
Bunker Hill, 81
Bunker Hill Road, *see* Walker family home
Burnham, Carrie, 147–148
Burnside, Ambrose, 40, 72
Burditt, Luther I., 77
Burlington Hawk Eye, 162
Butler, Benjamin F., 139
Butler, Mrs. R. M., 109
Butterfield, Daniel, 270n1

Cain, Superintendent of Police, 123
California, 149–150, 227
Calvert, TX, 124
Cambridge University, 99
Cameron, Simon, 32
Camp Casey, VA, 44
Camp William, 33
Canada, 11, 16
Canastota, NY, 20
Canby, Edward R. S., 48
capital punishment, MEW on, 84–85, 172–173, 197–198, 199, 200, 202–203, 222–224, 227, 228, 234, 251. *See also* crime and criminals; insanity
Carlisle, Scotland, 95
Carnegie, Andrew, 219
Carpenter, Mrs. Herbert, 249
Carrell, Mary E., 243
Carrier, Ella M., 167
Carson, Sarah J., 139
cartes de visite, 54, 76, 116
Cary, Alice, 20
Castle Thunder Prison, 58–61, 63, 69, 75–76, 104, 239, 262n19
Catholics, 3
Catt, Carrie Chapman, 214, 237, 249
Centennial Exposition, 150–151
Central Woman's Suffrage Bureau (CWSB), 112, 116, 134–135
Chaffee, Mrs. E., 188
Chambers, Sir Thomas, M.P., 84–85
Chancellorville, 45
Chapman, B. F., 29, 31, 107
Chapman, John, M.D., 94
Chapman, Maria Weston, 5
Charité Hospital, 98–99
Charles, S. R., 209
Chart, Mrs. Ormiston, 182
Chase, Kate, 48, 260–261n37
Chase, Salmon P., 81, 143, 260n37
Chattanooga, TN, 46, 50–51, 54, 62, 64, 73, 228
Chicago, IL, 194–195, 244–246
Chicago Tribune, 209, 218, 229, 240
Chickamauga, 46–47, 52, 54, 55, 62
Child, George, 151
Child, Lydia Maria, 5, 126
Childs, Harry, 178
Church, Ella, 182
Churchill, Mrs. Frank, 160
Cincinnati, OH, 14, 72, 113, 119, 179, 234
Cincinnati Commercial, 51–52
Circular, The (Oneida) 80, 82, 114
Civil War, 27, 30, 31, 111; ambulance services, 36; amputations, 34–35; Colored Troops, 44, 63; Confederate Army, 40, 45, 54, 55–57, 58–61, 99, 228, 261n11; Confederate supporters, 63, 68; culture of honor, 36; demoralized troops, 34, 45; deserters, 37, 63–64; diseases, 33, 40; freedmen, 70; hospital matrons, 71; hospitals, battlefield, 37–38, 40, 41, 42–43, 46, 49–50, 64; hospitals, Washington, 32, 36–37, 45, 49–50; international relations, 98; Medical Boards, 50–51, 52, 57, 73, 96; Medical Department, Union Army, 50, 51, 96; nurses, 32, 34, 42, 50, 51, 71, 127, 138–139, 140, 239, 246, 276n41 (*see also* Barton, Clara);

Civil War *(continued)*
  physicians, military, 32–33, 35, 42, 50, 51, 53, 57, 60, 64–68; physicians, volunteer, 32–37, 90; postwar transitions, 75–76, 99; prisoners, 45, 47, 58–61, 62, 63, 64–67, 75–76, 99, 207; prisons, 37, 45, 47, 58–61, 64–67; refugees, 62, 67–68, 70; relief societies, 35, 48–49; review of the videttes, 54; Secret Service, 57–58; spies, 57–58, 59; Union Army, 39–40, 41–42, 45, 46, 54–56, 57–58, 61; veterans, and MEW, 35, 41, 75–76, 137, 167, 207, 208, 235, 239, 242, 252; veterans' pensions, 127, 161, 186. *See also* African Americans; antislavery; Sanitary Commission; Walker, Mary Edwards; *individual battles by site name*
Claflin, Tennessee, 125
Clark, James Beauchamp, 250
Clarke, John A., 216
Clarksville, TN, 67–68; Clarksville Episcopal Church, 68
Clawyer, William, 44
Clayton, Henry D., 243
Cleveland, Grover, 179, 182, 194–195
Cleveland, OH, 118, 126
Clews, Jane M., 11, 16, 17
Clinedinst, Barnett McFee, 230, 282n9
Clinton, DeWitt, 13
Clinton, LA, 121
Coate, Holmes, M.D., 86
Coats, Lyman, 15, 69, 137
Coats, Vesta Walker, *see* Walker Coats, Vesta
Cody, William ("Wild Bill"), 45
Colby, Clara, 250
Collamer, J., 72–73
Colombia, 231
Columbian Law School, 71
Columbus, OH, 14, 257n32
Commonwealth, The, 90
Comstock, Anthony, 157, 167, 170, 208, 237
Concord, NH, 203
Congregationalists, 3
Congressional Union, 244
Conklin, Cary, 66, 144
Conklin, Elizabeth, 33
Connecticut, 100, 104, 164, 190, 202
Conscience Fund, 140
consumption, *see* medicine: tuberculosis
Conway, Moncure, 86, 98
Cooke, Sarah, 86
Cooley, Miss, 29
Cooper, Ann, 91
Cooper, Ashley, Earl of Shaftesbury, 84, 97
Cooper, Ellen, 91
Cooper, George, M.D., 51, 57, 67–68, 73, 261n45

Cooper, J. B., M.D., 123
Cooper, James Fenimore, 17
Cooper, Mary, 123
Cooper Institute, 49
Cornish, Harry S., 222, 223
Cortland, NY, 222
Cosmopolitan, 182
Counsel to Parents on the Moral Education of their Children (Elizabeth Blackwell), 156–157
Court Journal, The, 85, 88
Couzens, Phoebe, 151–152, 182
Cox, Miss, 91
Cox, Walter, 172, 216–217
Coyer, A. J., 108
Coyer, Dora, 108
Coyle, Colonel, 65–66
Craig, D. H., 84
crematories, MEW on, 239
Creswell, Postmaster General, 116
crime and criminals: assassinations, 172–173, 227–228; bombing, 193–194; Charles Guiteau trial, 172–173, 274n20; Charley Ross kidnapping, 147, 165–166; Christie Warden murder, 189–193, 197–198, 200–201, 202, 277n23; "criminal conduct" (adultery), 92; criminal psychology, 84, 87, 147; and dress reform, 170–171; executions, 173, 228, 234; false confessions, 198; Florence Burns trial, 229; hangings, 203–204; Harry K. Thaw trial, 237; Henry Manzer trial, 234; and militant suffragists, 246, 247, 250; murder, 189–193, 197–198, 222–224, 229, 233; other trials, 273n5; penal institutions, 226, 236; prevention, 208; Robert B. Molineux trial, 223–224; Russell Sage bombing, 193–194, 198; at Social Science Congress, 84–85; and U.S. imperialism, 213, 222, 227; youthful offenders, 236. *See also* capital punishment; *National Police Gazette*; Walker, Mary Edwards: arrests for clothing
Crimean War, 11, 88
Cromwell, Mrs. Napoleon, 160
"Cry from the Females, A" (Greeley), 115
Cuba, 217, 218, 219, 220
Culpepper, 54
Cumberland, *see* Department of the Cumberland
Cunningham, Dr., 29
Cutter, Calvin, M.D., 7
Czolgosz, Leon Franz, 227, 228

Daily Northwestern, 206
Daily People and Patriot, 198, 199
Daily Star, 161
Dall, Caroline, 182

INDEX

Dallin, GA, 58
Danville, NY, 20, 179
Daughters of the American Revolution (D.A.R.), 215, 217, 220, 250
Daull, Samuel, 228
Davies, Emily, 86
Davis, Andrew Jackson, 4
Davis, Joseph J., 272n50
Davis, Pauline Wright, 8
Davis, Webster, 215
Day, J. F. Preston, 38, 143, 144
Debs, Eugene V., 202
Declaration of Independence, 69, 151, 240
"Declaration of Sentiments" (1848), 6–7
Deeds of Valor (Beyer and Keydel), 226
De Foe, Edwin, 54
DeLarge, Robert C., 140–141
Delaware County, IA, 95
Delhi, IA, 28
Democratic Party: conventions, 194, 232; and MEW, 63, 141, 172, 177, 184, 188, 194, 207, 232–233, 244, 247, 250; in New York, 63, 194; opposition to Civil War, 63; party platforms, 63; presidential politics, 100, 151, 152, 169, 184, 207, 225, 232, 244; pro-slavery sentiment, 63; and race, 101, 184; and suffrage, 101, 117, 151, 172, 233
Denison, Rev. Charles, 91
Denison, Mary Palmer, 91
Department of Justice, 128
Department of the Cumberland, 51, 67
Department of the Interior, 174, 176
Department of the Treasury, 72, 117, 134, 144, 153–154, 156
Dependent Pension Act, 186
Dewey, George, 221–222, 225
Dickens, Charles, 88–89, 189
Dickinson, Anna, 53, 157
Dilke, Charles, 184
Dilke, Lady Ashton (Mary), 182, 184
Dillon, M. F., 200
dime museums, 180–181, 185, 189, 191
District Woman Suffrage Association, 247, 249
divorce, *see* Stanton, Elizabeth Cady: on divorce; Walker, Mary Edwards: divorce; women's rights movement
Dix, Dorothea, 34
Dix-Hill Plan, 59
Dodds, Andrew, 84
Dodds, Susannah Way, M.D., 84, 91
Dodge, Mary Abigail, *see* Hamilton, Gail
Doe, Charles, 193
Dole, Sanford B., 211, 212, 214
Donaldson, Professor, 99
Donnelly, Mary E., 82

Dornbusch, George, 86, 99
Douglas, Joseph, 165
Douglas Hospital, 50
Douglass, Frederick, 5, 49, 106, 115, 126, 135, 177, 184
Dow, Neal, 8, 95
Downing, George T., 110–111
Dred Scott v. Sanford, 18, 106
Dreger, Alice, 272n54
"Dress of Women, The" (Gilman), 180
dress reform: cane as symbol, 114; conventions, 20–21, 27, 28, 79, 113–114, 179; economics of, 17; generational changes, 180; in Great Britain, 86, 87; and health, 218 and higher education, 114; international, 218; and New Woman, 250; opposition to by the press, 19, 60, 82, 87, 113, 162; opposition to by women, 19–20, 34, 109, 146; organizations, 19; versus popular fashions, 17, 79, 80–81, 114, 159, 182–183, 241; styles, 18, 180; support of by men, 21, 77, 79, 86; support of by the press, 80–81, 82, 96, 114; in western states, 18, 221; and women physicians, 20, 75, 79, 84, 146 (*see also individual physicians by name*); and women's health, 18, 19, 37, 98; and women's mobility, 25; and women's rights, 19–20, 109. *See also* Anthony, Susan B.; dress reformer, MEW as; *Lily, The*; *Sibyl, The*; Stanton, Elizabeth Cady; suffrage movement: organizations; women's rights
dress reformer, MEW as, 125, 128; attacked physically, 9, 102, 125, 178, 192–193, 209, 246–247; attacked verbally, 9, 102, 125, 146–147, 168, 209, 269n5 (*see also* newspapers and books, attacks on MEW); "Chamber of Horrors," 251; in Civil War, 36, 38–39, 42; and *A Colony for New Women*, 206; at conventions, 20–21, 27, 28, 44, 79, 113, 179; on cross-dressing women and men, 226, 234–235, 282n11; emotional impact, 186; in Great Britain, 88, 91–92, 97; growing acceptance, 209, 221, 229, 235, 241; and liberty, 212; medical bases for, 8, 85, 103, 114, 144, 241; and military pension, 187–188; as a moral issue, 81, 159, 196; officer of organizations, 19–20, 44, 79, 113–114; outfits, 8–9, 15–16, 42, 56–57, 59, 70, 80, 114, 136–137, 145, 155–156, 167, 182, 209, 218, 230, 245, 249, 257n24; prize for best dressed woman, 242; reenergized movement, 113–115, 209. *See also* Walker, Mary Edwards: arrests for clothing; Walker, Mary Edwards: sexuality
Dress Reform Association, 19. *See also* National Dress Reform Association

"Dress Reform Dip," 248
Drexel, A. J., 151
Dreyfus Affair, 221, 223
"Dr. Mary Walker's Reforms Finally Win Recognition" (*Post*), 242
Dudley, W. W., 176
Duffield, H. M., 237
Dundee, Scotland, 95
Durkee, Charles, 112
Dwyer, Mrs. Frank, 252

Earl of Shaftesbury, *see* Cooper, Ashley
East Feliciana Patriot, 121
East Orleans, MA, 267n16
Eclectic Magazine, 105–106
Eclectic Medical and Surgical Journal, 10
Eclectic Medical College of New York, 102
Eclectic Medical Society, 102
eclectic medicine: and allopathic medicine, 9, 51, 102; and dress reform, 19; and germ theories, 208; materia medica, 11; as medical reform, 9, 101–102; organizations, 9, 10, 103; popularity of, 51; treatments, 144. *See also* American Eclectic Medical Association; medicine; Walker, Mary Edwards: physician
Edelweiss Swiss Choir, 208
Edinburgh, Scotland, 93, 94–95, 182
Edmunds, James, M.D., 90–91, 95, 97
Edson, Susan, M.D., 112, 143, 172
education, MEW on, 24, 126, 205–206; women's 21–22, 126
Elder, Robert H., 226
Elmira, NY, 228
Emancipation Proclamation, 43, 63
Emerson, Ralph Waldo, 89
Enforcement Act, 123
England, 84–99, 130, 133
Enterprise Club of Working Girls, 208
Episcopalians, 68
equality, MEW on, 24, 85, 88, 118, 120, 122, 125, 129, 136, 158, 199; *See also* abolition; Walker, Mary Edwards: as suffragist; women's rights
Erie Canal, 3
eugenics, 156–157
Evans, Commissioner, 228
Evans, Maria P., 189
Evarts, William M., 187
Evening Post, 80–81
Everson, Dr., 226
Executive Mansion, *see* White House receptions
Exposition Carnival, 230

Fairleigh, Colonel, 65–66

Fall, Anna Christy, 207
Fall, George H., 207
Falley Seminary, 7–8
Faneuil Hall, 203
Farmer, Mrs. E. A., 95–96
Farmers' Agricultural and Horticultural Society, 167
Farmers' Club of Oswego, 4, 136
farming, 70, 80, 167, 206, 225, 239. *See also* Walker family home
Farnsworth, John Franklin, 50
Farragut, David, 113
fashion, 17, 79, 80–81, 95, 114, 159, 182–183, 241. *See also* dress reform; dress reformer, MEW as
Father's Story of Charley Ross, The (Christian Ross), 165
Fay, Annie Eva, 174
Female Medical Society, 87, 91, 97
Female Military Prison, 62, 64–67
Femmes Docteurs en Mèdicine, Les (Fontanges), 226
Fenton, Reuben E., 72
Ferguson, Champ, 55–56, 89
Fern, Fanny, 19–20
Fernandina, FL, 126
Ferry, Thomas, 151
Fetter Lane Chapel, 91
Field, P. P., M.D., 203
Fifteenth Amendment, 115, 123, 126, 160
Finley, Clement A., 51
Finsburg Chapel, 95
First Spiritualist Church, 250
Fish, Secretary, 116
Fisher, A. N., 175
Fisk, James, 270n1; Fisk-Gould scandal, 270n1
Fitchburg, MA, 202
Flannery, Lawrence, 164
Flint, Mr. and Mrs., 191, 277n23
Florence, Thomas B., 136
Florida, 212
Folkmar, Elnora, M.D., 249
Fontanges, Harriet, 226
Ford's Opera House, 174
Forrest Hall Prison, 37
Forsyth, Dr., 84
Fort Barnard, VA, 44
Fort Ontario, NY, 251
Foster, Abby Kelly, 118
Foster, Charles, 225
foundling hospitals, 25–27, 48
Fourteenth Amendment, 78, 83, 101, 105, 106, 126, 160
Fowler, Lydia Folger, M.D., 10
Fowler, Susan P., 113, 230, 233, 235, 241

INDEX

Franklin, Benjamin, 144
Fraser's Magazine, 89
Fredericksburg, 41–42, 55, 62
free love, 27, 77, 125, 160
Freedman's Aid Society, 122
Freedmen's Bureau, 70
Freeman, Delphine, 69, 92
Freeman, Mary Wilkins, 225
Free National University, 134
Frémont, John C., 39, 63
French, Henry F., 272n50
French and Indian War, 4
French Economist, The, 85–86
French government, 98
Fuller, Frank, 76
Fulton, MO, 120
Fulton, NY, 136
Fugitive Slave Law, 5
Furer, Charles, 121

Gage, Frances D., 118
Gage, Matilda Joslyn, 137, 141, 149, 151, 166, 171, 181, 182, 184, 274n16
Gaine, Mary, 139
Gaines, Edmund Pendleton, 117
Gaines, Myra Clark, 117, 189
Galveston, TX, 124
Galveston News, 116
Gardner, Lella Crum, 146–147
Garfield, James, 169, 172–173, 175
Garfield, Mrs. (Lucretia), 174
Garrett, Elizabeth, L.S.A., M.D., 85, 86, 87
Garrison, Helen White, 105
Garrison, William Lloyd, 159
Gates, Susan Young, 220
Georgetown, 37
George Washington University School of Law, 71
Georgia, 55; Georgians, 56–57
Gettysburg, 169
Gibson Girl, 237
Gillespie, Elizabeth, 150–151
Gilman, Charlotte Perkins, 180
Gitt, D. L., 174–176
Glasgow, Scotland, 84, 94–95, 99
Glen Haven Water Cure, 20
Goldman, Emma, 227
Gompers, Samuel, 219
Gordon's Mills, GA, 52, 54–58, 262n19
Gould, Charles, 66
Gould, Jay, 194, 270n1
Grand Hotel, Paris, 98
Grant, Ulysses S.: in Civil War, 58; on dress reform, 113; inauguration, 113; presidency, 41, 100, 107, 116, 134, 141, 144, 145, 231, 270n1, 272n44; and MEW, 113, 134, 141, 145

Graves, Robert, 186–187
Gray, John, M.D., 173
Great Debates in American History, 152
Greeley, Horace, 106, 115, 141, 142
Green, J. N., M.D., 32–33, 72, 96
Greenwich, MA, 2, 22, 162, 204, 207
Greenwich Methodist Church, 2
Greenwood, Grace, 109, 110, 135, 171
Griffin, Walter, 189
Griffing, Josephine, 70, 105, 109, 111, 112, 117, 126, 135
Grimké, Angelina, 5, 21, 49
Grimké, Sarah, 5
Griswold, Luna Walker, *see* Walker Griswold, Luna
Griswold, Wickham, 15
Guam, 220
Guiteau, Charles, 172–173, 251

Haiti, 184
Hale, Edwin M., M.D., 178, 275n30
Hale, Mrs., 178
Hall, Harriet Walker, 14
Hall, Murray, 226
Hall, Susan, 64
Halleck, Henry Wager, 57–58
Hamilton, Gail (Mary Abigail Dodge) 147, 226; *Gail Hamilton's Life and Letters*, 226
Hamilton, Mary Morris, 21
Hamilton, Scotland, 95
Hammerstein's Victoria Theater, 247
Hammond, J. H., 64, 65, 262n26
Hanaford, Phebe A., 118
Hancock, Winfield, 169
Hanover, NH, 190, 191, 197, 199, 203
Hardwick, MA, 2
Hardy, Maria, 92
Harlan, John Marshall, 184
Harman, Ellen Beard, M.D., 20, 38, 103, 109, 112, 117
Harrington, Stephen R., 103–104, 177
Harper, Frances Watkins, 115, 125
Harper, Ida Husted, 249
Harper's Ferry, 29–30
Harper's Weekly, 22–23
Harris, Fidelia R., M.D., 20
Harris, Susanna, 242
Harrison, Mrs., 214
Harrison's Landing, VA, 68
Hart, Isabelle Kingsbury, 242
Hartford, CT, 104
Hartford Courant, 140
Hasbrouck, John S., 19
Hasbrouck, Lydia Sayer, M.D., 19–20, 17, 30, 32, 36, 37, 43, 46, 79, 113–114
Hastings, Etta, 249

Haven, M. Z., 232
Hawai'ian annexation, 210, 211–214, 216–217, 220, 222
Hawley, Joseph R., 140
Hayes, Rutherford B., 152–153
Henry, Patrick, 13
Hepburn-Dolliver Bill, 231
Hewitt, Charles, 191, 192
Higginson, Thomas, 106, 115
Hill, Alberta, 249
Hill, Daniel Harvey, 58, 194–195
Hillman House Hotel, 169
History of Woman Suffrage (Anthony, Stanton, Gage), 109, 139, 171, 274n16
Hitchens, Addie, 70
Hoar, George F., 219
Hodges, Henrietta, 97
Holmes, Major, 55
Holmes, Oliver Wendell, 54
Holt, Joseph, 45, 72, 73
Homeopathic College of Cleveland, 118
homeopathy, 9, 19, 51, 118, 144, 178, 208
Homer, NY, 18
honor, MEW on, 36
Hooker, Isabella Beecher, 126, 136, 137–138, 139, 148, 159
Hopkinton, IA, 28
Horan, Harry, 235
Hornellsville Weekly Tribune, 186–187
Hôtel Dieu Hospital, 98–99
Hotel Gerard, 243
House, A. E., 28
Houston, TX, 123–124
Howe, Julia Ward, 115, 150, 225
Hoyt, Harrison, 201
Hubbell, Algernon Sidney, 24
Huerta, Victoriano, 247
human rights, MEW on, 131, 137. *See also* women's rights
Human Rights Party, 244
Human Sexuality (Parke), 235
Hunt, Dorothy, 244, 283n9
Hunt, Mr. and Mrs. F. L., 244
hydropathy, 11, 19, 20, 38, 79, 84
Hygeio-Therapeutic College, 37–38, 103, 267n18
hygiene/hygenics, 8, 37–38, 103, 146. *See also* dress reform: and women's health; Hygeio-Therapeutic College; Trall, Russell, M.D.; Walker, Mary Edwards: physician

Illinois, 103
imperialism, U.S., *see* anti-imperialism; Walker, Mary Edwards, writings: *Isonomy*
Imperial Music Hall, 196
India, 130, 182
Indiana, 32, 111, 124, 190
Indiana Hospital, 32, 36, 39, 53, 62
infanticide, MEW on, 26, 85, 123
Ingalls, Ethel, 182
Ingersoll, Robert, 4
Inslee, W. D., 206
International Cutters' Association, 248
International Order of Good Templars, 95–96
Invalid Corps, 50
Iolani Palace, 213
Iowa, 28
Ireland, 91, 182
Irving, Washington, 17

"J'accuse!" (Zola), 221
Jackson, James C., M.D., 79, 113
Jackson, MS, 121
Jack the Ripper, 87
Jamaica, 96
James, William, 219
Japan, 219, 233, 236–237, 250
Jeanne d'Arc Suffrage League, 243
Jenks, Thomas P., 122
Jenkins, Lorrie, 246, 252
Jewett, Sarah Orne, 225
Joan of Arc Magazine, 243
Johns Hopkins Medical School, 208
Johnson, Albert, 215–216
Johnson, Andrew, 51, 70, 72, 73–75, 96, 98, 100, 144
Johnson, Bishop, 184
Johnson, Officer, 80
Johnston, Joseph E., 58
Jones, A. J., 184
Jones, Rosalie, 249
Journal of Nervous and Mental Disease, 173
Juarez, Benito, 98
Julian, George W., 111, 153, 272n44
Junction City, KS, 120
jurors, women as, 229
justice, as principle, 12, 199–201; MEW on, 65–66, 120, 212, 213, 214

Kansas, 100, 101, 111, 118, 120
Kansas City, MO, 120
Kehoe, J. D., 193
Kensington Society, 86
Kentucky, 2
Key, Francis Scott, 22
Key, Phillip Barton, 22–24
Keydel, O. F., 226
Kilmarnock, Scotland, 95
King, Julia, 209

insanity, 87, 173, 174, 199, 200, 227, 237; MEW on, 87, 164–165, 166, 173, 200, 234, 237

INDEX

King, Preston, M.D., 42, 96
"King Cotton," 31
Kirkwood, Margaret, 93–94
Knickerbocker Athletic Club, 222
Kortright, Fanny, 94

labor, 80, 93, 97, 178, 207, 244; activism, 71, 90, 97, 116–118, 125, 248; hired, 190, 195–196, 197–198, 199; MEW's views on, 47, 53, 90, 97, 120, 126, 131–133. *See also* Walker, Mary Edwards, writings: *A Colony for New Women*; *individual organizations by name*
Ladies' Mount Vernon Association, 21
Lady Maccabees, 242
Lady's Own Paper, 91
La Follette, Fola, 249
Laidlaw, W. R., 194
Lake, Anna Easton, M.D., 179, 275n33
Lake Pleasant, MA, 162, 168
Lamouche, Frances, 234, 235
Lancet, The, 96
Landis, Charles K., 233
Landis, Lillian E., M.D., 192
Landis, Simon Mohler, 192
Langston, James, 184
Lankester, Edwin, M.D., 85, 87
Lankester, Gay, 87, 91
Lansing, William, 140
Latimer, Henry R., 124
Law, Harriet, 97
Lawrence, KS, 120
Lawrence, William, 127
laws, 18, 22–24, 28, 29, 92 193, 195, 274n20. *See also* crime and criminals; Walker, Mary Edwards: as lawyer; Walker, Mary Edwards, writings: *Isonomy*
Leader Theater, 242
League of Nations, 250; MEW supports, 250
Leavenworth, KS, 120
Lectures of Lola Montez, 25, 258n18
Lee, Robert E., 99
legislative hearings, MEW's testimony at, 78, 105, 160, 168, 182, 196, 223, 224, 231, 241, 243, 246, 250
Leroy, KS, 120
lesbianism, 94, 107
Leslie, Mrs. Frank, 218
Liberty (Mill), 94
Liberty Party, 5
Libby Chronicle, 58
Libby Prison, 58, 59, 60
Life magazine, 179
Lili'uokalani, queen of Hawai'i, 211–214, 216–217, 219, 220
Lily, The, 15, 18, 19

Lincoln, Abraham, 43, 45, 49–50, 61, 63, 68, 70, 72, 81, 128, 144, 239, 251
Lind, Jenny, 8
Lind, John, 247
Literary Institute, 95
Livermore, Mary, 102, 113, 118, 209
Liverpool, England, 84
Lockwood, Belva Bennett McNall: fame, 195, 240; family, 103; friendship with MEW, 103, 114, 136, 146–147, 184, 189, 242–243; intelligence, 103; as lawyer, 144, 189; as lecturer, 209; marriage, 103; as peace activist, 245, 250; personality, 103, 266n37; photograph with MEW, 242; residence, 103, 156; speeches, 139, 142; as suffragist: and CWSB, 112, 134–135, 249; and District Woman Suffrage Association, 249; legislative activities, 136; and NWSA, 137, 138, 139, 141, 142, 151; and UFA, 103, 105; on voting at polls 143; as teacher, 103; as temperance advocate, 103
Lockwood, Ezekiel, 103, 113, 135, 136, 138, 148
Locomotive Firemen's Magazine, 202
Logan, Mary Cunningham, 244
Lohman, Caroline, 26, 258n20
London, 86–87, 91, 209
London Anglo-American Times, 91
London Dialectic Society, 97
London Globe, 85
London Temperance Hospital, 91
Los Angeles, CA, 217, 229
Louisiana, 2, 100, 118, 120, 121–123, 152, 212
Louisville, KY, 61–62, 64–67
Louisville Daily Journal, 67
Love, Alfred H., 111
Lozier, Clemence, M.D., 160
Luce, B. F., 124
Ludwig I, king of Bavaria, 25
lynching, MEW on, 234

Mackenzie, J. M., M.D., 32, 72, 96
Madison, Dolley, 225
Madison Square Garden, 237
Maher, John, 222–223
Maine, 92
Maine (ship), 218, 219
Malden, MA, 207, 208
Manchester, England, 84–85, 86
Manchester National Society for Woman's Suffrage, 86
Manierre, Police Commissioner, 81
Manila Bay, 221–222
Mansfield, Judge, 80, 81
Manzer, Henry, 234
Marion, OH, 161
Marlborough, NH, 92

marriage, MEW on, 15, 22, 24–25, 105, 133, 179–180, 231
Maryland, 100
"Mary Walkers," 217
Massachusetts, 111, 177, 202
Maximilian, Archduke, 98
May, Rev. Samuel J., 15, 21, 126
McCarthy, Charlotte, 94
McCarthy, John B., 249
McCarthy, Justin, 89, 94, 99, 121, 269n5
McClellan, George B., 63
McCook, Daniel, Jr., 52, 54–55, 56, 61
McDonald, John, 230
McGovern, S. W., 221
McKinley, William, 208, 212, 218, 219, 222, 225, 227, 228, 231
McNall, Lura, 103
McNoughton, Clara, M.D., 249
Mecklenburg Declaration of Independence, 240
Medal of Honor, 73–74, 251. *See also* Walker, Mary Edwards: Medal of Honor
Medical Press & Circular, 93
medical students, and MEW, 87–88, 93, 95
Medical Times and Gazette, 88, 89
Medical Women's National Association, 230
medicine: clitoridectomy, 93, 96; diseases of women and children, 10; Flexner Report, 208; laparotomy, 230; Medical Reformers movement, 9, 101–102; medical students, 88–87, 93, 95, 98–99; medical training, 9–11, 91; midwives, 91; neurology, 173; obstetrics, 10; sexuality, 235, 267n18, 272n54; sexually transmitted diseases, 108, 158, 267n18; smallpox, 33, 144; tuberculosis, 208, 217, 225, 234, 235, 242. *See also* allopathic medicine; eclectic medicine; homeopathy; hydropathy; Walker, Mary Edwards: medical training; Walker, Mary Edwards: as physician; women physicians
Mesmer, Franz, 256n10
Methodist Episcopal Church, 199
Methodists, 2, 3, 4, 168
Metropolitan Magazine, 206
Mexico, 98, 247
Mexico, NY, 195
Michigan, 45
Middlesex Hospital, 87, 96
Middletown, NY, 19
Milbourne, Randolph, 234
Mill, John Stuart, 94, 97, 128
Miller, Albert E.: adultery, 27–28, 31, 69, 76, 92, 107, 108; children, 92; criminal charges, 92; death, 267n16; divorce, 27–28, 69, 70, 76–77, 107, 267n16; as free love advocate, 77; graduation speech, 12, 13; and hypnotism, 256n10; as lecturer, 31, 92; liberalism of, 11–12, 13, 24, 27; marriage to Delphine Freeman, 92, 107, 267n16; marriage to MEW, 14, 15, 18, 27–28, 69, 70, 77, 92, 257n33; medical training, 11–12; morality, 27–28; private practice, 15–16, 92, 267n16; residences, 15–16, 267n16; as state legislator, 267n16
Miller, Charles Ransom, 275n25
Miller, Elizabeth, 82
Miller, Elizabeth Smith, 18, 38
Miller, Mrs. E.V.C., 184
Miller v. Miller, 92
Millerites, 3
Milton, John, 89
Minetto, NY, 8
Minneapolis Tribune, 209
Minor v. Happersett, 150
miscegenation, 60
Mississippi, 100, 118, 120–121
Missouri, 63, 100, 118, 120, 214
Mitchell, Edward P., 271n26
Mitchell, Maria, 225
"M.M.G.," 11–12
modesty, women's, MEW on, 34, 85
Molineux, Robert B., 222–224
Montague, Lord Robert, 85
Montez, Lola 25, 258n18
"Montrose" (pseud.), 51–52
Moore, Alice, 182
Moore's Garden Theater, 245
morality, MEW on, 24, 36, 81, 146, 157–158, 163
Morgan, George W., 72
Morgan, Middy, 271n26
Mormons, 220–221, 231–232
Morning Star, 89
Morrill, Lot M., 153
Moseman, William B., 82
Mosher, William, 165
Mott, Lucretia, 49, 76, 78, 109, 110, 111, 136, 138, 159
Muir, G. W., 95, 265n26
Mutual Dress Reform and Equal Rights Association, 113–114

Napoleon III, emperor of France, 98
Nashua Telegraph, 199
Nashville, TN, 67
Nation, Carrie, 227, 238–239
Nation, The, 82
National American Woman Suffrage Association (NAWSA), 201–202, 214, 239, 240, 244–245, 246, 250
National Antislavery Society, 43

National Association for Equal Suffrage, 246
National Citizen and Ballot-Box, 166
National College Equal Suffrage League, 250
National Congress of Mothers, 208, 220
National Convention of Colored Men, 111
National Council of Women, 220
National Dress Reform Association, 19, 20, 28 44, 79. *See also* Dress Reform Association
National Free Press, 183
National Labor Congress, 117, 167
National Police Gazette, 23, 93, 96, 162, 165–166, 177, 258n20
National Reformer, 89, 90
National Republican, 61, 142, 151
National Sanitation Convention, 146
National Temperance League Rooms, 99
National Vigilance Association, 184
National Woman Suffrage Association (NWSA): conservative elements, 182; and constitutional amendment, 110, 142–143, 150, 181–182; conventions, 125, 136, 137–138, 140, 141–142, 146, 147–148, 150, 151–152, 155, 159–160; and dress reform, 182, 272n40 (*see also* Anthony, Susan B.; dress reformer, MEW as; Stanton, Elizabeth Cady); generational differences within, 151–152; legislative activities, 137–138, 160; and MEW, 116, 136, 137–138, 143, 147–146, 151–152, 155, 159–160; national vs. state approach, 115, 150; and other suffrage organizations, 115, 125, 139, 171, 278n30; and presidential politics, 140; and race, 115–116, 125, 142; and voting and registration at polls, 137, 150; and working-class women, 115–116. *See also* suffrage movement; Walker, Mary Edwards: as suffragist
National Women's Party, 244
National Women's Rights Convention, 78
Native Americans, 17
Navy Department, 219
Needham, MA, 267n16
Nesbit, Evelyn, 237
Newcastle, England, 182
New England Woman Suffrage Association, 106
New Hampshire, 192, 197, 198, 199, 200, 202, 203–204, 205
New Hampshire Supreme Court, 199
New Haven, CT, 24
Newington, England, 97
New Jersey, 33
New London, CT, 24
New Orleans, LA, 117, 122–123, 189
Newport, RI, 110, 177, 239

newspapers and books, attacks on MEW: on her activism, 230–231; advocate violence against her, 162, 227; on her anti-imperialism, 227–228; and Christie Warden case, 191; on her clothing, 146, 146, 161, 170–171; and *A Colony for New Women*, 206–207; for discussing sexuality, 150, 171; false reports of her violence, 135–136, 153–154; on her government employment, 175–176; on her offer to sell finger, 242; on her pension, 140, 161, 166, 227–228; as a physician, 170–171, 232, 265n27; on her sanity, 177; on her sexuality, 156, 162, 170–171, 177, 179, 235; on *Unmasked*, 167. *See also* Walker, Mary Edwards: sexuality
newspapers and books, support of MEW: of her activism, 186–187, 189, 204, 225, 228, 232, 244, 249; of her anti-imperialism, 211, 212, 228; of her clothing, 166, 202, 209, 217, 242; and *A Colony for New Women*, 206; of her D.A.R. application, 217; defend against false reports, 168–169, 170; on eightieth birthday, 244; of her eloquence, 215, 216; of her labor activism, 248; of her medical work, 239, 242; obituaries 252; of her offer to sell finger, 242; of her rights, 140, 146, 155, 166, 215–216; of her strength, 244; of suffrage, 140, 141, 155, 215
New Woman movement, 126, 218, 221, 241, 250; and MEW, 127, 204–207, 208, 209, 224, 235–236. *See also* Walker, Mary Edwards, writings: *A Colony for New Women*
New York City, 69, 71, 78, 79–83, 100, 113–114, 125, 164–165, 196, 229
New York Express, 24
New York Herald, 113, 114, 117, 155, 230–231
New York Infirmary for Women and Children, 27
New York Medical Journal, 15, 93, 96
New York Round Table, 93
New York State: Assembly (legislature) 23, 76–77, 79, 196, 235, 241; central region, 1, 2–3, 17, 136, 195, 243; in Civil War, 44, 46, 49; congressmen, 140; courts and trials, 227; governors, 46, 63, 72; grange, 193; Judiciary Committee, 77, 241; laws, 26, 28, 29, 31, 81, 92, 227; medical facilities, 20, 27, 102; medical societies, 10, 102; reform movements in, 37, 83, 100; Supreme Court, 92, 107; women's rights activists in, 3, 6–7, 76, 83, 104–105, 125, 241 (*see also* antislavery movement; *individual names*)
New York State Eclectic Medical Society, 10
New York State Historical Society, 247, 250
New York Sun, 153–154, 271n26

New York Times, 80, 82, 94, 154, 162, 170, 172, 175–176 194–195, 223, 275n25
New York Tribune, 42–43, 45–46, 82, 120, 271n26
New York Volunteers, 44
New York World, 80, 155, 196
Nicholas II, czar of Russia, 224, 233
Nicholas, Princess Fredericka, 244, 246
Nightingale, Florence, 11, 86
Nimmo, Mr., 265n15
Nineteenth Amendment, 253
Nobel Prize for Peace, 236
Norcross, Henry, 193–194, 198, 199, 200–201
Norgren, Jill, 266n37
North American Journal of Homeopathy, 178
North Carolina, 166, 171
Northern Pacific Railroad, 76
Norwich, CT, 104
Nye, Bill, 206, 209

Oakland, CA, 149
Oasis, The, 17
O'Donnell, Mary Eleanor, 240
O'Donovan, John, 113
Ogden, UT, 149
O'Gorman, James R., 225
Ohio, 58, 60, 70, 100, 113, 118, 127, 225
Ohio State Woman's Suffrage Society, 119
Ohio Volunteers, 58, 60
Old Settlers Society, 167
"Olivia," *see* Briggs, Emily
Olmsted, Frederick Law, 34
Oneida Community, 80
Oneida County Agricultural Society, 239
"Only Self Made Man in America, The" (Nye), 209
Osawa, IA, 38
Oswego, NY, 39, 44; economy, 1, 3; grange, 193; intellectual life, 3, 17, 103, 204; newspapers, 44, 137, 239; organizations, events, 136, 137, 230; political activities, 63, 232–233, 250; population, 3; reform movements in, 5
Oswego and Syracuse Railroad, 3
Oswego Commercial Advertiser, 137
Oswego County, NY, 63
Oswego Female Institute, 103
Oswego Times, 45, 63, 113, 172, 221
Oswego Town, NY, 1, 2–3, 136–137, 206, 227, 239, 252. *See also* Walker, Mary Edwards: as physician; residences
Oswego Town Farmers' Club, 167
Ould, R. S., 167

Page, Dr. Huldah, 37
Painter, Hetty K., M.D., 42
Painter, L. M., 42
Painter, Mrs., 42
Pall Mall Gazette, 90
Palmer, Mrs. Potter, 195
Palmoni, Crypti, 169
Panama, 231, 232
Panama Canal, 230–231
Panama-Pacific Exposition, 250
Pan American Exposition, 227
Pankhurst, Emmeline, 247
Paris, France, 86, 92, 98, 99, 182
Paris Exposition, 86, 92, 98, 99
Park Theater, 226
Parke, Joseph, M.D., 235
Parker, Alton Brooks, 233
Parliament, British, 86, 90
Patent Office, 32, 33, 102
Paul, Alice, 244, 245
peace movement, 111, 112, 208, 236–237, 250
Peck, Charles, 195, 196
Peel Grove Institute, 92
penal servitude acts, 84
Pennsylvania, 2, 100
Pennsylvania Medical College, 42
pension, Civil War, 71, 75, 127, 169, 194, 231, 248. *See* Civil War: veterans' pensions
People of the Period (Pratt), 209
People's Party, 203
Perin, G., M.D., 51, 52, 96, 261n45
"Persecuting Dr. Mary Walker" (A. Johnson), 215–216
Peru, 219
"Petition for Woman's Rights" (1846), 6
petitions, 212. *See also* suffrage movement; Walker, Mary Edwards: petitions; women's rights movement
Phelps, Edward, M.D., 64, 66, 67, 72, 73, 96
Philadelphia, 70, 71, 117, 150–151, 181
Philadelphia Inquirer, 230
Philadelphia Press, 109
Philippines, 220, 222, 227, 232, 233
Phillips, Wendell, 49, 78–79, 106, 184
Phrenological Journal, 103, 129
phrenology, 129, 225
"Physical Culture" (J. King), 209
physicians, *see* allopathic medicine; British physicians; Civil War: physicians, military; Civil War: physicians, volunteer; eclectic medicine; homeopathic medicine; physio-medical practitioners; Walker, Mary Edwards: as physician; Walker, Mary Edwards, writings: *Unmasked*; women physicians
physiology, 8, 105, 114. *See also* Walker, Mary Edwards: lecturer; women physicians
physio-medical practitioners, 102
Pickett, Patrick H., 79–80, 81, 82

INDEX

Piedmont, VA, 42
Pillsbury, Parker, 115
Pinkerton, Allen, 57
Pinkerton's Female Detective Bureau, 57
Pinkerton's National Detective Agency, 57, 165
Pittsburgh, PA, 178
Pittsburgh Dispatch, 178
Plummer, John, 91
political corruption, MEW on, 128, 153–154, 166, 230, 250
polygamy, MEW on, 111–112
Pomeroy, Samuel Clarke, 111
Port Gibson, MS, 120–121
Port Jervis Evening Gazette, 124
Potomac, 33, 36, 40
Potter, Stephen H., M.D., 10, 14
Poughkeepsie, NY, 4
Poynter, Lida, 266n37
Prairie Farmer, 114
Pratt, A. T. Camden, 209
Presbyterian Hospital, 243
Presbyterians, 3, 22
Preston, Ann, M.D., 71–72
Principles of Nature, The (Davis), 4
prostitution, 23, 48, 65, 92, 156, 158. *See also* "Social Evil"
Providence, RI, 177
public diary, 99, 266n37
Public Ledger, 151
Puck, 179
Puerto Rico, 220, 233
Pulaski, NY, 195
Purvis, Charles, M.D., 110–111, 112
Purvis, Harriet, 125

Quartermaster's Bureau, 49, 54
Queen, 95, 96, 97, 265n27, 266n31

race, MEW on, 110–11, 125, 137, 188, 212–213, 234, 267–268n27. *See also* abolition
rape, 24, 32, 46, 58, 157–158, 159
Raymond Street Jail, 226
Raynor, Solicitor, 156
Ream, Vinnie, 128
"Reasons for the Enfranchisement of Women" (Bodichon), 85
Reconstruction, 75–76, 100, 141
Reed, Mary L., 120
Reese, B. M., 146
Reformer, The, 20, 103
Reform Medical Society, 102
Refuge House, 67–68
Rehoboth, MA, 2
Remond, Sarah, 125
Remonstrants, 168

Republican Party: antislavery sentiment, 46; candidates, 63, 184; and MEW, 46, 63, 90, 143, 188; in New York, 63, 230; presidential politics, 63, 100, 152–153, 169, 184; and race, 101; and suffrage 101, 106, 117, 143, 152, 169
Restell, Madame, 26
Revolution, The, 112, 125, 269n13
Rhode Island, 137
Richards, Edward M., 91–92
Richardson, W. A., 145
Richmond, VA, 59–61, 69, 105, 106
Richmond Enquirer, 59
Richmond Examiner, 59
Riddle, Haywood Yancey, 160
Right of Women to Vote, The (Lockwood, Winslow, and Edson), 143
"rings," political, 128, 154, 230
Roberts, Brigham H., 220
Robinson, M. S., 181
Robinson, Police Inspector, 191
Rochester, NY, 44, 138
Rochester Post-Express, 228
Rome, NY, 15, 20, 24, 29, 207, 239
Rome Sentinel, 27, 207
Roosevelt, Franklin Delano, 247
Roosevelt, Theodore, 227, 230–231, 232, 233, 236, 237, 244, 247
Rose, Ernestine, 49
Rosencrans, William S., 46
Ross, Charley, 147, 165–166
Ross, Christian, 165, 273n5
Ross, L. A., 54
Ross, Police Officer, 145–146
Royal College of Surgeons, 239
Royal Infirmary of Glasgow, 84
Rucker, Daniel H., 49
Rushmore, Mary D., M.D., 230
Russell, William E., 207
Russo-Japanese War, 236–237
Rutland, VT, 244, 246

Sacramento, CA, 32
Sage, Russell, 193–194, 198, 201
Salladin, A., Jr., 225
Salter, Dr., 46
San Antonio, TX, 124, 202
Sand, George, 18, 25, 106, 121, 138
San Francisco, CA, 25, 149–150, 179, 250
Sanitary Commission, 34, 35, 51
Santa Rosa, CA, 149
Santo Domingo, 134
Sarasvati, Pundita Ramabai, 182
Saturday Evening Post, 177
Savannah, GA, 127
Schenectady, NY, 104, 105
Schurz, Carl, 219

Scotland, 84, 94
Scoville, Frances, 173, 174
Scoville, George, 173, 174
Second Great Awakening, 4
Secular League, 250
Seekonic, MA, 2
Seneca Falls Convention, 6
Severance, Caroline, 115
Sewall, May Wright, 220
Seward, Cameron, 57
sexuality, MEW on, 105, 108, 150, 157–159, 272n54. *See also* Walker, Mary Edwards, writings: *Unmasked*
Seymour, Horatio, 46, 63
Shaklett, Misses, 42
Shaw, Rev. Anna Howard, M.D., 238, 239, 242, 249
Sheldon, George T., 139–140
Shepard, Lewis, 228
Sherman, John, 153–154, 184
Sherman, Mildred, 225
Sherman, William Tecumseh, 54, 57, 61–62, 63, 73, 113
Shoreham Hotel, 211
Sibley Memorial Hospital, 236
Sibyl, The, 19–27, 29–30, 36, 38, 46, 47, 79, 85, 91, 131
Sickles, Daniel, 22–24, 116, 258n23
Sickles, Teresa Bagioli, 22, 23–24, 116
Sing Sing Prison, 223
Sisters of Mercy, 50
Smith, Gerrit, 3, 5, 18, 21, 106, 126
Smith, Justice, 202
Smith-King, Cora, M.D., 249
Smithsonian Institute, 39
Smoot, Reed, 231–232
Snoad, Arthur D., 190–191, 193, 197, 198, 199–201, 202
Snoad v. Walker, 199–201
"Social Evil," 157, 158
social science, and MEW, 84–85, 86, 156
Social Science Association, 86
Social Science Congress, 84–85, 86
Soldier's Letters, 222
Sons of Jonadab, 248
South Carolina, 152, 184
"Southern Bastille," 58
South Newbury, OH, 114
Southworth, E.D.E.N., 135
Spain, 116, 218, 219, 220
Spanish-American War, 134, 217–220, 231, 280n18
Speare, Mrs. H. E., 138–139
"Special Session of Congress, The" (Clinedinst), 230
Spectator, The, 95, 96, 97

Spencer, Charles S., 81
Spencer, Sara Jane Andrews, 135, 141, 160, 249
Spinner, Francis E., 144–145
Springfield, MA, 202
Springsteen, Alexander, 44
St. Bartholomew's Hospital, 86, 239
St. Francisville, LA, 121, 122
St. Francisville Democrat, 121
St. James Hall, 87–88, 89, 90, 91, 93, 95, 265n15
St. Louis, MO, 84, 230, 232, 250, 271n27
Stanton, Edwin M., 37, 46–47, 49, 72, 73, 100, 140
Stanton, Elizabeth Cady: children, 268n39; in Civil War, 49; and constitutional amendments, 105, 106, 115; on divorce, 110, 125; and dress reform, 18, 19, 21, 38–39, 84, 101, 142, 148, 272n40; editor, *The Revolution*, 115, 125; in England, 184; fame, 240; leadership qualities, 83, 117, 127, 149, 184; lecturer, 118, 268n39, 269n11; legislative activities, 182; marriage, 125–126, 268n39; as martyr, 142; and peace movement, 111; as political candidate, 83; and presidential politics, 140, 141; and race, 78, 101, 106, 109, 111; relationship with Anthony, 83, 136, 147, 151; relationship with MEW: antagonistic, 83, 101, 138, 141–142, 146, 182–184; cooperative, 102, 105, 106, 118, 127, 136; relationship with other suffragists, 115, 137, 141–142, 147–148, 166, 182–184, 270n8; at Seneca Falls Convention, 6; at suffrage conventions, 78, 106, 109, 136, 137–138, 141–142, 146, 147–148, 151, 160, 182; on voting at polls, 143; and Wendell Phillips, 78; on women's rights, 128; writings, 21, 109, 139, 142, 171 (*see also History of Woman Suffrage*)
Stanton, Emily, 111
Stebbins, J. H., 12–13
Stephenson, Lieutenant, 65–66
Stevenson, Adlai E., 195
Stewart, Maria, 5
Stillman, H. C., 137
Stockley, William, 151
Stockwell, E. W., M.D., 14, 72, 96
Stone, Lucy: and AERA, 105; at conventions 109, 113, 119, 126; and dress reform, 142; on dress reform, 19, 38; father's opposition, 6; leadership, 18, 49, 106; marriage, 125–126, 257n33; relationship with Anthony and Stanton, 115, 118, 141, 171; relationship with MEW, 102; on women in politics, 119. *See also* American Woman Suffrage Association; Walker, Mary Edwards: as suffragist

INDEX

Stowe, Harriet Beecher, 225
Strowbridge, Lydia, M.D., 79, 103, 222
Sturge, Ella, 188
Subjugation of Women, The (Mill), 128
suffrage movement: advancements, 83, 100, 101, 105, 106, 112, 113, 115, 125, 133, 184, 237, 246; and Centennial Exposition, 150–151, 155; and citizenship, 78, 83, 105, 150, 201 (*see also* U.S. Constitution; Walker, Mary Edwards: as suffragist); and civil rights, 49, 141; and constitutional amendment for women suffrage, 20, 110, 126, 181–183, 201, 238; in crisis, 18, 78, 141–142, 184, 244; and Democratic Party, 112, 172, 244; and divorce, 125–126; at fairs, 242, 249; and Fifteenth Amendment, 115, 123, 126; and Fourteenth Amendment, 78, 83, 106, 110, 123, 126, 135; generational differences, 184; in Great Britain, 85, 86, 94, 97, 182–183, 184, 244–245, 247; hoaxes, 120–121; international cooperation, 249; on labor, 141; legislative activities, 137–138, 243; marches and parades, 245–246, 249, 250; militancy, 244–245, 247; Nineteenth Amendment, 253; opposition to, 6; opposition to, by men, 106, 115; opposition to, by other women, 94, 160, 168, 182; opposition to, by the press, 95, 116, 162, 168, 240; petitions and bills, 105, 112, 135, 136, 241, 250; postwar transition, 78, 79, 83; and presidential politics, 134, 137, 141; publications, 20, 128, 141; and race, 78, 83, 101, 105, 109–111, 112, 115–116; and Republican Party, 78, 100, 106; and the South, 120–125; state voting rights, 160, 246; support from other reformers, 69, 97, 111, 112; Taylor-Dilke dispute, 184; and universal suffrage, 78; on voting at polls, 20, 86, 106, 126, 138, 141, 143, 169, 245; in the West, 250; and working-class women, 117–118 (*see also* labor). *See also* Fifteenth Amendment; Fourteenth Amendment; Walker, Mary Edwards: as suffragist; women's rights movement
suffrage organizations: compatibility between, 105, 112, 250; internal dissension over leadership roles, 100–101, 106, 125–126, 147–148, 151–152, 184, 244; internal dissention over policy differences, 83, 100–101, 110, 112, 115–116, 119, 125, 141–142, 147–148, 151–152, 182–183, 184, 237–238, 244–245, 246; internal dissention, race-related 18, 106. *See also individual organizations*
"Suffragettes of Yesterday and Today" (O'Donnell), 240

Sumner, Charles, 81, 143, 147. 180–181, 183, 226
Supreme Court, U.S., 144, 150, 193, 217
Swedenborg, Emanuel, 4
Sydenham Lecture Hall, 91
Syracuse, NY, 1, 2, 179, 194, 199, 200, 226, 237, 242, 249
Syracuse Evening Telegram, 225, 232
Syracuse Medical and Surgical Journal, 11
Syracuse Medical College, 9–14, 38, 72, 257n31
Sweet, Assemblyman, 241
Sweet, Cora, 234

Taft, William Howard, 242
Tampico Incident, 247
Tarbox, Jerome, 76
Taylor, Bayard, 25
Taylor, Helen, 184, 269n5
Teller, Henry Moore, 176
temperance movement, 6, 7, 8, 20, 83, 95–96, 208, 231, 242, 248. *See also* Walker, Mary Edwards: as temperance advocate
Temple, The (London), 86, 95
Tennessee, 2, 55
Texas, 100, 118, 120, 123–124, 202, 212
Thaw, Harry K., 237
theater, MEW on, 196, 208, 226
Thomas, Charles S., 247
Thomas, David Morgan, 95, 97
Thomas, George H., 46, 52, 54, 57, 58, 62, 72, 73, 113
Tilden, Samuel J., 152, 155, 162, 164
Tillotson, Mary, 113, 159, 160, 233, 272n40
Tilton, Theodore, 78, 126
"Tingwick Girl," 185
Toledo Bee, 221
Topeka, KS, 120
Townsend, Edward D., 62
Trades Demonstration, 90
Train, George Francis, 101, 112, 125, 174
Trall, Russell, M.D., 37–38, 86, 92, 97, 103, 267n18
Treaty of Portsmouth, 236
Trumbull, Lyman, 137–138
Truth, Sojourner, 125, 142
Truth and The Removal, The (Guiteau), 173
Truth Seeker, 167
Turkey, 130
Twain, Mark, 219
typhoid fever, 40
Typographical Union, 117

Underground Railroad, 5
Union League, 45, 48
Union League Hall, 103, 105

Union Woman Suffrage Society, 125
Uniontown, IA, 96
Universal Franchise Association (UFA), 105, 106, 109, 111, 112, 116; and MEW, 109–110, 143
Universal Peace Society (Union), 111, 178, 209, 267n24
Universalists, 3, 176–177
University College, 94
University of Chicago, 245
unwed mothers, MEW on, 25–27, 48, 85, 157
U.S. Army, 222. *See also* Civil War
U.S. Colored Troops, 44
U.S. Constitution: and women as citizens, 83. *See also* Walker, Mary Edwards: as suffragist
U.S. General Hospital, 251–252
U.S. Law Library, 156
U.S. War Senate, 219–220
U.S. Volunteers, 33, 237
Utah, 111, 112, 125, 231
Utica, NY, 77, 104, 107, 237
Utica State Hospital, 173

Vance, Zebulon Baird, 166
Van Hoosen, Bertha, M.D., 245, 252
Van Slingerland, Nellie B., 243–244
Vaughan, Mary, 83
Vermont, 72
Vibbert, George H., 115
Vicksburg, LA, 121
Victoria, queen of England, 95, 264n5
Victoria League, 137
Victoria Magazine, 91, 97
Vineland, NJ, 106, 233
Virginia, 33, 61, 86, 103, 111

Wade, Benjamin F., 100, 105, 111
Waldorf, Mrs. Reginald, 241–242
Walker, Abel (brother), 2
Walker, Abel (great-grandfather), 2
Walker, Abel II (grandfather), 2, 20
Walker, Alvah (father), 14; abolitionist, 5, 8; antitobacco, 84; childhood, 2; death, 167–168; dress reform advocate, 5, 6, 7; education, 2; founds free school, 5, 241; health, 5–6; influence on MEW, 5–6, 20, 168; inventor, 33, 137, 179; legal documents of, 15, 156, 169; medical interests, 5–6, 7, 38; MEW visits, 136; occupations, 2, 4, 5; religion, 4, 5, 17, 168; residences, 1, 2, 77, 156, 169–170; support of MEW's actions, 9, 168, 172
Walker, Alvah, Jr. (brother): agnosticism, 168, 256n9; alienated from family, 168, 169–170, 178–179, 187, 274n13; birth, 1; death, 187; inventor, 33, 179; marriage, 4, 257n32; military service, 68; on his parents, 275n32
Walker, Cynthia, 1, 15
Walker, Ebenezer, 2
Walker, Mary (aunt), 1, 162, 204, 229
Walker, Mary (criminal), 94
Walker, Mary (Spiritualist), 94
Walker, Mary Edwards:
  adolescence, 7–8
  aids poor, 71 (*see also* Walker, Mary Edwards, as physician: patients)
  arrests for clothing, 79–83, 120, 123, 145–146, 164–165, 177–178, 245
  bequeathed money, 177
  birth, 1
  as businesswoman, 77, 89, 91, 218, 229, 265n15, 265n26
  as candidate for U.S. Senate, 171–172, 188
  carries a gun, 35, 55, 77
  childhood, 3–7
  death, 252
  divorce, 27–28, 29, 31, 32, 69, 76–78, 79, 92, 103, 107, 109, 130–131
  and dress reform (*see* dress reformer, MEW as)
  education: Bowen Collegiate Institute, 28–29; at home, 4, 5, 6, 17–18; Falley Seminary, 7–8 (*see also* Walker, Mary Edwards: medical training)
  fame: desire for, 17; as dress reformer, 18, 242; international, 85–86, 87, 96, 142, 226, 239; national, 99, 105, 116, 120, 133, 135, 150–151, 168, 188–189, 195, 211, 225, 226, 227, 230, 237, 242; as pioneer, 233, 237–238, 241–252; teaspoons with her image, 283n1; from war service, 30, 31, 33, 35, 45, 54, 63, 64, 75, 76, 128, 226, 237, 239
  family scrapbooks, 17–18
  fear of rape, 55, 58
  female-identified, 108–109
  founding institutions, 25–27, 48–49, 85, 126, 127, 168, 174, 208, 217, 223, 224–225, 232, 236, 247–248
  friendships: with dress reformers, 19, 113, 230, 233; in Great Britain, 84, 86, 87, 94, 97, 118, 120, 121; in Oswego, 28, 232, 246; with physicians, 11, 17, 19, 38, 64, 72, 120, 123, 135, 143, 178, 179, 222, 226, 245, 249; with suffragists, 109, 136, 143, 242–244; in Washington, D.C., 102–104, 109, 177, 243 (*see also* Lockwood, Belva)
  government appointments, 116–117, 144–145, 174–176, 272n50 (*see also* Walker, Mary Edwards: as physician)
  hairstyles, 54, 56, 71, 145, 250

INDEX

health: chronic bronchitis, 215, 236, 243; disability, from imprisonment, 60–61, 69, 74, 78, 140, 146, 148, 215, 236; failing, 251–252; heart disease, 215; hospitalizations, 162, 236, 243, 245, 251–252; leg injury, lameness, 186, 215; robust, 9, 150, 192, 206, 207; stress-related illness, 175; throat problems, 97; tubercular, 224, 226

inheritance, 15

interviews: on actresses and the theater, 196; on being a physician, 186–187, 207; on capital punishment, 202, 237; on *A Colony for New Women*, 206; on Dewey, 221–222; on dress reform, 209, 218, 221; on the Dreyfus Affair, 221, 223; on labor, 178; on her life, 209; on her political activism, 199, 209, 218, 232; on President Arthur, 179, 186, 248; on her sexuality, 218; on U.S. imperialism, 217, 221

as inventor, 179

as lawyer: association with other lawyers, 86, 134, 195, 200; legal training, 29, 71, 145, 164, 166, 243; practice, 45, 71, 123, 136, 177–178, 202, 278n31, 280n27

letters from: John W. Bell, 128; Charles and Selena Bracebridge, 86; C. B. Brockway, 76; Mary Baird Bryan, 208; Civil War acquaintances, 64, 75–76; Dr. Jane Clews, 17; Dr. George Cooper, 68–69; A. J. Coyer, 108; "Doc," 66–67, 177; Professor Donaldson, 99, 266n37; dress reform supporters, 114; Mrs. E. A. Farmer, 95–96; George M. Gamwell, 281n1; R. Garner, 116; Dr. Ellen Beard Harman, 117; Dr. Lydia Sayer Hasbrouck, 69–70; Dorothy Hay, 252; Charles Herron, 116; Henrietta Hodges, 97; Lorrie Jenkins, 246, 252; Abraham Lincoln, 50; Belva Lockwood, 134, 244; Charlotte McCarthy, 94; J. Morgan, 95; Aurora Pankhurst, 252; B. M. Reese, 146; Edward M. Richards, 91–92; G. Richmond, 75–76; soldiers and their families, 63–64; Dr. Lydia Strowbridge, 79; David Morgan Thomas, 95, 97; veterans, 75–76, 116; D. A. Weber, 122; Bradley and Josephine Wightman, 122; Alfred Williams, 140–141; Woman's National Democratic League, 252

letters to: Czarina Alexandra of Russia, 236; Mrs. Astor, 194; John W. Bell, 128; Charles and Selena Bracebridge, 86; Mary Baird Bryan, 208; Colonel Coyle, 65–66; Professor Donaldson, 99; family 32–33, 59–60, 77; George M. Gamwell, 281n1; Rutherford B. Hayes, 152–153; Abraham Lincoln, 49–50; Belva Lockwood, 134, 136; Charlotte McCarthy, 94; New Hampshire governor, 197; New Hampshire secretary of state, 197; Czar Nicholas II of Russia, 233; Russell Sage, 194; soldiers and their families 33, 63; Edwin M. Stanton, 46–47; David Morgan Thomas, 97; Samuel J. Tilden, 162, 164; Andrew Warden, 191; D. A. Weber, 122; Woodrow Wilson, 251 (*see also* Walker, Mary Edwards, writings: letters to the editor)

love of dancing, 91, 139–140, 248

love of poetry, literature, 17, 31, 49, 149, 206

marriage to Albert Miller, 14, 15, 18, 69, 77, 107 (*see also* Walker, Mary Edwards: divorce; Walker, Mary Edwards: romantic relationships)

marriage, false rumors of, 155–156, 209, 267n17

Medal of Honor, 72–74, 75, 78, 81, 91, 96, 100, 207, 218, 237, 251, 252, 284n23

medical training: Alumni Society, 12–13, 14; Bellevue Hospital clinics, 38; challenges to, 8; graduates with honors, 12; graduation speech, 13–14, 17; Hygeio-Therapeutic College, 37–38; internship, 11; self-taught, 7, 88; Syracuse Medical College, 6, 9–14, 18, 88, 157 (*see also* Walker, Mary Edwards: as physician)

meeting Queen Victoria, 95

missionary goal, 7

offers to sell finger, 241–242 (*see also* Walker, Mary Edwards: as physician: sanitarium development)

at Oswego Town fair, 136–137

in Paris, 98–99

at Paris Exposition, 86, 251

patriotism, 30, 39, 43, 60, 68, 69, 98, 213–214, 215, 230, 240, 246

as peace activist, 111, 178, 233, 236–237, 244, 245, 247, 250, 251

pension, military, 58, 78, 140, 144, 146, 147, 160–161, 166, 174, 186–189, 215, 219, 227–288, 281n36 (*see also* Walker, Mary Edwards: petitions)

personality, 63; anger, 28–29, 82, 114, 136, 140, 194; charm, 85, 89, 97, 168–169; conspiracy theories, 189–190, 198, 202, 204, 215, 218; ego, 101, 182, 183, 221, 230, 233, 236–237, 242, 243, 244; endurance, 117, 220; honor, 36; independence, 77, 89, 98, 107, 129, 179, 196, 240, 248; intellectualism, 3, 4, 25, 109, 213, 244; leadership qualities, 17, 54–55, 101; performative nature, 54, 155–156, 177, 218;

Walker, Mary Edwards *(continued)*
  persecution fears, 189–190; private vs. public persona, 27; self-confidence, 13, 17; self-promotion, 50, 89, 120, 196, 207, 239; self-sacrifice, 116; strong will, 83, 175, 244; wit, 82, 85, 102, 114, 124, 129, 196
petitions, memorials, bills: for Almy reward, 199–201, 202, 203–204; against capital punishment, 173, 223, 228, 235; for clerkship pay, 145; on Mormons' rights, 220–221; for nurses' pensions, 127, 139, 140; for her pension, 166–167, 187–188; for poor women and children, 174; for postal reform, 176; on slander, 196; for women's rights, 71, 166, 196, 235, 247; for women's suffrage, 139, 152, 247, 250
philosophy of: democratic values, 101, 111; gender and reason, 44–45; living one's principles, 13, 38–39, 70, 79, 186, 189, 242; medical, 129 (*see also* dress reformer, MEW as; Walker, Mary Edwards: as physician; Walker, Mary Edwards: as suffragist)
photographs and portraits of, 54, 116, 128, 150, 155, 177, 209, 221, 230, 240, 242, 264n5, 283n9
as physician: advocates eclectic medicine, 9–14, 243; advocates women's exercise, 231, 235; aids other physicians, 87; aids soldiers and families, 35–36, 37, 40, 43, 44, 45, 46–47, 48–49, 63–64 (*see also* Civil War: veterans); aids strangers, 235; amputations, 34–35, 42–43, 259n10; applies for ship's surgeon, 84; on the battlefield, 39–43, 49, 51–52, 53, 61, 62, 70, 72, 73–74, 75, 81, 88, 260n23; in Civil War, as volunteer surgeon, 30, 32–35, 36–37, 39–43, 46–47, 49, 53, 73–74; consulting, 29; at Female Military Prison, 62–67; at Indiana Hospital, 32, 36, 39, 53, 62; interests in hygiene, 8; as laborer, 53; licensed, 207, 208; and male medical students, 87–88, 93, 95, 98–99; at medical conventions, 230; on medical issues, treatments, 33, 41–42, 108, 144, 208, 233, 242, 267n18; and medical jurisprudence, 173; night calls, 77; patients, 16, 33, 34–35, 40–41, 46, 53, 55, 70, 93, 124–125, 144, 150, 224, 246; on phrenology, 129; police surgeon offer, 161–162; preventive medicine, 208, 225, 243; private practice in New York, 206, 229; private practice in Rome, NY, 14, 15–16, 18, 27–28, 31, 88, 122; private practice in Washington, DC, 42, 45, 69, 70, 75, 101, 105, 149, 164, 229, 248; at Refugee House, 67–68; sanitarium development, 208, 224–225, 234–235, 236, 241–242, 246; seeks military commission, 61–62, 70, 72, 75; and self as patient 224, 236, 243; and sexual knowledge, 150 (*see also* Walker, Mary Edwards, writings: *Unmasked*); Union Army contract surgeon, 30, 31, 33, 42, 45–47, 49–52, 53–69, 73–74, 96, 251, 262n19; visits European hospitals/clinics, 84, 86–87, 98–99 (*see also* Walker, Mary Edwards: medical training; Walker, Mary Edwards: as prisoner of war; women physicians)
and police, 48
police officer application, 161–162
as political force in Washington, D.C., 43, 113, 116 (*see also* legislative hearings, MEW's testimony at)
postwar transition, 75–83
as prisoner of war, 45, 58–61, 66, 69, 74, 75–76, 78, 99, 104, 205, 228, 239, 261n11, 261n19
public protests, 29
relationship with brother, 169, 274n13 (*see also* Walker, Alvah, Jr.)
religious beliefs, 4, 5, 120, 130, 131, 133, 162–163, 174, 176–177, 199, 201, 203
as reporter, 113, 116, 136, 229, 271n26
residences: Brooklyn, NY, 226; Delhi, OH, 18; New York City, 76, 77, 78, 82; Oswego Town, NY, 1, 3, 70, 156, 167, 197, 217, 223, 234–235, 236, 239, 246, 251, 252, 255n5, 282n11; Rome, NY, 15, 77; Washington, DC, 39, 48–49, 69, 70, 100, 156, 165, 208–209
romantic relationships, 11–12, 66–67, 97, 103–104, 107–108, 179 (*see also* Walker, Mary Edwards: marriage)
seeks national political office, 171–172, 188, 194
seeks state political appointments, 225, 232–233, 250
sexuality, 93, 94, 102, 107–108, 116, 218 (*see also* Walker, Mary Edwards: marriage; Walker, Mary Edwards: and undoing gender)
as spy for Union Army, 46
as subscription agent, 11, 35
as suffragist: advocates universal suffrage, 78, 109, 110, 141, 240; advocates voting at polls, 20, 86, 106, 123, 126, 136, 169, 184–185, 245; attempts to vote and register, 101, 135, 169; and British suffragists, 85, 86, 105, 182–183, 245–246; at conventions and congresses, attempts to silence MEW, 119, 138, 181–183, 185, 214, 215; hoaxes, 120–121, 155–156; leadership standing, 117, 233, 246, 247–248, 249;

INDEX   305

legislative activities, 135, 136, 137–138, 139, 160, 182; on militancy, 244–246; opposes Constitutional amendment 110, 123, 126, 137, 160, 238, 244 (*see also* Edwards, Mary Walker, writings: *Crowning Constitutional Argument*); in parades, 249, 250; parents' support, 6; predictions about, 85; and the press, 120–121; relationship with Anthony (*see* Anthony, Susan B.); relationship with other suffragists, 108–109, 119, 135, 136, 137, 139, 142, 151–152, 160, 166, 171, 180, 182–183, 214, 238–240, 244, 245–246, 250; relationship with Stanton (*see* Stanton, Elizabeth Cady); and suffrage organizations, 83, 105, 108–109, 115–116, 134–140, 141–144, 146–149
as teacher, 8, 9
as temperance advocate, 17, 90, 92, 95, 99, 125, 182, 208, 231, 235
and undoing gender, 30, 107–108, 132, 177, 218, 234–235, 267n19 (*see also* dress reformer, MEW as; Walker, Mary Edwards: hairstyles; personality; sexuality)
vegetarianism, 86
visits Rome, NY, 239
as women's rights activist: on constitutional rights, 142; frustration with poor advancements, 168; in Great Britain, 84–99; lifelong, 17, 69; and taxation, 208; as U.S. Senate candidate, 171–172, 185; on women's public speaking, 128; on woman's sphere, 185; and working class, 204–207, 208 (*see also* dress reformer, MEW as; Walker, Mary Edwards, lectures; Walker, Mary Edwards: as suffragist; Walker, Mary Edwards, writings)
as writer, 28; and fame, 17; on medicine, 102, 144, 235; on political issues, 149; processes, 20–21; proposed articles, 167; on reform, 144; self-publication, 279n5; on suffrage, 184–185, 239–240 (*see also* Walker, Mary Edwards: letters from; petitions; Walker, Mary Edwards, lectures; Walker, Mary Edwards, writings
Walker, Mary Edwards, lectures, 28, 29, 75, 125, 136
on agricultural issues, 239
on American independence, 167, 240
on Anthony Comstock, 248
"Beauties, Uses and Injuries of Tobacco," 181
benefit lectures, 92, 95, 208, 225, 226
for the Betterment League on the Prevention of Disease, 243
"Causes of Unusual People," 181

on crime and criminals, 147, 202
"Crinoline," 85
"Curiosities of the Brain," 181
at dime museums and theaters, 180–181, 185, 247
on divorce, 248
on dress reform, 15, 21, 70, 85, 90, 99, 113–114, 149, 155, 164, 179, 181, 185, 196, 221, 230, 248 (*see also* dress reformer, MEW as)
"Dr. Mary E. Walker, Her Capture by the Confederates, and Four Months' Detention as a Prisoner of War," 89
"Experiences of a Female Physician in College, in Private Practice, and in the Federal Army, The," 87–88
at Exposition Carnival, 230
at fairs, 202, 239, 242
"Fairwell Lecture to the Ladies of London, on Dress Reform," 99
at Faneuil Hall, 203
on fashion, 128, 149, 241
at Fourth of July celebrations, 104
in Great Britain, 61, 84–99, 104
"Great Labor Question, The," 181
on greenbacks, 164
"Human Electricity," 181, 230
on human nature, 49
"Human System, The," 105
"Influenza, Improperly Called the Grip," 226
"Justice to All," 120
on labor, 120, 137, 164, 174, 178, 181
on the law, 207, 208
and male medical students, 87–88, 93
on marriage and trial marriages, 105, 112, 157–159, 179, 248
on medical issues, 105, 120, 174, 181, 185, 226, 230, 232, 242, 248 (*see also* Walker, Mary Edwards: as physician: sanitarium development; Walker, Mary Edwards, lectures: on dress reform; on women physicians)
"Men's Rights, Women's Wrongs, and Women's Suffrage," 122
on nudity and the female body, 248
"On Washington," 39
at Oswego society circus, 230
on the peace movement, 250
"Physical Health," 120
at political rallies, 63, 113
"Prevention of Throat and Lung Troubles," 174
"Pure Love and Sacred Marriage" (title varies), 105, 112, 150
"Reform in Women's Dress, The," 154

Walker, Mary Edwards, lectures (*continued*)
"Science of Dress," 181
on science, 178, 266n37
on Spiritualism, 180
spontaneous speeches: in government buildings, 185, 193, 197; on labor issues, 208; on McKinley's assassination, 227; at political rallies, 135, 194; on suffrage, 142, 148, 239–240; on a train, 168; on U.S. imperialism, 218, 219, 227; on women's rights, 160
on suffrage, 97, 105, 119–120, 122–123, 136, 137, 164, 177, 184, 243, 244, 245, 247
on temperance, 90, 92, 95, 99, 120, 125, 248
tours, 61, 69, 70, 104–105, 118, 119–125, 144, 149–150, 151, 164, 179, 180–181, 202, 244, 246
on U.S. imperialism, 211
for veterans, 208
on her war experiences, 39, 45, 49, 63, 69, 86, 87, 88, 89, 92, 104–105, 119–120, 208
"Who Dare?" 151
"Woman," 150
"Woman's Franchise," 181
"Woman Suffrage," 125
"Women's Dress and Men's Rights," 146
on women in politics, 119
on women physicians, 86, 87, 90, 91, 92
"Women's Dress in Relation to Strong Men," 230
on women's rights, 49, 90, 123–124, 160, 180, 202, 248
for working classes, 91, 92–93, 180
at World's Food Fair, 202
Walker, Mary Edwards, writings:
articles in *The Sibyl*, 19, 20–28, 29–30
articles in *Washington Sunday Gazette*, 136, 146
autobiographical narratives, 72, 187–188, 239
autobiographical petition, 187–188
"A Bloomer in the Street," 21, 131
A Colony for New Women, 127, 204–207, 208, 209, 224
Consumptive School Sanitarium, 224–225
Crowning Constitutional Argument, 142–144, 147, 148, 152, 171, 181, 183–184, 237–239, 243, 247, 249
"Dress Reform Convention," 20–21
"Dr. Mary Walker's Love Story," 11–12, 257n25
"Dr. Mary Walker's Views Regarding Proper Masculine Attire," 229–230
Hit, 128–133, 136, 137, 150
"Home to the World," 251
"Hotel de Castle Thunder," 61
"Incidents Connected with the Army," 258n10
Isonomy, 213–214
letters to the editor: Algiers, LA, newspaper, 123; *Morning Star*, 99; *National Republican*, 53; *New Orleans Republican*, 123; *Oswego Palladium*, 227, 249; *Oswego Times*, 227; *Philadelphia Inquirer*, 189; *The Sibyl*, 20–21, 36, 38–39, 43–45, 46; *The Spectator*, 96; *Washington Post*, 211–212
"Mistaken Identity," 197
"Moral Statues," 146
"Mount Vernon Association," 21
"New York State Foundling Hospital," 26–27
"N. York State Foundling Hospital," 25–26
poetry, 17–18, 251
"Positions that Women ought of Right to Occupy," 47
"Punching the Bag Makes Pale Cheeks All Abloom," 235
satiric petition for national costumer, 188
"The Secessionists," 38
"Sickles and Key Tragedy," 23–24
"Smallpox and Dress," 144
"Synopsis of a Sermon," 21
"The True Spirit; Go on Faithfully," 43–44
Unmasked; or, The Science of Immorality, 108, 150, 156–159, 161–162, 164, 171, 182, 267n18
"Welcome Home," 241
"What Can Woman Do?" 36
"Why Women Should Wear Trousers," 196–197
"Woman's Mind," 44–45
"Women Soldiers," 29–30
Walker, Mary S., 94
Walker, Mary Snow, 2
Walker, Philip, 2
Walker, Vashti, 162, 204, 207, 229
Walker, Vesta Whitcomb (mother): abolitionist, 5; death, 178–179; dress reform advocate, 5, 7; founds free school, 5, 241; health, 5, 178, 274n13; inheritance, 204; influence on MEW, 20, 38; letter to *The Sibyl*, 22; marriage, 2, 4; medical interests, 38; MEW visits, 136; MEW's support of, 169–170; occupations, 4, 5; parents, 2; personal traits, 2; religion, 4, 5, 22; residences, 1, 2, 22, 77, 169–170; support of MEW's actions, 9, 59–60; women's rights advocate, 22
Walker, Widow (ancestor), 2
Walker Coats, Aurora Borealis (sister): birth, 1; death, 225; education, 7; as educator, 9, 241; fair exhibitor, 137, 167; health, 225; inheritance, 15; marriage, 15, 225; occupation, 5; relationship with MEW, 225; tribute from MEW, 240

Walker family home (Bunker Hill Road), 1, 3, 22, 156, 169–170, 255n5. *See also* Oswego Town; Walker, Mary Edwards: residences
Walker Griswold, Luna, 1, 7, 15, 241
Walker Lodge, I.O.G.T., 95–96
Walker Worden, Vesta (sister), 1, 5, 15, 233, 241
Walker's U.S. Patriots, 46–47
Wall, Amanda, 135
Wall, S. B., 184
Walling, George, 164–165
Walrath, D. D., 31
Warden, Andrew, 191, 197–198, 202
Warden, Christie, 189–193, 197–198, 200–201
Warden, Fannie, 190
Warden, Louisa, 190, 191, 197–198, 202, 203
Warden, Oscar, 191–193, 197, 202
War Department, 37, 41, 42, 45, 49
Warner, Charles Dudley 140
Warrenton, VA, 40, 41, 62, 186–187
Washington, D.C., 71; City Hall, 48; in Civil War era, 31–37, 39, 43, 45, 47–49, 64, 69; conventions in, 105, 106, 112; courts and trials in, 22–24, 45, 117, 172–173, 189–194, 216; government, 70; hospitals, 236; home rule, 135; police force, 161–162; political organizations, 45, 100, 247; reform movements in, 100, 103, 112
Washington, George, 21
Washington, Martha, 225
Washington Chronicle, 102, 145, 146
Washington Gazette, 134, 136
Washington Post, 161, 162, 167, 215–216, 217, 233, 242, 248
"Washington Scare, The," 154
Washington Times, 229
water cure, *see* hydropathy
Water-Cure Journal, 3
Watkins Glen, NY, 149
Wayman, Bishop, 113
Waymouth, Dr., 86–87
Weber, D. A., 122
Weedsport, NY, 188
Wellesley College, 114
Wells, Samuel R., 103
Welsh, John, 151
Westbury, NY, 208
Westervelt, William, 165
Westminster Review, 94
West Point, 71
Wheelock, Julia S., 139
"When Mary Walker is a Policeman," 162
Whitcher, Professor, 203
Whitcomb, James, 2
Whitcomb, Polly Hinds, 2
White, Stanford, 237
Whitehouse, Mrs. Norman De R., 249
White House receptions, MEW at, 43, 173–174, 182, 212, 242
White Mountains, 168
Whitman, George, 41
Whitman, Walt, 35, 41, 151
Whittier, John Greenleaf, 20
Whittlesey, Nelson, 92
Wightman, Bradley, 122
Wightman, Josephine, 122
Wilcox, Hannah Tyler, M.D., 146, 271n27
Wilhelm, kaiser of Germany, 251
Willard, Frances E., 182, 209, 220
William Austin's Nickelodeon, 185
Williams, Alfred, 140–141
Williams, Frank, 234
Williams v. The State of Mississippi, 243
Willimantic, CT, 104
Wilmot, Sir Eardley, 85
Wilson, Henry, 40–41, 111
Wilson, Henry Lane, 247
Wilson, Woodrow, 244, 247, 248, 250
Wilton, NY, 199
Winder, John H., 58, 59, 60
Winslow, Caroline, M.D., 112, 135, 143, 182
Wisconsin, 20
Winslow, Forbes, Dr., 87
Wollstonecraft, Mary, 138
Woman's Campaign, 141
Woman's Centenary Association, 177
Woman's Christian Temperance Union, 177, 182, 208
Woman's National Loyal League, 49
Woman's New York State Temperance Society, 83
"woman's sphere," 27, 47
women physicians: and abortion, 26; and appropriate patients, 62; in Civil War, 32–37, 42, 47; in Great Britain, 85–86, 87, 239; internationally, 226; and medical colleges, 9–14, 20, 26, 37–38, 42, 71, 87, 91, 118, 203, 245; MEW on, 26, 128; mutual support, 11, 16, 17, 23–24, 71–72, 85, 120, 179 (*see also* Walker, Mary Edwards: friendships); opposition to, by general public, 75; opposition to, by male physicians, 9, 64–65, 87, 93, 96; opposition to, by male medical students, 10, 11, 87–88, 93, 95; opposition to, by military, 32, 49, 51–52, 64–67; opposition to, by newspapers, 88–89, 170–171; opposition to, by other women, 19–20, 56, 64–67; organizations, 230, 245; preferred by women, 93; as professors, 37, 245; and suffrage, 112, 249; support for, 51–52, 67, 86–87, 89, 90–91, 93, 96, 98–99; in the White House, 172, 179. *See also individual physicians by name*

women's congresses, 114, 176–177; MEW at, 103, 208, 220, 247
Women's Declaration of Independence, 151
Women's Federal Suffrage Association, 249
Women's International Council, 182–183
Women's Medical College of Pennsylvania, 11, 71
Women's National Democratic League, 247
Women's National Labor League, 174
Women's Political Union, 249
Women's Relief Association, 48–49, 53
Women's Relief Corps, 242
Women's Rights Association of New Orleans, 123
women's rights movement: and animal rights, 220; and antislavery movement, 18; and antiwar proclamations, 220; and civil rights, 49; conventions, 30, 78, 220; and divorce, 28, 77–78, 110; and dress reform, 115; and education, 21; in Great Britain, 86, 97; and guardianship of children, 125; and labor, 20, 102, 174; male support of 15, 54, 86, 89, 94, 121, 141; and marriage, 22, 125–126; petitions, 49; postwar transition, 75; and property rights, 125; and racial equality, 49; and sexuality, 94; and Spiritualism, 4; and taxation without representation, 6, 20, 30; and temperance movements, 20; and U.S. presidents, 113. *See also* dress reform; suffrage movement
Women's Society, 121

Wonderland museum, 181
Wood, Robert C., M.D., 50, 64–65, 66, 73, 96, 262n26
Woodhull, Victoria, 123, 125, 127, 135, 136, 137–138, 140, 147, 160, 270n8
Woodrow, Mrs. Wilson, 250
Wooll, J. H., 64
Worcester, MA, 202
Worden, Byron, 230, 251
Worden, Lyman J., 27, 77, 258n23
Worden, Vesta Walker, *see* Walker Worden, Vesta
Worden, Willet, 15
working classes, *see* labor
workingmen's organizations, 71
World Health Association, 103
World War I, 249, 251
World's Fair (Chicago, 1893), 195
World's Food Fair, 202
Wren, Lieutenant, 35–36
Wright, Fanny, 5, 138
Wright, Martha Coffin, 142
writers' retreat, 149
Wu, Madame, 218
Wu, Tingfang, 212, 218, 230
Wyman, Treasurer, 154
Wyoming, 125

Yates Hotel, 226

Zola, Émile, 221

About the Author

SHARON M. HARRIS is a professor of English and the director of the Humanities Institute at the University of Connecticut. She is author of several books, including *Executing Race: Early American Women's Narratives of Race, Society, and the Law*; and of numerous editions and collections, including *U.S. Letters and Cultural Transformations, 1760–1860*, coedited with Theresa Strouth Gaul, and *Rebecca Harding Davis: The Civil War Years*, coedited with Robin Cadwallader. She is advisory editor for *Legacy: A Journal of American Women Writers* and founding president of the Society for the Study of American Women Writers.